TRENDS IN TESTOSTERONE RESEARCH

TRENDS IN TESTOSTERONE RESEARCH

RAYMUND E. VERITOS
EDITOR

Nova Science Publisher, Inc.
New York

For permission to use material from this book please contact us:
Telephone 631-231-7269; Fax 631-231-8175
Web Site: http://www.novapublishers.com

Library of Congress Cataloging-in-Publication Data
Trends in testosterone research / Raymund E. Veritos (editor).
p. ; cm.
Includes bibliographical references and index.
ISBN 978-1-60456-127-2 (hardcover)
1. Testosterone. I. Veritos, Raymund E.
[DNLM: 1. Testosterone--physiology. 2. Research--trends. WJ 875 T794 2007]
QP572.T4T76 2007
612.6'1--dc22 2007046485

Published by Nova Science Publishers, Inc. ✦ New York

Contents

Preface

This new book presents important and recent research on testosterone which is a steroid hormone from the androgen group. Testosterone is primarily secreted in the testes of males and the ovaries of females although small amounts are secreted by the adrenal glands. It is the principal male sex hormone and an anabolic steroid. In both males and females, it plays key roles in health and well-being. Examples include enhanced libido, energy, immune function, and protection against osteoporosis. On average, the adult male body produces about twenty times the amount of testosterone that an adult female's body does.

Chapter I - Prostate cancer is the leading cause of malignancy among American men and the third leading cause of cancer deaths. Approximately 42% of men will progress following local definitive therapy, with either rising PSA or metastatic disease. Androgen-deprivation therapy (ADT) is the primary treatment for metastatic prostate cancer. Although it is increasingly used in different disease stages and patient populations, there is still controversy regarding its use in patients whose sole determinant of disease progression is rising PSA. Various treatment modalities have been studied in combination with ADT to determine their overall efficacy and benefit in terms of progression-free and overall survival, leading to the use of ADT in selected patient populations. However, ADT is not without side effects. Different dosing strategies, such as intermittent ADT and rapid hormonal cycling, are being employed to determine how to administer ADT for maximum benefit and minimal toxicity. For the many patients who will eventually develop incurable, often debilitating metastatic castrate-resistant disease, strategies for directing novel therapies at the androgen-receptor signaling pathway and apoptotic genes hold future promise. This chapter discusses the clinical applications, side effects, and overall effects of ADT, clinical studies that support or controvert its use in selected patient populations and stages of prostate cancer, and the biology of castrate-resistant prostate cancer and novel approaches to its treatment.

Chapter II - This review investigates whether lowering gonadotropin levels using leuprolide acetate would be preferable to testosterone (T) treatment for men with Alzheimer's disease (AD). There is considerable evidence from animal and cell culture studies that high gonodatropin and low T levels may have detrimental effects on the brain. Several observational studies have also reported low levels of T and high levels of gonadotropins in men with AD. Chemical castration using leuprolide acetate in men with prostate cancer has shown some improvements, but also significant decline in memory functions. Limited data suggest that this effect may be worse in older men. However, the authors only found high gonadotropin levels in older (80+ years), but not younger AD cases. Possibly, increased gonadotropin levels may be an adequate, if failed, response to earlier lowered levels of T in the disease. As T treatment also decreases gonadotropin levels, is neuroprotective and has shown positive effects on cognition in AD, it might be a more suitable alternative than leuprolide acetate. Age, genetics, prior levels of T and estrogens may all play a role in determining optimal levels of T to improve cognition in AD.

Chapter III - Stress that can be exerted in various ways, including immobilization (IMO), induces a rapid increase in glucocorticoid secretion (in rodents, corticosterone, CORT) and a parallel decrease in circulating testosterone (T) levels. At the same time, nitric oxide (NO), a reactive free radical and fast acting neurotransmitter that is thought to be produced at higher rates in some tissues during stress, has been shown to suppress the biosynthesis of T by Leydig cells. Assessment of the respective roles of CORT and/or NO in acute stress-mediated reduction of T production is an ongoing area of research. The pharmacokinetics and pharmacodynamics of CORT have been studied in IMO-stressed wild type (WT) and inducible nitric oxide synthase knockout (iNOS-/-) mice. Notably, similar basal plasma and testicular T levels are present in both genotypes and their exposure to 3 h of IMO results in a marked elevation in plasma CORT and a dramatic reduction in T concentrations. In addition, testicular T levels exhibit the same pattern while the concentrations of nitrite and nitrate, the stable metabolites of NO in testicular extracts did not differ. Studies performed using WT mice have shown that the changes in CORT and T levels are very rapid. Together, these findings raise the issue of what role, if any, NO has as a mediator of stress in mammals. This question has additional relevance in that the presence of the NO synthase (NOS) enzyme family members in Leydig cells, which has also been reported, is subject to doubt. The authors will show in the present chapter that testicular expression of NO synthase (NOS) isoforms that catalyze synthesis of NO is not linked to stress physiology. In tissues such as brain or adrenal glands, NOS isoforms may act as mediators of enzymatic activity and hormone release, thereby modulating the response of the testis to stress.

Chapter IV – Follicle stimulating hormone (FSH) and testosterone have been described as necessary factors for proliferation of Sertoli and germ cells, as well as having a role in apoptosis. However, their role in germ cell differentiation has not been studied in detail. FSH is a proteic hormone produced in the anterior hypophysis and has receptors located in Sertoli cells, which in turn function as nurse cells for germ cells in the seminiferous epithelium. The expression of FSH receptors changes during the cycle of seminiferous epithelium. Germ cells in consecutive steps of differentiation are located in each progressive stage of the seminiferous epithelium, indicating a role for FSH signaling in the differentiation of germ cells. CREB (CRE-protein binding) is a transcription factor involved in differentiation of germ cells and it is modulated by FSH. Some CREM-regulated products have been shown to participate in germ cell differentiation. Recent studies have focused on the intracellular signaling after FSH joins with its receptor, and how it influences germ cell differentiation. Testosterone-stimulated germ cell development occurs via paracrine communication with Sertoli cells. The androgen receptor is expressed in a stage-specific manner during the seminiferous epithelium cycle. Recent studies on gene expression show a number of genes modulated by testosterone, many of which do not follow the traditional pathway of androgen/receptor/gene expression, but are activated by another signalization pathway. This chapter begins with the background necessary to understand the general role of FSH and testosterone in seminiferous epithelium and then addresses the molecular signaling initiated by these chemical messengers.

Chapter V - Animal research demonstrated a link between reductions in testosterone (T) levels, the development of the amyloid beta (Aβ) and tau (τ) proteins, and the presence of the APOEε4 allele. The Aβ and τ proteins are neuropathological characteristics whereas the APOEε4 allele is a risk factor for Alzheimer's disease (AD). On the other hand, several studies performed in men showed that a decline in T correlates with aging. Given that the risk to develop AD increases with age, some researchers proposed a relationship between the development of AD and reductions of T. Should this hypothesis be true, links should exist between aging, AD, cognitive deficits and depletion of T, and between T substitution treatment and cognition in elderly hypogonadal and AD men. The goal of this chapter was therefore to critically review the studies examining, in elderly hypogonadal and AD men, the T levels and cognitive functioning, and the effects of T substitution treatment on cognition. Method: A search of MEDLINE and PsycInfo databases was conducted in order to identify articles published between 1994 and 2006. The key terms included "testosterone", "male hormone", "androgens", "gonadotropin", "cognition", "cognitive function", "Alzheimer's disease", "dementia", "aging", and "men". English-language, peer-reviewed articles were included. The populations of the reviewed studies were men aged of 50 years and greater. The studies assessing cognition and T levels had to use standardized measures, and were required to present diagnostic and/or control group comparisons. The treatment studies had to use at least placebo-control designs. Human single-cases were excluded. Results: Analyses of the reviewed data showed that T levels were generally lower in the AD than healthy groups, and that elderly men with high T levels had better cognition than those with low T levels. Some studies however did not report any relationship between T levels and cognition. T substitution treatments generally yielded improvement in memory, executive and visuospatial functions in healthy elderly and AD men with and without hypogonadism. Conclusion: Methodological limitations of the existing data include the lack of longitudinal studies, and small sample size in clinical trials for AD. However, there seems to be a relationship between pathological aging, cognitive impairment and reductions of T.

Chapter VI - Standard animal lab chow is soy-based, and diets rich in soy protein contain estrogen-like compounds called phytoestrogens. The purpose of this study was to explore the hormonal effects of a soy versus a soy-free diet on testosterone levels in male hamsters. In Experiment #1, thirteen adult male hamsters (110-125 g) were individually-housed, and then divided into a soy and a soy-free group. All hamsters had continuous access to food and water, and they were sacrificed after seven weeks. Blood was collected to measure testosterone levels and the testes were removed to analyze the morphology. There was a significant difference in testosterone levels between the Soy (9.11±1.26 ng/ml) and the Soy-Free group (3.89±0.27 ng/ml)[$t(11)=3.74$; $p<0.005$]. There was no difference in testes weight, but the dimensions were different between the Soy (251.2±6.9 mm2) and the Soy-Free group (229.5±6.8 mm2)[$t(13)=2.2$; $p<0.05$]. In Experiment #2, twenty adult male hamsters (110-125 g) were individually-housed and then divided into four groups: 1) Castrate+Soy; 2) Castrate+Soy-Free; 3) Sham Castrate+Soy; and 4) Sham Castrate+Soy-Free. Animals were sacrificed seven weeks after surgery and the diet manipulation. There were no detectable levels of testosterone in castrated males. However, the Sham+Soy (12.21±2.95 ng/ml) had significantly higher levels of testosterone compared to Sham+Soy-Free (3.92±0.8 ng/ml)[$t(9)=2.95$; $p=0.01$]. In sum, the authors have demonstrated that a soy-free diet lowered endogenous levels of testosterone, and they recommend that investigators evaluate the impact of phytoestrogens when investigating behavioral experiments that involve neurosteroids.

Chapter VII - As outlined in a later chapter in this collection, the association between testosterone, aggression and anger in humans has been the focus of substantial research attention over the last number of decades (e.g., Archer, 1991; Archer, Birring & Wu, 1998; Dabbs, Jurkovoic & Frady, 1991; Harris, 1999; O'Connor, Archer, Hair & Wu, 2002; O'Connor, Archer & Wu, 2004; Pagonis, Angelopoulos, Koukoulis & Hadjichristodoulou, 2006). Generally, these studies have either involved comparisons of testosterone levels and self-reported aggression between violent and non-violent groups or have been correlational in nature, investigating the degree of association between endogenous testosterone levels, aggression and hostile feelings in various samples of men.

Chapter VIII - Steroids produced in the periphery have long been of interest to reproductive biologists. The emergence of neuroendocrinology as a dominant subfield of behavioral studies appeared to demote steroids to a lesser status than the exciting neuropeptides that clearly interacted with many regions of the brain. Seminal findings in recent years, however, have propelled the study of steroids back onto center stage. In this chapter the authors identify the seminal findings and describe why they are revolutionary. These new findings have demonstrated steroids have the capacity to modify the structure and function of brain regions both related to and unrelated to reproduction. The consequences on behavior are likely to be profound. This chapter focuses on one steroid, testosterone, because it occupies a strategic position in the metabolic cascade of the sex steroids. It is a position that can influence the actions of androgens and estrogens, as well as the adrenal precursors of testosterone and the recently identified neurosteroids, on the brain and behavior. The authors believe future research will reveal testosterone to have behavioral effects extending well beyond those related to reproduction. Still, the massive literature on testosterone – sociosexual behavior provides a solid background on which to begin that work.

In: Trends in Testosterone Research
Editor: Raymund E. Veritos

ISBN: 978-1-60456-127-2

Chapter I

Androgens, Androgen Suppression, and Prostate Cancer: Recent Preclinical and Clinical Findings and Implications

***Jeanny B. Aragon-Ching*[1], *Nima Sharifi*[1,2] *and James L. Gulley*[3]**
[1] Medical Oncology Branch, [2] Cancer Stem Cell Section, Laboratory of Cancer Prevention,
[3] Laboratory of Tumor Immunology and Biology,
Center for Cancer Research, National Cancer Institute,
National Institutes of Health, Bethesda, MD

Abstract

Prostate cancer is the leading cause of malignancy among American men and the third leading cause of cancer deaths. Approximately 42% of men will progress following local definitive therapy, with either rising PSA or metastatic disease. Androgen-deprivation therapy (ADT) is the primary treatment for metastatic prostate cancer. Although it is increasingly used in different disease stages and patient populations, there is still controversy regarding its use in patients whose sole determinant of disease progression is rising PSA. Various treatment modalities have been studied in combination with ADT to determine their overall efficacy and benefit in terms of progression-free and overall survival, leading to the use of ADT in selected patient populations. However, ADT is not without side effects. Different dosing strategies, such as intermittent ADT and rapid hormonal cycling, are being employed to determine how to administer ADT for maximum benefit and minimal toxicity. For the many patients who will eventually develop incurable, often debilitating metastatic castrate-resistant disease, strategies for directing novel therapies at the androgen-receptor signaling pathway and apoptotic genes hold future promise. This chapter discusses the clinical applications, side effects, and overall effects of ADT, clinical studies that support or controvert its use in selected patient populations and stages of prostate cancer, and the biology of castrate-resistant prostate cancer and novel approaches to its treatment.

Introduction

Since Huggins and Hodges established a link between prostate cancer and androgens in 1941 [1], androgen-deprivation therapy (ADT) in the form of chemical or surgical castration has become a cornerstone of treatment for metastatic prostate cancer. The rationale behind the use of ADT in prostate cancer derives from the interdependent actions of various hormones and their effects on the prostate gland (figure 1).

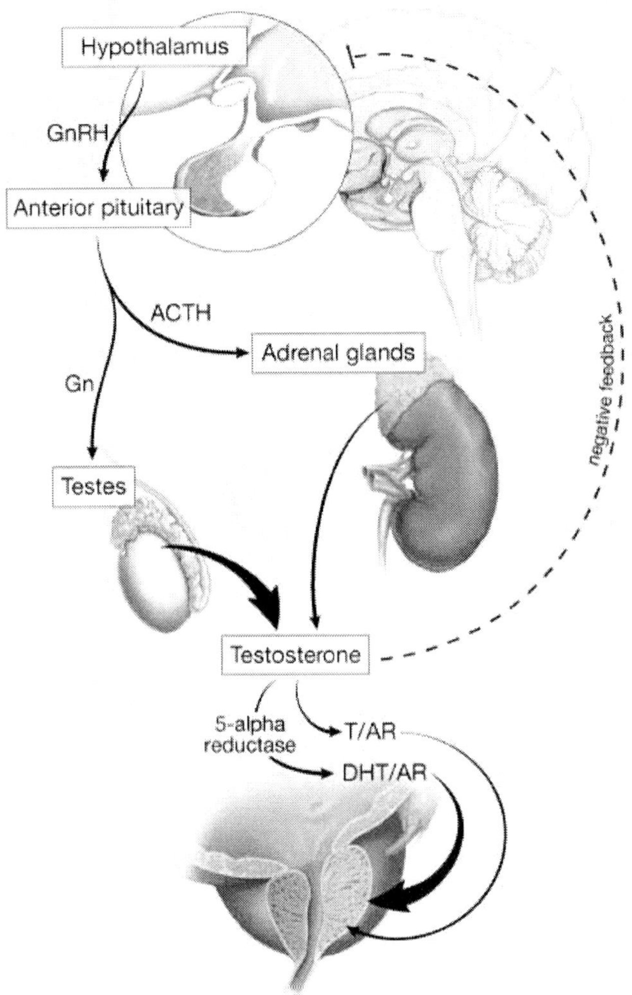

Figure 1. Hypothalamic-pituitary-gonadal axis. The hypothalamus/pituitary/testes endocrine loop is shown above. Gonadotropin-releasing hormone (GnRH) stimulates the secretion of gonadotropic hormone (Gn) from the anterior pituitary, and Gn in turn stimulates the production of testosterone. Circulating testosterone (and estrogens) acts in a negative feedback loop to down-regulate the expression of GnRH. Adrenocorticotropic hormone (ACTH), also made by the pituitary, stimulates androgen synthesis in the adrenal gland. Testosterone (T) and dihydrotestosterone (DHT) bind to the androgen receptor (AR), causing increased expression of androgen-responsive genes and leading to cell growth.

The hypothalamus initiates a series of events that lead to the secretion of testosterone, a hormone required by the prostate to develop into and remain a functional gland. Gonadotropin-releasing hormone (GnRH), also known as luteinizing hormone-releasing hormone (LHRH), is produced in the neurosecretory cells of the hypothalamus in a physiologically pulsatile manner. These neurons terminate in the hypothalamic-hypophysial portal system, a unique vascular bed that shuttles GnRH directly to the anterior lobe of the pituitary. In response to GnRH, the anterior lobe of the pituitary secretes luteinizing hormone, perhaps more accurately known as gonadotropic hormone (Gn), which enters the circulation and exerts an effect on the testes.

The testes contain a network of seminiferous tubules that produce sperm. In between these tubules are the interstitial cells of Leydig, which have high-affinity receptors on their plasma membranes to which the Gn binds. Leydig cells produce testosterone as a result of enzymatic conversion of cholesterol upon stimulation by Gn. Testosterone then enters the blood stream and the cells of the prostate, where it may be converted by 5-alpha reductase into dihydrotestosterone (DHT). Both DHT and testosterone can directly bind to the cytoplasmic androgen receptor (AR) and initiate growth, although DHT binds with greater affinity. The adrenal cortex plays a lesser role in prostatic growth, producing only a small proportion (about 10% to 15%) of total testosterone. These androgens, which are essential for normal glandular growth, are also implicated as growth factors in the development of prostate cancer. As in other endocrine systems, negative feedback control is fundamental. When testosterone (or estrogen) levels in the blood stream increase, the hypothalamus reduces the secretion of GnRH, which in turn inhibits the secretion of Gn from the pituitary gland. The overall effect is a net decrease in the amount of Gn that can stimulate the Leydig cells, thus decreasing testosterone production.

Androgens are the hormones that primarily regulate the growth, proliferation, and differentiation of prostate cancer cells. Since AR is expressed in almost all prostate cancers, this expression is the basis of the initial response of prostate cancer to ADT. AR is a 919 amino acid member of the steroid receptor transcription factor superfamily and has incorporated within its protein structure an N-terminal regulation domain, a central DNA binding domain, and a C-terminal domain, which includes the ligand binding domain [2]. In the absence of stimulation, AR resides in the cytoplasm. Once activated, it localizes to the nucleus within a few minutes [3], where it regulates the transcription of numerous genes [4]. When androgens bind to AR, AR protein is stabilized and levels increase [5]. AR is critical for normal male development, and its role in the physiology and health of the adult male is best illustrated by the adverse effects of ADT described later in this chapter. The role of AR in development is probably best illustrated by some loss-of-function AR mutations, which can result in complete androgen insufficiency syndrome, including a superficial female habitus and lack of a prostate [6].

ADT, also known as androgen-suppression therapy, derives from the basic principle that androgens stimulate the growth of prostate cancer. Androgen deprivation is achieved by various methods, including surgical castration with bilateral orchiectomy, or medical castration in the form of GnRH agonists (GnRH-A) or antagonists, estrogens, androgen-receptor antagonists or antiandrogens, ketoconazole, and aminoglutethimide (see table 1 for FDA-approved hormonal agents and their dosing). The first large-scale study on the effectiveness of orchiectomy showed that patients with advanced prostate cancer had a 73% one-year survival and a 35% 5-year survival following orchiectomy, compared to 66% and 20% respectively for placebo [7]. Although orchiectomy is a relatively simple procedure with minor operative risks and low physical morbidity, it has fallen out of favor because of its psychological effect on the patient, and because medical alternatives to achieving androgen suppression are now available [8, 9].

Table 1. FDA-approved hormonal therapy agents and their dosing

Hormonal Therapy	Dosing	Manufacturer
GnRH agonists		
Lupron Depot® (leuprolide acetate for depot suspension)	7.5 mg s.c. q mo 22.5 mg s.c. q 3 mos 30 mg s.c. q 4 mos 45 mg s.c. q 6 mos	TAP Pharmaceuticals, Inc.
Zoladex® (goserelin acetate implant)	3.6 mg s.c. q mo 10.8 mg s.c. q 3 mos	Astra-Zeneca Pharmaceuticals
Viadur® (leuprolide acetate implant)	yearly implant	ALZA Corporation under license to Bayer Corporation
GnRH antagonist		
Plenaxis® (abarelix)	100 mg i.m. days 1,15, 29, q 4 wks thereafter	Praecis Pharmaceuticals
Antiandrogens		
Casodex® (bicalutamide) tablets	50 mg daily	Astra-Zeneca Pharmaceuticals
Eulexin® (flutamide) capsule	250 mg p.o. t.i.d.	Schering-Plough Pharmaceuticals
Nilandron® (nilutamide) tablets	150 mg p.o. daily	Aventis

s.c. = subcutaneous; i.m. = intramuscular; q = every; mo = month; p.o. = per orem; t.i.d. = 3x per day.

Diethylstilbestrol (DES) is a synthetic estrogen that blocks Gn and follicle-stimulating hormone (FSH) via a negative feedback loop (figure 1), resulting in complete testosterone suppression. DES was the first alternative to orchiectomy and was commonly used for androgen suppression through the late 1970s. Although estrogen treatment resulted in improved cancer-specific survival compared to placebo, as established in the Veterans Administration Cooperative Urological Research Group Study, it was accompanied by side effects including nausea, vomiting, fluid retention, gynecomastia, and most significantly, serious cardiovascular events [7, 10, 11]. In 1971, Schally et al. successfully isolated and identified the decapeptide GnRH, which has a unique primary structure that is able to regulate production and secretion of Gn and FSH [12, 13]. However, a shortcoming of this form of GnRH is its half-life of 2 to 4 minutes, which precludes its therapeutic usefulness. Subsequent cloning studies were undertaken with single amino acid substitutions that identified compounds with longer half-lives. Substituting the amino acid positions 6 and 10 led to the development of superagonists 50 to 100 times more potent than the native peptide [14].

GnRH-A supplants the effect of physiologically pulsatile endogenous GnRH, producing steady-state levels of GnRH and desensitizing the pituitary. This causes down-regulation of receptors in the pituitary and arrests pituitary secretion, thereby decreasing testicular function. Testosterone production in the gonads decreases within 3 weeks, with a subsequent decrease in the growth of androgen-dependent tissues [15-17]. Available formulations can be administered every 1, 3, 4, 6, or 12 months. An initial increase in the level of testosterone causes an acute stimulation of prostate cancer growth and may result in a "flare" reaction of increased bone pain in patients with metastatic prostate cancer. This effect can be alleviated by androgen-receptor antagonists [18]. It is recommended that an androgen antagonist be administered prior to initiation of treatment with a GnRH-A and continued for 2 to 4 weeks to block the effect of the testosterone surge on peripheral AR [19]. In clinical practice, this regimen is often reserved for patients with significant metastatic disease that may become more symptomatic with the testosterone surge.

As an alternative method of medical castration, a GnRH antagonist has the benefit of obviating the acute testosterone surge. However, abarelix, the only GnRH antagonist approved in the United States, caused an immediate-onset systemic allergic reaction in 1.1% (15/1,397) of patients [20, 21], and the cumulative risk of this adverse event increased with the duration of treatment. As a result, GnRH antagonists are no longer available in the U.S. for new patients.

A number of studies have examined the efficacy of medical vs. surgical castration for advanced prostate cancer, including 10 randomized trials comparing GnRH-A and orchiectomy. A published meta-analysis of all of these trials found equivalence between GnRH-A and orchiectomy in terms of survival, progression-related outcomes, and time to treatment failure [22]. Given a choice between bilateral orchiectomy and GnRH-A therapy, only 22% (32/147) of patients in 2 clinical studies elected to undergo bilateral orchiectomy [23].

Other classes of agents used clinically to block the effects of androgen are AR antagonists such as flutamide, bicalutamide, and nilutamide, which are often used alone or in combination with castration to block the effects of adrenal androgens. Other adrenal-ablating drugs, such as ketoconazole, inhibit cytochrome P450 enzymes that are required for synthesis of androgens and other steroids. Another class of drugs is the 5-alpha reductase inhibitors, which inhibit the enzyme responsible for the conversion of testosterone to DHT, the potent activator of AR. While 5-alpha reductase inhibitors currently have no role in the treatment of advanced prostate cancer, they may have a role in prevention [24].

Regardless of the means, the goal of androgen blockade is to achieve the lowest possible serum testosterone level in order to minimize stimulation of prostate cancer cells. Castration is generally achieved when the serum testosterone level falls to less than 50 ng/dL [25]. However, since most men who undergo surgical castration achieve levels below 20 ng/dL, reassessment of the definition of castrate levels has been proposed to reflect this threshold [26]. This chapter will address the indications and clinical settings for ADT, and the studies and issues that support or controvert its use, as well as the biology of castrate-resistant prostate cancer (CRPC).

Prevention Studies

5-Alpha Reductase Inhibitors

5-alpha reductase enzymatically converts testosterone into DHT, the most active androgen in the prostate. Two 5-alpha reductase enzymes have been isolated: type 1 is the predominant enzyme located in extraprostatic tissues such as the skin and liver; type 2 is predominantly expressed in the prostate [27]. Recent findings that may have important implications in the choice of drug treatment suggest that there is a shift in isozyme expression from type 2 to type 1 in recurrent prostate cancer, as well as in androgen-stimulated benign prostate and prostate cancers [28]. Two FDA-approved 5-alpha reductase inhibitors are currently available: finasteride and dutasteride. Finasteride, a selective inhibitor of type 2 5-alpha reductase, decreases levels of serum DHT by about 70%, reducing gland size by 20% to 30% and improving urinary symptoms for patients with benign prostatic hypertrophy [29]. The Prostate Cancer Prevention Trial (PCPT) demonstrated that 7 years of prophylactic finasteride decreased the incidence of prostate cancer by 6% (24.4% in the placebo group vs. 18.4% in the finasteride group). However, there was a statistically significant 1.3% absolute increase in the incidence of high-grade tumors (Gleason score 7 to 10) in the finasteride group, with 6.4% of men in the finasteride group and 5.1% of men in the placebo group having this pathology [24, 30]. One possible explanation for the increase in high-grade tumors in the finasteride group is that finasteride causes shrinkage of the normal prostate gland [29] that may be out of proportion to the tumor, and may cause more shrinkage in lower-grade tumors than in more aggressive-appearing tumors. This could lead to relative oversampling of tumors in the finasteride-treated patients. In the PCPT, the prostates of finasteride-treated men were about 25% smaller than the prostates of placebo-treated men. This effect of finasteride may have increased sampling bias by increasing the likelihood of detecting prostate cancer by needle biopsy. Another possible explanation for the absolute increase in high-grade cancer in the finasteride group is that increased sensitivity of the PSA test used in the finasteride group led to greater detection of prostate cancer in this group [31].

Dutasteride, another 5-alpha reductase inhibitor, has also been used in a chemoprevention trial. Whereas finasteride primarily inhibits type 2 5-alpha reductase, dutasteride inhibits both 5-alpha reductase isoenzymes and reduces DHT by > 90% [32]. Retrospective analysis of data from several early trials of dutasteride in benign prostatic hyperplasia indicated a lower incidence of prostate cancer with the use of this agent [33]. The Reduction by Dutasteride of Prostate Cancer Events (REDUCE) trial, a 4-year, international, multicenter, randomized, double-blind, placebo-controlled study, will evaluate the efficacy and safety of oral dutasteride 0.5 mg/day in men aged 50 to 75 who are at increased risk of developing prostate cancer. The target enrollment is 8,000 men, who will be randomized 1:1 to receive dutasteride or placebo for 4 years. Enrollment of approximately 4,000 participants per treatment group will provide over 90% overall power to detect the superiority of dutasteride 0.5 mg treatment vs. placebo after 4 years. Eligibility criteria include PSA of between 2.5 and 10 ng/mL for men aged 50 to 60, or between 3.0 and 10 ng/mL for men older than 60, and a free PSA of 25% or lower at initial screening. Enrollees must have no histological evidence of prostate cancer, based on a negative 6 to 12 core biopsy within 6 months prior to enrollment. Prostate biopsies will be performed at 2 and 4 years to evaluate for prostate cancer. PSA, genetic, and protein markers will also be obtained. The primary endpoint is biopsy-determined prostate cancer after 2 and 4 years of treatment. Several secondary endpoints will also be assessed, including overall survival [34].

A large chemoprevention trial that does not utilize a testosterone-lowering approach is the Selenium and Vitamin E Cancer Prevention Trial (SELECT) [35]. This clinical trial will attempt to confirm the findings of previous studies that suggest that selenium and vitamin E may reduce the risk of developing prostate cancer [36, 37]. SELECT closed to accrual in 2004 with an enrollment of over 35,000 men from various ethnic groups.

Treatment Studies

Role of ADT in Early Prostate Cancer

ADT is most commonly used to treat metastatic prostate cancer. However, there is emerging evidence that using ADT as a neoadjuvant, or as an adjuvant combined with local definitive therapy, in the treatment of localized disease can provide clinically significant outcomes in selected patient populations. Neoadjuvant therapy is therapy administered after diagnosis but before definitive local treatment. Surgery and radiotherapy (RT) are generally effective in treating localized disease. However, as a cure for patients with apparently localized disease, surgery may fail if the cancer is incompletely resected due to understaging of the tumor or the existence of micrometastases prior to surgery. The addition of systemic therapy is therefore appealing.

ADT Combined with Radiation

Combining RT and hormonal therapy has the potential benefits of decreasing prostate volume, diminishing the number of cancer cells, improving tumor oxygenation, and eliminating micrometastases. One of the first trials to indicate the benefit of combining RT with ADT was the Radiation Therapy Oncology Group trial (RTOG 83-07) [38]. Comparison to a historical control group showed that 2 different hormonal strategies—megestrol acetate and DES—had equivalent efficacy in patients with clinical stages T2B or T3 prostate cancer. Although the primary objective of this trial was to evaluate the relative effectiveness and toxicity of megestrol acetate vs. DES as neoadjuvant therapies to RT, this initial combination of hormonal agents with RT led to succeeding trials that examined the overall survival benefit of adjuvant ADT with RT.

Several randomized phase III trials have shown an overall survival benefit of RT plus ADT compared to RT alone for patients with locally advanced extracapsular or node-positive disease. (See table 2 for a list of selected studies combining ADT with RT.) A trial by the European Organisation for Research and Treatment of Cancer (EORTC) showed an overall survival benefit following 70 Gy RT plus 3 years of ADT compared to 70 Gy RT alone for patients with locally advanced and high-grade clinically localized prostate cancer [39, 40]. In the EORTC trial, 412 analyzable patients with T1 to T2 tumors of World Health Organization (WHO) class 3 (Gleason score 8 to 10) or T3 to T4, N0 to N1 M0 tumors were randomly assigned to receive RT alone (50 Gy delivered to the pelvis over 5 weeks, and 20 Gy over 2 weeks as a prostatic boost) or RT plus immediate treatment with goserelin (3.6 mg subcutaneously every 4 weeks beginning on the first day of irradiation, with 150 mg oral cyproterone acetate (CPA) given for 1 month starting 1 week before the first goserelin injection). ADT was continued for 3 years in the combined arm. The primary endpoint was clinical disease-free survival. At 5 years, overall survival was 78% for the combined-treatment group and 62% for the RT-alone group ($p = 0.0002$). Five-year disease-free survival was 74% for the combined-treatment group and 40% for the RT-alone group ($p = 0.0001$).

The most compelling results from clinical trials combining hormonal therapy with RT are seen in patients at high risk for recurrent disease (table 3). In RTOG 85-31, patients with T3 or T1-2 with N1 disease were randomized to RT with adjuvant hormonal therapy, or RT alone with hormones initiated at relapse [41, 42]. Among 945 analyzable patients, improvement in overall survival favored the ADT arm, with an estimated 10-year absolute survival of 53% vs. 38% ($p < 0.0043$) [43]. When these results were updated, they still showed an absolute survival rate at 10 years of 49% vs. 39% ($p = 0.002$) favoring the adjuvant vs. RT-alone arm [44]. All other parameters, including local failure rate, incidence of distant metastases, and disease-specific mortality, favored the adjuvant arm. Further subset analysis showed ADT improved survival in patients with involved regional lymph nodes [45]. A prospective randomized controlled trial by D'Amico et al. that looked at 70 Gy 3-dimensional conformal RT (3D-CRT) with or without 6-month ADT using GnRH reported evidence of extraprostatic disease, as measured by a PSA of at least 10 ng/mL [46]. Patients enrolled in the trial had clinically localized prostate cancer with high-risk features, including Gleason score of at least 7. After a median follow-up of 4.52 years, patients randomized to receive 3D-CRT plus ADT had a significantly higher survival rate of 88% vs. 78% for the 3D-CRT-alone group ($p = 0.04$), lower prostate cancer-specific mortality ($p = 0.02$), and higher survival free of salvage ADT of 82% vs. 57% ($p = .002$). A similar suggestion of benefit was observed in a cohort of 241 men with clinically localized prostate cancer and pretreatment PSA velocity of > 2 ng/mL/year (which is increasingly identified as another feature of high risk) who underwent 6 months of ADT with RT vs. RT alone [47]. Treatment with RT and ADT compared to RT alone was associated with a longer time to PSA recurrence (adjusted hazard ratio [HR] = 0.22; 95% confidence interval [CI]: 0.14 to 0.35; $p < 0.001$), prostate cancer-specific mortality (HR = 0.23; 95% CI: 0.09 to 0.64; $p = 0.005$), and all-cause mortality (HR = 0.30; 95% CI: 0.16 to 0.58; $p < 0.001$). Conversely, the RTOG 86-10 trial of 471 men with stages cT2-4 prostate cancer indicated no difference in 5-year overall survival, but improved progression-free survival (36% in ADT plus RT vs. 15% in RT alone [$p < 0.001$]), as well as local control (46% in ADT plus RT vs. 71% in RT alone [$p < 0.001$]) [48]. In this trial, ADT was given 2 months prior to and throughout the duration of RT. Updated results at 8 years of follow-up showed an improvement in overall survival (70% vs. 52%; $p = 0.015$) favoring the short-term androgen ablation arm only for patients with Gleason scores of 2 to 6, and no benefit in overall survival or locoregional control in patients

Table 2. Selected studies utilizing ADT with RT

Study	Study design	No. of patients	Population	Study intervention	Median follow-up (mos)	Results
Bolla et al. [40]	Randomized phase III	415	T1/T2 high-grade, T3/T4 any grade, N0-N1, M0	Definitive RT vs. RT + goserelin on day 1 x 3 yrs	66	Benefit in RT + ADT: 5 yr OS 78% vs. 62% ($p = 0.0002$); 5 yr DFS 74% vs. 40% ($p = 0.0001$)
Lawton et al. [42]	Randomized phase III	977	Node-positive or clinical stage T3	Definitive RT vs. RT + goserelin on last week of RT	96	No OS benefit at 8 yrs: 49% vs. 47%; improved local control with RT + ADT (failure rate 23% vs. 37%)
Pilepich et al. [49]	Randomized phase III	471	T2-T4, node-negative or -positive	Definitive RT vs. RT + CAB 2 mos prior and 2 mos during RT	96	Improvement with ADT in all endpoints: local control, DFS, cause-specific mortality, biochemical DFS, and OS (70% vs. 52%; $p = 0.015$) at 8 yrs only in patients with Gleason score 2–6
Hanks et al. [268]	Randomized phase III	1,500	T2C-T4	CAB 2 mos prior and during RT followed by 2 yrs CAB vs. no CAB	58	No difference in OS between LTAD-RT vs STAD-RT (80.0% vs. 78.5% at 5 yrs; $p = 0.73$), but improved in Gleason 8 to 10 group (80% vs. 69%; $p = 0.02$)
D'Amico et al. [269]	Retrospective cohort	1,586	T1-T2c	1,310 men got RT but no ADT; 276 got ADT 2 mos prior, 2 mos during, and 2 mos after RT	23-30	Decreased risk of biochemical failure for ADT + RT (88% vs. 62%) in intermediate-risk and 68% vs. 43% in high-risk group
D'Amico et al. [46]	Prospective randomized	206	T1b-T2b	70 Gy 3D-CRT vs. 70 Gy 3D-CRT + 6 mos GnRH-A + flutamide	54	Higher survival ($p = 0.04$), lower prostate cancer-specific mortality ($p = 0.02$), higher survival free of salvage ADT ($p = 0.002$)

RT: radiotherapy; OS: overall survival; DFS: disease-free survival; ADT: androgen-deprivation therapy; CAB: combined androgen blockade; 3D-CRT: 3-dimensional conformal radiation therapy.

with Gleason scores > 8 [49]. Further secondary analysis of RTOG 86-10 showed that 54% (n = 247) developed relapse and required subsequent salvage hormonal therapy. Overall survival and disease-specific survival were compared with the extent of disease progression (manifested by presence or absence of distant metastasis) at the time salvage ADT was initiated. Both were reduced in patients with distant metastasis, but a statistically significant increase in disease-specific survival ($p = 0.045$) was observed among 143 patients with no known distant metastasis but in whom PSA was < 20 ng/mL, compared with those in whom PSA was ≥ 20 ng/mL at the time of initiation of salvage ADT [50]. Although the optimal duration of ADT in these studies has not been determined, evidence suggests that hormonal therapy in combination with RT is beneficial. However, it is important to note that none of these adjuvant studies involving radiation included an arm using hormonal therapy alone [51].

Table 3. Risk categories for PSA failure after definitive treatment

	Low	Intermediate	High
Stage	T1c, T2a	T2b	T2c
PSA	< 10	10-20	> 20
Gleason	≤ 6	7	≥ 8
Qualifier	and	or	or
5-year risk of biochemical failure	< 25%	25% to 50%	> 50%

*Adapted from Gulley JL, Dahut WL. Novel schedules of hormone therapy for prostate cancer. In: Devita V, Hellman S, Rosenberg S, eds. *Progress in Oncology*. Boston: Jones and Bartlett; 2004:236-253.

ADT Combined with Surgery

Neoadjuvant ADT has been used to downstage primary tumors and to potentially improve outcome by decreasing tumor burden. However, data indicate that neoadjuvant ADT prior to radical prostatectomy (RP) provides no long-term overall or disease-free survival benefit (table 4). In a multicenter phase III study involving 282 patients, there was an apparently significant decrease in positive surgical margins after 3 months of neoadjuvant ADT prior to RP (18% in the neoadjuvant group vs. 48% in the RP-alone group [$p < 0.001$]). However, this did not translate to improved biochemical recurrence rate or disease-free survival rate at 5 years of follow-up (64.8% in the neoadjuvant group vs. 67.6% in the RP-alone group [$p = 0.663$]) [52]. In a study of 156 nonrandomized patients comparing shorter and longer durations of neoadjuvant ADT prior to RP, there was an overall PSA recurrence rate of 12% at 5 years of follow-up after 8 months of neoadjuvant ADT for clinical T3 disease [53]. This risk was proportional to known adverse risk factors such as higher pretreatment PSA, higher Gleason score, and higher pathologic stage. A randomized multicenter trial by the Canadian Uro-Oncology Group has reported interim data on 500 patients with T1c-T2 tumors, equally stratified to 3 months vs. 8 months of neoadjuvant complete androgen blockade prior to RP [54]. The percentage of patients with undetectable PSA prior to surgery (3-month: 75% vs. 8-month: 43%; $p < 0.0001$) and the rate of positive margins (3-month: 23% vs. 8-month: 12%; $p = 0.016$) favored the 8-month group. There was a higher incidence of hot flashes and newly reported adverse events in the 8-month neoadjuvant group. However, follow-up was too short to draw any definitive conclusions. Because there are insufficient data to support either overall or disease-free survival, there is currently no definitive role for neoadjuvant ADT prior to RP, unless micrometastasis is suspected.

The role of ADT after definitive curative surgery is also controversial. However, for patients with the highest risk of recurrence, such as those with positive lymph nodes, ADT seems strongly indicated [55]. A prospective randomized trial by the Eastern Cooperative Oncology Group (ECOG) examined the effect of early ADT on outcomes for men with pelvic lymph node involvement who had undergone RP. Fifteen percent (7/47) of men in the early-ADT arm died after a median follow-up of 7.1 years vs. 35% (18/51) of men in the observation arm ($p = 0.02$). Furthermore, 36 men (77%) in the early-ADT arm were alive and disease-free with undetectable PSA levels vs. 22 men (43%) in the observation arm ($p < 0.001$) [56]. In a retrospective study from a single institution, data from 3,663 patients who underwent RP and bilateral pelvic lymphadenectomy for prostate cancer were examined. Patients with multiple regional lymph node metastases had increased risk of death from disease, whereas patients with single lymph node involvement appeared to have a more favorable prognosis after RP and immediate adjuvant ADT [57].

ADT for Patients Ineligible for Local Definitive Therapy

For patients deemed ineligible for definitive local therapy because of increased comorbidities, decreased life expectancy, advanced local tumor stage or other existing malignancies, or who refuse local therapy for any reason, ADT remains a viable treatment option. A prospective randomized Swiss trial (SAKK 08/88) with a total of 197 patients attempted to determine if immediate ADT had an advantage over deferred treatment in newly diagnosed asymptomatic prostate cancer patients who were not candidates for curative local treatment [58]. Although the study showed no statistically significant difference in overall survival between the 2 arms ($p = 0.09$), it was underpowered to conclude equivalence. Recently, EORTC 30891, a randomized trial involving 985 patients with newly diagnosed prostate cancer, demonstrated statistically significant improvements in subjective and objective disease progression and in overall survival of men with nonmetastatic prostate cancer who were not candidates for local therapy but who were treated with immediate ADT, compared to men not treated until they were symptomatic [59]. Interestingly, the significant survival benefit was apparently due to fewer nonprostate cancer deaths and not to prostate cancer-related deaths. It may be that patients with less aggressive cancers, who might therefore respond better to early ADT, have a better chance of disease-specific survival.

Table 4. Selected neoadjuvant ADT followed by radical prostatectomy (RP)

Study	Study design	Population	No. of patients	Study intervention	Median follow-up (mos)	Results
Gleave [53]	Nonrandomized	T1c-T3a	156	32 wks CPA + DES or CAB followed by RP	54	PSA recurrence rate 12.2%
Schulman [270]	Prospective randomized	cT2-cT3 PSA<100	402	12 wks CAB followed by RP	48	PFS 26.4% vs. 32.5% (p=0.19)
						Decrease in positive margins in cT2 (p<0.01) and cT3 (p=0.01)
Soloway [52]	Prospective randomized	cT2b, PSA<50	282	12 weeks CAB followed by RP	60	5 yr DFS 67.6%(RP only) vs. 64.8% (p=0.663)
Aus [271]	Prospective randomized	T1b-T3a	126	3 wks CPA + 12 wks GnRH-A followed by RP	82	7 yr DFS 51.5% (RP) vs. 49.8% (p=0.588)
Gleave [54]	Prospective randomized	T1c-T2	500	12 wks vs. 32 wks CAB followed by RP	24	Positive margin rate 12% (8-mo group) vs. 23% (3-mo group), p=0.016
						Undetectable PSA rate before RP 75% (8-mo group) vs. 43% (3-mo group), p=0.0001

CPA: cyproterone acetate; RP: radical prostatectomy; CAB: combined androgen blockade; DFS: disease-free survival, equivalent to biochemical recurrence rate; PFS: progression-free survival, equivalent to PSA progression-free survival; PSA: prostate-specific antigen; GnRH: gonadotropin-releasing hormone agonist; DES: diethystilbestrol.

Alternatively, the finding of increased cardiovascular mortality in the control arm may be attributed to increased thrombotic events secondary to more advanced cancer [60]. It is important to note that, in this study, early ADT did not lead to earlier symptomatic or radiographic progressive disease with CRPC. The finding that there was no difference in time to progression after CRPC further allays concerns that earlier ADT would likely result in earlier development of hormone-refractory disease. This study therefore provides persuasive evidence that, for patients with nonmetastatic prostate cancer who are otherwise not good candidates for local therapy, immediate ADT provides meaningfully improved overall survival, with no decline in quality of life and no earlier time to progressive CRPC [61].

Role of Continuous ADT in Biochemical Recurrence of Prostate Cancer

Adoption of routine PSA testing after primary local therapy with surgery or RT has helped to identify a greater number of patients with PSA-only disease, also referred to as serologic or biochemical recurrence. The definition of biochemical recurrence is dependent on the treatment modality, since detectable PSA post-surgery indicates residual disease [62], while a PSA nadir post-RT can last as long as 18 months [63]. Although biochemical recurrence is considered a legitimate endpoint for defining treatment outcome, its clinical significance remains unclear [64]. One retrospective study of 1,997 men, of whom 315 (15%) developed biochemical recurrence after RP without hormonal therapy, revealed a median actuarial time to metastasis of 8 years after PSA elevation was noted, and a median of 5 years from metastasis to death [65]. However, of the subset of patients with Gleason scores > 8 and biochemical recurrence within 2 years of prostatectomy, only 53% remained free of metastasis at 3 years. A retrospective study with a larger cohort (379 analyzable patients out of 5,096 who underwent RP) and a longer median follow-up of 10 years showed that clinical parameters such as faster PSA doubling time (< 3 months), higher Gleason score (> 8), and shorter time from surgery to biochemical recurrence (< 3 years) were significant predictive risk factors for time to prostate-specific mortality [66]. [Note: PSA doubling time can be calculated by the natural log of 2 (0.693) divided by the slope of the relation between the log of PSA and the time of PSA measurement [67].] Several studies have examined various PSA dynamics, including doubling time, PSA response to salvage ADT, and PSA velocity, as indicators of which patients would develop clinically significant disease following biochemical recurrence after primary surgery or RT [68]. A PSA doubling time of < 3 months after RP or RT has consistently been shown to be associated with higher prostate cancer-specific mortality [69, 70]. Numerous treatment options are available for men with biochemical recurrence, including salvage RT or surgery (depending on the primary modality used), ADT, cryotherapy, brachytherapy, or observation. However, patients who present with biochemical recurrence may not be suitable candidates for salvage local therapy because of associated metastatic disease. ADT has been used in this treatment setting, but its value is unknown because there have been no randomized trials specifically for men with biochemical recurrence following local therapy. Researchers can only extrapolate from data on the use of

ADT in patients with more advanced disease or high-grade disease, which demonstrate a survival advantage for adjuvant ADT.

Early Versus Late Therapy

The question of whether to begin ADT early or late in the course of disease is in constant debate. The issue of timing stems from 2 hypotheses regarding the sensitivity of prostate cancer to hormonal ablation. The first hypothesis (the adaptation model) assumes that androgen-resistant clones of a homogeneous cell population develop through adaptive transformation after castration [71]. It would therefore be prudent to withhold androgen therapy for as long as possible. The other hypothesis (the clonal selection model) assumes that prostate cancer becomes heterogeneous soon after malignant transformation because of inherent genetic instability. Therefore, combining definitive local therapy (either surgery or radiation) with adjuvant ADT destroys the primary tumor when the percentage of androgen-resistant clones is still small and susceptible to eradication [72]. These and other hypotheses will be discussed further in the section on castrate resistance.

Several randomized trials have studied the use of early vs. delayed ADT in men with locally advanced or metastatic disease, but none of these trials has included patients with true PSA-only or biochemical recurrence. A retrospective, observational, multicenter database analysis of 5,382 men who underwent primary RP demonstrated that early hormonal therapy in patients with biochemical recurrence after RP was an independent predictor of delayed clinical metastasis only for high-risk cases. This delay in clinical metastasis was seen in patients with a pathological Gleason score > 7 or a PSA doubling time of ≤ 12 months (HR = 2.12; $p = 0.01$) [73]. The British Medical Research Council conducted a randomized trial of early vs. late ADT in more than 900 patients with M0/M1 locally advanced or asymptomatic metastatic disease [74]. Early reports showed a survival benefit for M0 patients in the immediate-treatment arm (71% vs. 62%; $p = 0.001$), but the benefit disappeared after follow-up report [75]. Immediate treatment was associated with disease-specific survival and decreased incidence of ureteric obstruction, spinal cord compression, and transurethral resection of the prostate, but also with an increased number of deaths from nonprostate cancers. Immediate ADT was not associated with an increase in cardiovascular deaths. The reduction in overall survival on long-term follow-up may be a result of prolonged hormonal treatment contributing to greater nonprostate cancer-related mortality. The study did not report on patient quality of life or bone pain, either of which could influence the decision to begin ADT early or late in the course of disease.

ADT should be used judiciously, taking care not to overtreat patients. Disease progression after biochemical recurrence can be long and variable, and the 8-year median time to metastasis may be even longer in patients treated with ADT. Therefore, any potential benefits of early ADT should be weighed against the adverse effects of long-term ADT. Such caution is especially important for patients with rising PSA but no radiographic evidence of metastatic disease, for whom the potential harm from long-term ADT may be substantially greater. A large systematic review of 4 trials involving 2,167 patients was conducted by Cochrane Database. The review showed an overall survival favoring the early-treatment group that was significant only at 10 years, when few patients had survived. Although these randomized controlled trials varied in study design, stage of cancer, subjects enrolled, and specific treatment utilized, the available information suggests that early androgen suppression for treatment of advanced prostate cancer reduces disease progression and its accompanying complications, and may provide a small but statistically significant improvement in overall survival at 10 years (odds ratio (OR) = 1.5; 95% CI: 1.04 to 2.16) [76].

Peripheral Androgen Blockade

Peripheral hormonal therapy for biochemical recurrence of prostate cancer has been tested in small studies. In a recent study, 98 evaluable patients with rising PSA after definitive local therapy were put on an oral regimen of finasteride 5 mg/day and flutamide 250 mg 3 times/day [77]. PSA was reduced by > 80% in 91 of 94 (97%) patients, with a median time of 1 month to a PSA level of < 1 ng/mL; 76 patients achieved a median time of 3.2 months to PSA nadir of < 0.2 ng/mL. After 59 months of follow-up, 48 patients were still undergoing treatment. Of these patients, 15 had documented disease progression that was responding to further hormonal manipulation. Toxicity was reportedly mild, with few reported grade 3 or 4 adverse events. Peripheral androgen blockade using finasteride and flutamide has fewer side effects than conventional ADT, especially in terms of sexual potency and libido. However, the long-term efficacy of this approach is currently unknown.

Role of Continuous ADT in Advanced Disease

Huggins and Hodges established prostate cancer's dependence on hormones over 50 years ago [1, 78]. In the setting of metastatic disease, ADT produces clinical response rates of 70% to 80% [79]. Early randomized controlled trials comparing orchiectomy to DES have demonstrated equivalent efficacy [7] and overall survival [80]. A systematic review and meta-analysis of 10 trials involving 1,908 patients reported no significant difference in overall survival between ADT and orchiectomy. The hazard ratio showed GnRH-A to be essentially equivalent to orchiectomy (HR = 1.1262; 95% CI: 0.915 to 1.386) [22]. The 3 GnRH-A used in these studies were associated with similar overall survival, although CIs were wider for leuprolide (HR = 1.0994; 95% CI: 0.207 to 5.835) and buserelin (HR = 1.1315; 95% CI: 0.533 to 2.404) than for goserelin (HR = 1.1172; 95% CI: 0.898 to 1.390). Bilateral orchiectomy or chemical castration with GnRH are thus the recommended initial treatments for patients with metastatic prostate cancer. Different approaches to delivering ADT have been studied in the setting of advanced prostate cancer and will be reviewed here.

Table 5. Selected studies comparing combined androgen blockade (CAB) with conventional ADT

Study	Study design	No. of patients	Tumor stage	Study intervention	Max/med follow-up (mos)	Results
Crawford et al. [83]	Randomized double blind	603	D2	Leuprolide + placebo vs. leuprolide + flutamide	48	Improved PFS and length of survival in CAB group (16.5 vs. 13.9 mos; p = 0.039 and 35.6 vs. 28.3 mos; p = 0.035, respectively)
Denis et al. [272]	Randomized phase III	327	M1	Orchiectomy alone vs. goserelin + flutamide	84	Improvement with CAB in OS (p = 0.04), time to death from malignant disease (p = 0.008), time to first progression (p = 0.009), and PFS (p = 0.02)
Janknegt et al. [85]	Randomized double-blind	457	M1	Orchiectomy alone vs. orchiectomy + nilutamide	35–54	Improvement with CAB in PFS (20.8 vs. 14.9 mos; p = 0.005) and median time to death (30.0 vs. 37 mos)
Eisenberger et al. [87]	Randomized	1387	M1	Orchiectomy + flutamide vs. orchiectomy + placebo	84	No difference in OS (p = 0.14)
Tyrrell et al. [273]	Randomized double-blind	571	M0 and M1	Goserelin vs. goserelin + flutamide	56.2	No difference in PFS and OS
Iversen et al. [274]	Randomized	264	M0 and M1	Orchiectomy vs. goserelin + flutamide	57	No difference in PFS (16.8 vs. 16.5 mos) and OS (27.6 vs. 22.7 mos)
Boccardo et al. [275]	Randomized	304	C and D	Goserelin vs. goserelin + flutamide	24	No difference in PFS (24 vs. 17 mos; p = 0.09) or OS

PFS: progression-free survival; CAB: combined androgen blockade; OS: overall survival.

Combined Androgen Blockade

ADT remains the primary systemic treatment for advanced prostate cancer. Testosterone produced by the testes supplies around 90% of the body's androgens, with the rest produced by the adrenal glands. Labrie et al. introduced complete blockade of the effects of both testicular and adrenal androgens through the use of nonsteroidal antiandrogens (AAs), a practice now known as combined or complete androgen blockade (CAB) or maximal androgen blockade (MAB) [81]. The rationale is that low concentrations of androgens of adrenal origin can remain in the body after androgen suppression and exert a stimulatory effect on hormone-sensitive prostate cancer cells, and that any such residual effect can be reduced by the use of AAs.

There are 3 FDA-approved AAs in common use in the United States (table 1). These drugs competitively antagonize the binding of testosterone and DHT to the AR and thus block the androgens' growth signal. Since the early 1980s, numerous randomized trials have studied the efficacy of CAB [82]. Though the approach was initially promising and some trials suggested that CAB conferred a significant survival advantage [83-86], others showed no survival advantage [87, 88] (see table 5). Specifically, the largest prostate cancer trial (SWOG or INT-0105 trial), which compared 687 patients treated with orchiectomy plus placebo with 700 patients treated with orchiectomy plus flutamide, found no difference in overall survival ($p = 0.14$) [87]. CAB had no advantage over orchiectomy alone in terms of time to progression, even in patients with minimal disease. The only notable differences in the arm using CAB with flutamide were higher rates of diarrhea and anemia, and a higher rate of discontinuation from therapy because of this toxicity (5% vs. 1%).

The Prostate Cancer Trialists' Collaborative Group reviewed 27 trials of CAB vs. androgen suppression involving 8,275 men. The meta-analysis found that the addition of an AA to androgen suppression improved overall 5-year survival by about 2% to 3%, depending on whether the analysis included CPA, which conferred a slightly unfavorable outcome compared to nilutamide and flutamide [88]. A subsequent meta-analysis of 21 randomized trials with a total of 6,781 patients comparing ADT and CAB found no statistically significant difference in overall survival at 2 years (HR = 0.970; 95% CI: 0.866 to 1.087) [89]. However, based on more limited data, the meta-analysis found a statistically significant increase in overall survival at 5 years (total of only 10 trials, HR = 0.871; 95% CI: 0.805 to 0.942) for CAB minus CPA. This modest increase in overall survival should be weighed against the increased risk of adverse events that could affect the patient's overall quality of life. CAB with GnRH-A plus AA confers the highest estimated quality-adjusted survival, but at an incremental cost of over USD 1 million per quality-adjusted life-year over orchiectomy alone [8].

Antiandrogen Monotherapy

Nonsteroidal AAs are often used in conjunction with castration as a component of CAB. However, monotherapy with a nonsteroidal AA has also been explored as an alternative therapeutic approach. Nonsteroidal AAs act through competitive inhibition of androgen-binding at the receptor level, inhibiting the action of androgens from both the adrenal glands and the testes. Because of their mode of action, decreases in testosterone concentration are not seen after monotherapy with these agents. Instead, testosterone levels generally increase slightly, offering potential quality-of-life advantages over conventional ADT [90]. Flutamide has been used in AA monotherapy for the longest period of time. However, only 2 studies have reported survival data: one comparing flutamide monotherapy to orchiectomy (319 patients) and another comparing flutamide to CAB (104 patients). Neither study reported an overall survival or clinical progression-free advantage [91, 92].

Bicalutamide monotherapy has been most widely evaluated. Bicalutamide 150 mg/day was compared with flutamide 250 mg 3 times/day, in combination with an LHRH, in a study involving 220 patients. No statistically significant differences in overall or progression-free survival were noted between the 2 groups, although bicalutamide treatment fared better in terms of quality-of-life assessments, with fewer instances of diarrhea or withdrawal from study due to adverse events [93]. Lower doses of bicalutamide (50 mg/day) showed inferior overall survival compared to castration [94]. In PSA dose-response studies, bicalutamide at once-daily 150 mg was found to be an appropriate, well-tolerated dosage, prompting subsequent evaluation of bicalutamide in larger comparative trials. The clinical efficacy of bicalutamide 150 mg/day monotherapy for treatment of 480 patients with locally advanced M0 disease and 805 patients with M1 disease was studied in comparison with medical or surgical castration in 2 randomized phase III trials [95, 96]. Survival data from patients randomized to castration vs. bicalutamide after a follow-up of 1.9 years showed that bicalutamide was not as effective as castration. Further analysis of mature data at 6.3 years in patients with locally advanced nonmetastatic disease demonstrated no statistically significant difference in overall survival or time to progression [97]. An overall survival advantage of 6 weeks (42 days) was seen in favor of castration in patients with M1 disease ($HR = 1.3$; 95% CI: 1.04 to 1.65; $p = 0.02$). This advantage was observed only in patients with PSA levels of $\geq$ 400 ng/mL; for patients with M1 disease with PSA $\leq$ 400 ng/mL at baseline, bicalutamide 150 mg seemed just as effective as castration in terms of overall survival, which may have been due to differences in tumor burden in these groups of patients. Since AAs work by competitively inhibiting the AR binding site, it is conceivable that the total number of ARs present and the penetration of AA into the tumor, which vary according to tumor burden, dictate the clinical efficacy of AAs [98].

These trials further demonstrated that patients receiving bicalutamide had measurably greater physical capacity and sexual interest. This assessment, which covered most aspects of daily life, indicated that patients receiving bicalutamide monotherapy maintained a more normal lifestyle than those who underwent castration (table 6). In these trials, the most commonly reported adverse events with bicalutamide treatment were breast pain (40.1%) and gynecomastia (49.4%) (these figures were higher in the more recent Early Prostate Cancer (EPC) program involving bicalutamide [97, 99]), but withdrawal from therapy because of these adverse events was low. Prophylactic radiation at 12 to 15 Gy x 1 has been used to prevent this adverse effect [100]. Once gynecomastia has developed, estrogen antagonists and aromatase inhibitors may be effective complements to treatment, since gynecomastia is caused by an increase in the ratio of estrogen to androgen [101].

Table 6. Advantages and disadvantages of nonsteroidal AA monotherapy over GnRH-A

Advantages	Disadvantages
Less loss of physical capacity	Not FDA-approved
Less sexual dysfunction	Significant gynecomastia and mastodynia
No loss of BMD	4% to 10% withdrawal due to adverse events
Equivalent outcomes in D0 disease	Worse outcomes in metastatic D2 disease
Fewer hot flashes	Visual and respiratory disturbance and alcohol intolerance (nilutamide)

A major collaborative clinical trials program was set up to investigate the efficacy and tolerability of bicalutamide 150 mg combined with standard care (RP, RT, or watchful waiting) in patients with localized or locally advanced disease [102]. The bicalutamide EPC program consisted of 3 randomized, double-blind, placebo-controlled trials of similar design conducted in distinct geographical areas, including North America (Trial 23), Europe, South Africa, Mexico, Israel, and Australia (Trial 24), and Scandinavia (Trial 25). In the first analysis of the EPC program, after a median follow-up of 3 years, patients in the bicalutamide arm had 42% less objective disease progression compared with standard care alone ($p < 0.001$). Patients treated with watchful waiting had more disease-progression events than patients in the other groups. At the second analysis, after 5.4 years of follow-up, there were no overall survival differences, but improved progression-free survival with bicalutamide was seen in Trials 24 and 25 [103]. Of note were the differences in entry and selection criteria among the 3 trials. Trial 23 ($n = 3{,}292$) excluded patients with lymph node metastasis and had no watchful-waiting arm, while Trial 24 ($n = 3{,}603$) and Trial 25 ($n = 1{,}218$) included node-positive patients and those managed with watchful waiting. At a median follow-up of 7.7 years for Trial 23, no differences in the primary endpoints of objective progression-free survival and overall survival were seen between patients treated with bicalutamide and those treated with standard care alone, although once-daily bicalutamide 150 mg significantly improved time to PSA progression (HR = 0.80; 95% CI: 0.72 to 0.90; $p < 0.001$) [104]. In a combined analysis of all 3 trials at 7.4 years follow-up, adding bicalutamide to standard care for patients with localized disease offered no benefit in terms of progression-free survival and, in fact, trended toward decreased survival compared to patients undergoing watchful waiting alone (HR = 1.16; 95% CI: 0.99 to 1.37; $p = 0.07$) [99]. This was in contrast to patients with locally advanced disease, for whom bicalutamide significantly improved progression-free survival irrespective of standard care. Bicalutamide also improved overall survival in patients receiving RT (HR: 0.65; 95% CI: 0.66 to 1.01; $p = 0.03$), and appeared favorable to watchful waiting (HR = 0.81; 95% CI: 0.44 to 0.95; $p = 0.06$). The EPC program concluded that adjuvant bicalutamide provided no benefit to patients with localized prostate cancer, but did improve progression-free survival in patients with locally advanced disease, and appeared to increase overall survival in a selected group of patients. Another large trial conducted by the EORTC closed to accrual in February 2003. It is a randomized phase III step-up study on initial AA monotherapy compared to watchful waiting in asymptomatic T1 to T3 (any Gleason) N0 or NxM0 prostate cancer patients without local treatment with curative intent. Trial results have not been reported [105].

Based on current data, AA monotherapy, specifically bicalutamide 150 mg once daily, is an attractive alternative to castration for patients with locally advanced prostate cancer, especially those who wish to retain potency or those for whom quality-of-life issues are a major concern (table 6). Ongoing studies are needed to determine the exact role of AA monotherapy in the treatment of localized prostate cancer. Currently, the American Society of Clinical Oncology states that monotherapy with a nonsteroidal AA may be discussed with patients as an alternative to ADT, but steroidal AAs, which are currently not approved in the United States, should not be offered as monotherapy [8].

Antiandrogen Withdrawal

Another method of hormone manipulation in prostate cancer patients involves withdrawal of the use of AAs. This paradoxical response to flutamide withdrawal was recognized only recently, despite over 2 decades of use in patients with progressive prostate cancer [106]. Subsequent studies of this withdrawal syndrome found that it was not limited to flutamide, but was also observed with bicalutamide, another AA, and reported with nilutamide, ketoconazole, megestrol acetate, and CPA, suggesting that the phenomenon is more generalized than originally believed. The biochemical response can be achieved in approximately 15% to 20% of patients with CRPC on CAB upon AA therapy withdrawal [107]. In addition to PSA declines, tumor regression and resolution of tumor-related symptoms have also been documented, along with improvements in abnormal hematological parameters [108, 109]. It is believed that the mechanism of this withdrawal phenomenon is related to mutations in the hormone-binding domain on the AR. In addition, there may be a different binding site for each AA, turning the AA from an AR antagonist (AR corepressor) to an AR agonist (AR coactivator). In vitro studies have shown that the AR in prostate cancer cell line LNCaP contains a specific point mutation [110] that results in a paradoxical stimulation of growth following incubation of hydroxyflutamide, nilutamide, CPA, and progestins [111, 112].

Beyond the obvious advantages of lower toxicity and greater cost-effectiveness, AA withdrawal has important therapeutic implications for patients who are progressing on hormonal therapies despite castrate levels of testosterone [113], especially if they are enrolled in clinical trials. AA withdrawal should be considered before alternative strategies since some improvements, such as PSA levels, may be attributed to the study agent when, in fact, they are due to AA withdrawal. It is unknown at this point whether tumor-cell apoptosis in response to AA withdrawal is due to an in vivo step selection because of continual exposure to an AA, or whether it is a natural action of prostate cancer cells as they undergo androgen independence. Regardless of the mechanism of action, AA withdrawal may further delay progression of prostate cancer, allowing for consideration of alternative therapies.

Intermittent ADT

Intermittent ADT (or intermittent androgen suppression) is an alternative approach to treating hormone-sensitive prostate cancer. It involves administering hormonal agents for 2 to 3 months beyond "best response," then discontinuing hormonal therapy and restarting it at a predetermined time. This strategy evolved in response to concerns that early ADT could lead to androgen independence [114]. Studies using animal models have suggested that successive rounds of androgen withdrawal and replacement delay progression to androgen independence [115]. The underlying hypothesis is this: if prostate cancer cells that survive androgen deprivation are forced by androgen replacement to continue normal differentiation, then treatment-induced apoptosis may occur, androgen dependence may be prolonged, and progression to androgen independence may be delayed [116]. Other concerns about prolonged or continuous ADT include the side effects of prolonged hormonal ablation, as well as the cost of treatment as many more patients are being treated earlier in the course of disease [117].

Role of Intermittent ADT in Biochemically Recurrent Prostate Cancer

Intermittent ADT in the setting of biochemical recurrence has uncertain long-term efficacy. A 31-month interim follow-up of the European EC 507 phase III trial of intermittent vs. continuous ADT (RELAPSE study) for men with PSA relapse after RP showed no difference in progression-free survival between the 96 patients who received intermittent ADT and the 78 patients who received continuous ADT (1,234 days vs. 1,010 days; $p = 0.9852$). Progression was reported in 8.3% of those receiving intermittent ADT vs. 6.4% of those receiving continuous ADT (p = not significant) [118]. Although these results suggest equivalent efficacy between continuous and intermittent ADT in patients with biochemical recurrence, definite conclusions cannot be made because of early follow-up. One ongoing phase III trial sponsored by the National Cancer Institute of Canada is the PR.7 trial (available through Southwest Oncology Group (SWOG), Medical Research Council, and Cancer Trials Support Unit), which has the primary objective of comparing overall survival for intermittent vs. continuous ADT in men with biochemical progression after RT.

Understanding the kinetics of testosterone after GnRH-A therapy is an important tool in planning subsequent treatment and timing of intermittent ADT. In a randomized prospective phase III analysis of 80 men with PSA-only biochemically recurrent disease, treatment consisted of 6 months of either leuprolide 22.5 mg or goserelin 10.8 mg, after which patients received either thalidomide or placebo [119]. When PSA rose to $\geq$ 5 ng/mL or baseline without evidence of metastatic disease, patients received another 6-month course of GnRH-A and crossed over to the opposite oral therapy. Testosterone and DHT levels were obtained every 3 months on GnRH-A therapy and monthly on oral study drug; analyses of these levels were secondary endpoints of this trial. The median time to an increase of testosterone $\geq$ 50 ng/dL and DHT $\geq$ 212 ng/dL was 12.9 weeks and 16.6 weeks, respectively. Levels remained elevated and did not return to normal until a median of 14.9 weeks and 16.6 weeks, respectively. Understanding the kinetics of androgen normalization following GnRH-A therapy may help guide treatment decisions, especially where discontinuation of GnRH-A therapy is employed, as in the case of intermittent ADT.

The use of a predetermined PSA trigger point or threshold level as a basis to initiate therapy has also been studied in a prospective, noncomparative, multicenter phase II trial of 103 men with localized prostate cancer who had biochemical recurrence after external-beam radiation. Study subjects underwent cyclic ADT after 36 weeks of GnRH-A treatment [120]. If serum PSA was not < 4.0 ng/mL at 24 weeks and 32 weeks of treatment, patients were taken off study. Serum PSA and testosterone levels were monitored thereafter and ADT was resumed when PSA rose to ≥ 4.0 ng/mL. After a median follow-up of 4.2 years, the time off treatment averaged 53% of the total cycle time, but progressively decreased with each succeeding cycle, ranging from 63.7 weeks in cycle 1 to 25.6 weeks in cycle 5. The good response rates seen in this study again demonstrated the feasibility of cyclic ADT. Although the proportion of the total length of each cycle spent in the off-treatment phase became progressively shorter with time, the off-treatment interval remained appreciable, ranging from 65% in cycle 1 to 46% in cycle 5.

Role of Intermittent ADT in Locally Advanced or Metastatic Prostate Cancer

Data from a number of phase II trials have provided the basis for the current use of intermittent ADT (table 7). One of the first trials involved 12 patients with localized disease and 8 with metastatic disease who received DES and flutamide for a median of 10 months prior to halting treatment [121]. Disease progression was noted after a median of 8 months. In addition, 9 out of 10 patients who were rendered impotent by ADT resumed sexual activity within 3 months after going off treatment, and all patients who relapsed had a rapid response upon reinitiation of treatment. The use of PSA level to define an optimal trigger point or threshold was first described in a trial where 47 patients were treated with combined ADT for 24 to 32 weeks, when a PSA nadir in the normal range (≤ 4.0 ng/mL) was obtained [122]. Patients went off treatment until PSA rose to a mean value between 10 ng/mL and 20 ng/mL. The first 2 cycles were of 73 weeks and 75 weeks duration, with mean percentages of time off therapy of 41% and 45%, respectively. The mean time to achieve a PSA nadir was 20 weeks in cycle 1 and 18 weeks in cycle 2. Serum testosterone returned to normal pretreatment levels at a median of 8 weeks after stopping treatment. This normalization of serum androgens has been confirmed in a prospective analysis of a phase III trial utilizing ADT, where the median time to a testosterone level of ≥ 212 ng/dL was 16.6 weeks [119].

Several factors have been shown to predict the time off ADT in patients undergoing intermittent ADT [123]. Patients who had an undetectable PSA (< 0.05 ng/mL) within one year had a median off phase of 29 months vs. 8.5 months for those whose PSA did not become undetectable within one year ($p = 0.00002$). For patients who had biochemical recurrence without radiographic evidence of disease, median duration of the off phase was twice as long as it was for patients who had no prior definitive therapy (24 vs. 12 months; $p = 0.028$), which may be related to a higher disease burden in the former group. Finally, those patients whose testosterone recovered within 4 months after discontinuing ADT had a shorter median time in the off phase than those whose PSA did not recover within 4 months (10 vs. 25 months; p = 0.0022).

Table 7. Published reports of use of intermittent ADT with at least 50 patients

Author	Year	No. of patients	Treatment	Stage of disease (L/BF/M)	Median time on therapy (mos)	Median time off therapy (mos)
Bruchovsky [125]	1998	110	GnRH + AA	0/110/0	9	9
Bracarda [276]	1998	55	GnRH + AA	44/0/11	7	6
Theyer [277]	1998	52	GnRH + AA	15/0/37	6	16
Gleave [278]	1998	70	GnRH + AA	41/0/29	9	9
Crook [279]	1999	54	GnRH + AA	11/4/39	8	9
Strum [123]	2000	52	GnRH + AA	24/19/9	19	24
Grossfeld [280]	2001	61	GnRH + AA	34/27/0	9	6
Prapotnich [281]	2003	233	GnRH + AA	NR^	6*	13*
Tangen [282]	2003	663	GnRH + AA	0/0/663	NR	NR

L: localized; BF: biochemical failure without radiographic evidence of disease; M: metastatic; AA: antiandrogen; NR: not reported.

^All patients had either biochemical failure, PSA > 30 (without local therapy), or metastatic disease.

*Median for first cycle. Treatment was stopped when PSA was < 4 ng/mL and restarted when PSA was > 20 ng/mL.

**Adapted from Gulley JL, Dahut WL. Novel schedules of hormone therapy for prostate cancer. In: Devita V, Hellman S, Rosenberg S, eds. *Progress in Oncology*. Boston: Jones and Bartlett; 2004:236-253.

To address the effects of intermittent vs. continuous institution of CAB in patients with locally advanced or metastatic prostate cancer, a large phase III trial conducted on behalf of the South European Urooncological Group demonstrated no association between intermittent CAB and higher rates of subjective or objective disease progression (p = 0.32), and no evidence that intermittent ADT leads to a significantly elevated risk of death (p = 0.79) compared to continuous ADT, after a median follow-up of 4.3 years [124]. In this study, 766 treatment-naïve patients with advanced-stage or metastatic prostate cancer were treated for 3 months with hormonal therapy consisting of 2 weeks of CPA at 200 mg/day, followed by monthly depot injections of decaptyl plus CPA. Patients who achieved a PSA of < 4 ng/mL, or reduced their PSA level by 80%, were further randomized to continuous (n = 312) or intermittent (n = 314) CAB. In the intermittent arm, patients underwent treatment only when their PSA level was ≥ 10 ng/mL with symptoms, or ≥ 20 ng/mL without symptoms, or when they reached ≥ 20% of the nadir value. About 50% of patients were off treatment for a year after the first cycle of hormonal therapy; of those who had a nadir PSA < 2 ng/mL, the time off treatment was 74 weeks. After these patients returned to therapy, they had a median of 14 weeks of treatment, followed by a second period off treatment for a median of 70 weeks. The results of this study suggest the feasibility and equivalent outcome of intermittent CAB compared to continuous CAB in men with locally advanced or metastatic disease.

While there are definite benefits to the use of intermittent ADT, especially improved quality of life [125, 126], the overall survival benefit of intermittent ADT over CAB cannot be fully ascertained [127]. This is particularly true for patients with advanced prostate cancer who exhibit poor prognostic features and should not be considered for intermittent therapy [128]. An ongoing phase III trial that will attempt to address this issue is SWOG 9436, which is currently available via various cooperative groups [129]. Recent data published from SWOG 9436 and INT-0162 showed that D2 prostate cancer patients with a PSA nadir between 0.2 ng/mL and 4 ng/mL had one third less risk of death than those with a PSA nadir $\geq$ 4 ng/mL, and those with PSA nadir $\leq$ 0.2 ng/mL had less than one fifth the risk of death of patients with a PSA nadir of $\geq$ 4 ng/mL ($p < 0.001$). This translated to a median survival of 75 months in the $\leq$ 0.2 ng/mL PSA group compared to 44 months for the group with PSA between 0.2 ng/mL and 4 ng/mL, and only 13 months for the PSA > 4 ng/mL group [130]. All 1,395 eligible patients received 7 months of induction ADT using a GnRH-A and bicalutamide, of whom 81% (1,134) achieved a PSA of $\leq$ 4 ng/mL on months 6 or 7 and were randomly assigned to continuous vs. intermittent ADT on month 8. Four statistically significant ($p < 0.05$) risk factors predicting postinduction survival are performance status, Gleason score, bone pain, and PSA upon study entry. Although this study concluded that achieving a PSA of $\leq$ 4 ng/mL after 7 months of ADT is a strong predictor of survival, the primary objective of SWOG 9436 to compare overall survival between patients undergoing intermittent ADT vs. continuous ADT has not been reported.

Individual Dosing Based on Testosterone Levels

Taking an individualized approach to androgen suppression is an evolving strategy that appears to be safe and cost-effective [131]. For many men, testosterone suppression continues well beyond the scheduled readministration of GnRH-A [132], especially for those with a long history of GnRH use [133]. Thus, delaying readministration of a GnRH-A until testosterone suppression has abated to noncastrate levels might lead to significant cost savings, with no negative effect on outcomes. The feasibility of this approach was demonstrated by a small phase I study composed of 32 patients with stage T3N± M± or greater treated with a 3-month depot of leuprolide injection [134]. Serum testosterone and PSA levels were obtained every month beginning 3 months after the last leuprolide injection. The median duration of castrate-level testosterone was 6 months. Another study prospectively enrolled 22 patients in a control-crossover-designed trial of dosing depot GnRH-A based on serum testosterone [132]. The median duration of castrate testosterone was 5.5 months (range 3.5 to 10), but the primary outcome of the study was to examine the health-related quality of life of patients with prostate cancer undergoing this treatment strategy. Short-term overall health-related quality of life and patient satisfaction were significantly improved over baseline measurements, and the yearly cost of care was significantly decreased using the method of redosing based on serum testosterone (USD 3,567.90 vs. USD 7,135.80). A similar finding of castrate levels of testosterone lasting for 6 months after the last GnRH-A dosing was seen in a study involving 80 patients, all of whom were treated with 6 months of GnRH-A therapy, with testosterone levels obtained monthly [119]. These early results suggest that using serum testosterone levels as a guide in redosing GnRH-A may be a novel, cost-effective approach to administering intermittent ADT.

Rapid Hormonal Testosterone Cycling

Another evolving strategy being explored in patients with locally advanced or metastatic prostate cancer combines hormonal cycling and chemotherapy, the rationale being that cycling, rather than prolonged androgen deprivation, will induce multiple cycles of apoptosis [135]. In a trial consisting of 23 patients (18 with metastatic disease and 5 with biochemical recurrence), treatment involved a 3-month induction of GnRH-A monthly plus bicalutamide for a month, followed by monthly cycles of androgen repletion with topical testosterone for 7 days and a GnRH-A monthly [136]. No disease progression was observed, and 6 of the 15 evaluable patients achieved the study's primary endpoint of successively declining PSA troughs after androgen deprivation. To further improve responses with rapid hormonal cycling, addition of cytotoxic chemotherapy using docetaxel was studied in a total of 63 patients, 25 with biochemical recurrence and 38 with metastatic prostate cancer [137]. Six treatment cycles were given, each lasting for 4 weeks, consisting of GnRH-A plus docetaxel 75 mg/m^2 given on day 1 of week 1, followed by testosterone gel given for 7 days beginning on day 1 of week 4. The primary endpoint of the study was to determine the number of patients who achieved the following PSA levels: $\leq$ 0.05 ng/mL in those who had undergone prostatectomy; $\leq$ 0.5 ng/mL in those who had undergone radiation therapy; and $\leq$ 2.0 ng/mL in those with metastatic prostate cancer without local therapy. Results showed that 4 of 11 evaluable patients (36%) in the biochemical-recurrence group and 9 of 26 evaluable patients (35%) in the metastatic-disease group achieved the primary endpoint. A notable toxicity was grade 3 and 4 neutropenia, which occurred in 82% of the biochemical-recurrence group and 88% of the metastatic-disease group. These studies show that rapid hormonal cycling plus docetaxel is feasible. Longer follow-up is necessary to compare this treatment approach to standard hormonal therapy in patients with biochemical recurrence after primary therapy for prostate cancer. A phase II study of rapid hormonal cycling with testosterone and leuprolide in combination with docetaxel in patients with recurrent or noncastrate metastatic prostate cancer has closed to accrual with results pending [138].

Other Agents

After first-line ADT has failed, usually in the form of orchiectomy, GnRH-A therapy, CAB, and AA withdrawal, alternative second-line ADT may be considered. Second-line ADT has not been shown to provide an overall survival advantage, but it can decrease symptomatic disease and cause radiographic responses and PSA declines.

Ketoconazole

Ketoconazole, an oral imidazole antifungal agent, suppresses testicular and adrenal steroidogenesis and is associated with significant PSA declines when used as a second-line hormonal agent [139-141]. In vitro data with androgen-independent cell lines PC-3 and DU-145 suggest that ketoconazole may have direct cytotoxic effects as well [142]. A decline in PSA of at least 50% in 11 of 20 patients (55%) and a median duration of PSA response of 9 months was seen in one trial [143]. Castrate levels of testosterone may be seen after only 48 hours of therapy, making ketoconazole a treatment of choice in cases requiring urgent ADT, such as spinal cord compression or active disseminated intravascular coagulation [140, 144, 145]. In another study of 16 patients with D2 prostate cancer despite ADT in whom pain was a prominent clinical feature, 13 patients (81%) noted improvement in pain for periods of 1 to 8 months (median 3 months) [146]. Despite its advantages, ketoconazole can cause toxicity at high doses and requires glucocorticoid (e.g., hydrocortisone) supplementation to prevent adrenal insufficiency even at lower doses [141].

Aminoglutethimide

Aminoglutethimide, originally developed as an anticonvulsant, blocks adrenocorticoid synthesis by inhibiting the conversion of cholesterol to pregnenolone. One study showed a > 50% PSA decline in 37% of patients with CRPC treated with 1,000 mg/day aminoglutethimide and 40 mg/day hydrocortisone, with a median duration of response of 9 months and median survival of 23 months [147]. However, changes in androgen levels do not seem to correlate with tumor response. Aminoglutethimide has also been found to ameliorate bone pain and is used as a second-line hormonal treatment in patients with advanced disease [148, 149]. Like ketoconazole, it must be administered with glucocorticoid replacement. Although aminoglutethimide has largely been replaced by ketoconazole, it remains an active available agent and is a reasonable alternative for patients requiring a secondary hormonal approach. Aminoglutethimide is started at a dose of 250 mg 3 times/day for 3 weeks, then increased to 4 times/day [150].

Abiraterone Acetate

Abiraterone acetate is an oral 17-alpha hydroxylase/C17,20-lyase inhibitor developed as a steroidal inhibitor following observations that nonsteroidal 3-pyridyl esters had improved selectivity for inhibiting testosterone synthesis [151]. Several phase I studies evaluating the effects of abiraterone acetate have shown that enhanced testosterone suppression is achieved in castrate men [151, 152].

ADT Combined with other Modalities

ADT and Chemotherapy

As a prostate cancer treatment, chemotherapy alone has been shown to palliate symptoms of disease, but until the recent introduction of taxanes it has shown no survival advantage [153]. The success of chemotherapy noted in early trials by the National Prostatic Cancer Project (NPCP) in the 1980s caused enthusiastic speculation on the potential benefits of combining chemotherapy with ADT. It was suggested that multiply heterogeneous prostate cancer cells may be susceptible to both chemotherapy and hormonal therapy agents [154]. The first prospective trial by the NPCP randomized 246 newly diagnosed metastatic prostate cancer patients to orchiectomy or DES alone, DES plus cyclophosphamide, or cyclophosphamide plus estramustine phosphate (EMP) [155]. Overall response rates were similar for all 3 treatment arms, although there appeared to be significantly poorer survival in patients with painful metastasis compared to those who were asymptomatic. This led to a subsequent NPCP study (Protocol 1300) that randomized 319 men to ADT alone, a combination of ADT and chemotherapy (cyclophosphamide plus 5-fluorouracil), or EMP alone [156]. There were no significant differences between the groups in progression-free or overall survival. In another trial, 96 patients with locally advanced or metastatic prostate cancer were randomized to hormonal therapy with a GnRH-A and flutamide, with or without 4 cycles of adjuvant mitoxantrone [157]. Men with localized prostate cancer receiving adjuvant chemotherapy had a higher initial objective response rate (95% vs. 53%; $p = 0.008$) and median survival (80 vs. 36 months; $p = 0.04$) than patients treated with hormonal therapy alone. No advantage was observed with adjuvant chemotherapy in men with metastatic disease. The use of adjuvant chemotherapy in conjunction with other hormonal agents such as prednisone has been studied.

EMP, a synthetic drug with both nitrogen mustard and estrogenic properties, has been used in the treatment of prostate cancer since 1981. As a single-agent treatment for metastatic disease, radiographic improvement was noted in only 5% to 19% of patients [158, 159]. EMP is believed to target the microtubule-associated proteins alpha-tubulin and beta-tubulin. Preclinical data suggesting additive antitumor effects of combining EMP with microtubule-targeted agents such as taxanes, etoposide, and vinca alkaloids spurred clinical trials. Neoadjuvant chemotherapy, with or without EMP, has been examined [160-164]. In the 2 trials involving patients who were to undergo radical prostatectomy, combination chemotherapy with EMP and etoposide was given to 18 patients, and KAVE (ketoconazole plus adriamycin alternating with vinblastine and EMP) plus CAB was given to 27 patients. None of the patients had a pathologically complete response, although undetectable PSA was noted in all patients [160, 164]. Docetaxel and EMP combination was studied in 21 patients prior to local therapy with either RT or RP [165]. EMP was given over 3 days and therapy was repeated every 3 weeks. Clinical response was noted in all patients as measured by DRE, imaging, and PSA responses, and other pathologic endpoints, such as a negative margin rate of 70%, were favorable. All patients also achieved suppressed testosterone levels despite the short duration of EMP treatment. These improvements in radiographic and biochemical response rates in patients with advanced disease led to further phase III trials [166-168]. In the phase III SWOG 9916 trial that compared docetaxel and EMP with mitoxantrone and prednisone in patients with advanced CRPC, docetaxel and EMP improved median survival by nearly 2 months ($p = 0.01$) [169]. Patients in the docetaxel and EMP treatment groups also had a significantly higher PSA response rate (50% vs. 27%; $p < 0.0001$). There was, however, no statistically significant difference in bone-pain palliation or quality of life between the 2 treatment arms [170].

The TAX 327 trial compared docetaxel weekly, docetaxel every 3 weeks, and mitoxantrone plus prednisone every 3 weeks in men with CRPC. Compared with mitoxantrone plus prednisone, docetaxel every 3 weeks improved overall survival ($p = 0.009$), and both docetaxel regimens improved patient quality of life [171]. Because it has a similar survival advantage and fewer side effects than docetaxel and EMP, the combination of docetaxel and prednisone has become the standard of care for patients with metastatic CRPC [153]. An alternative treatment sequence utilizing cytotoxic chemotherapy with docetaxel followed by ADT has also been studied. Severe combined immunodeficient mice bearing human LNCaP prostate tumors were treated with docetaxel and/or surgical castration, applied singly, concurrently, or in different sequences. Initial observations showed that docetaxel followed by castration had the most potent antitumor effect [172]. The beneficial therapeutic effect of this treatment sequence is thought to be due to cytotoxic drugs known to be active in CRPC targeting the androgen-sensitive components of prostate cancer cells, since a subpopulation of tumor cells that are resistant to apoptosis, as demonstrated by an altered bax-to-bcl2 ratio, is believed to emerge within weeks of androgen ablation [173]. The feasibility of this treatment sequence was examined in 32 men with biochemical recurrence and 7 with metastatic disease [174]. When treatment was initiated with docetaxel at 70 mg/m^2 every 3 weeks for up to 6 cycles, followed by CAB for 12 to 20 months, 48.5% of patients (17/35) had a serum PSA decrease of $\geq$ 50%, and 20% (7/35) had a serum PSA decrease of $\geq$ 75%.

Taken together, these studies provide rationale and feasibility for the use of chemotherapy as an adjunct to localized treatment for a select group of high-risk patients. Ongoing studies will further evaluate clinical endpoints in patients treated with ADT alone vs. ADT with chemotherapy. TAX 3501 will randomize patients to observation, ADT, or ADT plus docetaxel every 3 weeks. SWOG 9921 will evaluate overall survival following hormone therapy alone and hormone therapy plus adjuvant chemotherapy with 6 cycles of mitoxantrone plus prednisone in men who have had RP for high-risk prostate cancer.

ADT and Vaccines

While numerous ADT regimens have been described, no standard therapy options involving ADT have been shown to prolong survival for prostate cancer patients with biochemical progression after localized therapy. The generally indolent nature of prostate cancer compared with other solid tumors and the low tumor burden seen with biochemical progression have spurred significant interest in the development of vaccines for this disease state, and in the potentially significant benefits of combining ADT with vaccines. Several lines of research have demonstrated the immunosuppressive effects of androgens. Both testosterone and DHT have been shown to increase levels of TGF-beta, which can negatively modulate the immune response [175-181]. Murine studies showed that androgen deprivation increased levels of T cells in peripheral lymphoid organs, and that T cells from these mice proliferated more vigorously with antigen stimulation [182]. There is also evidence of improved immunologic function following ADT. In a murine tumor-prevention model, Hsueh et al. showed that androgen ablation with an oral AR antagonist augmented immune responses, with a modest improvement in antitumor efficacy to a whole-tumor cell vaccine (B16) [183]. A similar augmentation of immune response was observed in a transgenic mouse model that stably expressed prostate antigen. Failure of immunotherapy usually stems from the rapid development of tolerance by prostate-specific T cells. This study found that androgen ablation brought about a decrease in tolerance of prostate-specific T cells [184].

These preclinical data linking castration to more potent immune response mirror findings from studies done in humans. Research on autoimmune disease in humans also supports the immunoinhibitory effects of androgens [185]. ADT induces profuse T-cell infiltration of benign glands and tumors in human prostates, which is readily apparent after 7 to 28 days of therapy [186]. Recruitment and activation of antigen-presenting cells in treated prostate tissues may also contribute to local T-cell activation. Androgen ablation therefore induces priming of T cells to prostate antigens. Blazar et al. showed that ADT increased circulating levels of T ($p \leq 0.01$) and NK ($p \leq 0.05$) cells in men [187]. In this study, 6 of 10 patients showed a substantial increase in absolute T-cell receptor rearrangement excision circles (TRECs), indicating an increase in thymic function. A larger study analyzed peripheral blood mononuclear cells from 83 patients who underwent either autologous or allogeneic bone marrow transplant for hematologic malignancies. Patients received either ADT or no ADT, along with high-dose myeloablative chemotherapy, followed by bone marrow transplant. While complete data from this trial are not yet available, interim results from a subset of 20 adult patients showed a significant increase in naïve CD4+ T cells and CD4+ TRECs in patients treated with ADT [188]. Results in these animal and human studies suggest that immunotherapy for prostate cancer may be most effective when administered following androgen ablation—thus forming the rationale for combining ADT and vaccines.

Several phase I trials have evaluated the safety and biological effects of vaccinia virus expressing human PSA in patients with prostate cancer [189-191]. In some patients, serum PSA stabilized for 6 to 11 months [190]. In a phase II trial designed to analyze the toxicity, immunogenicity, and time to treatment failure using vaccine, AA therapy, or their sequential use, 42 patients with CRPC and increasing PSA levels without radiographic evidence of metastatic disease (stage D0.5) were randomized (21 in each arm) to receive vaccine vs. AA therapy with nilutamide [192]. Nilutamide was chosen because clinical and biochemical responses have been reported with nilutamide after flutamide and bicalutamide failure [193, 194]. Median time to treatment failure for the vaccine arm was 9.9 months vs. 7.6 months for the nilutamide arm ($p = 0.28$). Eight patients in the combined AA/nilutamide arm who were given vaccine at the time of PSA progression had a median time to treatment failure of 5.2 months; 12 patients in the vaccine arm who had nilutamide added at the time of PSA progression had a median time to treatment failure of 13.9 months. Based on the potential synergy between ADT and vaccines, a randomized, double-blind, phase II trial of ONY-P1 vaccine vs. placebo in men with D0 prostate cancer following limited androgen ablation is underway that will determine if the vaccine can lengthen the time to PSA progression. It is hoped that these trials will determine whether there is a role for combination therapy in this patient population for whom there is currently no standard of care.

Adverse Effects of ADT

Skeletal Changes and Loss of Bone Mineral Density

As the number of prostate cancer patients being treated with ADT has increased, significant declines in bone mineral density (BMD) [195-197] and increased risk of fracture [198-200] have been reported (figure 2). A recent study of over 50,000 men from the Surveillance, Epidemiology, and End Results program (SEER) and Medicare databases compared the risk of fracture in men with prostate cancer who were treated with ADT vs. those not receiving ADT [197]. The study found that for men treated with ADT, the risk of fracture increased one year after diagnosis and rose with the number of doses of GnRH-A received. Several randomized trials of bisphosphonates for the treatment of ADT-induced osteoporosis have been published. A randomized trial of 47 men with nonmetastatic prostate cancer compared GnRH-A alone with GnRH-A plus 60 mg pamidronate given every 12 weeks. After 48 weeks, men in the GnRH-A-alone arm had a mean decrease in lumbar, trochanter, total hip, and trabecular lumbar spine BMD of 3.3% ($p < 0.001$), 2.1% ($p = 0.003$), 1.8% ($p = 0.005$), and 8.5% ($p = 0.02$), respectively. Mean BMD in the GnRH-A-plus-pamidronate group did not change significantly [201]. In a randomized trial of 106 men with nonmetastatic prostate cancer, men who were beginning ADT were randomly assigned to receive zoledronic acid or placebo every 3 months for a year [202]. Mean lumbar spine BMD decreased in the placebo group by 2.2%, but increased by 5.6% in the zoledronic-acid group ($p < 0.001$). In another study, 44 men with nonmetastatic prostate cancer who were receiving a GnRH-A were assigned randomly to receive zoledronic acid (4 mg IV × 1) or placebo [203]. At the end of 12 months, mean (± SE) BMD of the posteroanterior lumbar spine increased by 4.0% ± 0.9% in men treated with zoledronic acid and decreased by 3.1% ± 0.9% in men who received placebo ($p < 0.001$ for between-group comparison). BMD of the total hip decreased by 0.7% ± 0.6% in men treated with zoledronic acid and decreased by 1.9% ± 0.7% in men who received placebo ($p = 0.005$). Although these data suggest the feasibility of once-yearly dosing of bisphosphonates for patients undergoing ADT, it is too soon to recommend routine use of bisphosphonates as standard treatment for all men receiving ADT.

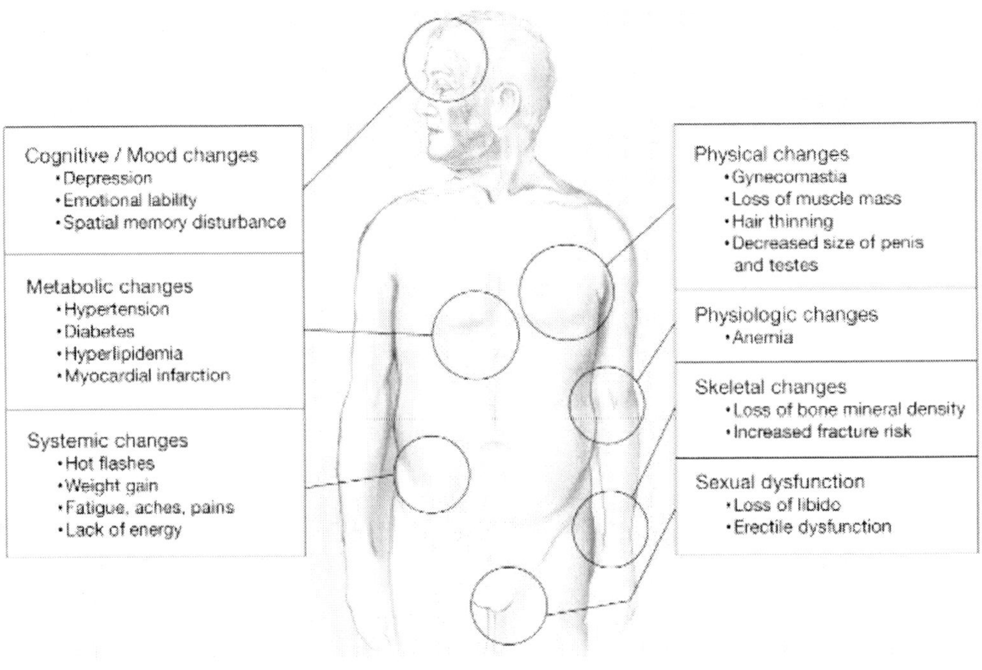

Figure 2. Adverse effects of ADT.

At present, no systematic guidelines have been published on diagnosing or managing osteoporosis in patients receiving ADT [204]. Furthermore, no trials of other interventions, including nonpharmacologic therapies, calcium, or vitamin D, have been performed in this setting. Based on available data, it is recommended that patients have a baseline evaluation of BMD before starting ADT and periodic follow-up assessments depending on baseline findings, and that patients already on ADT for prostate cancer undergo annual assessment of BMD [205]. Men should be counseled about calcium and vitamin D intake and behaviors that reduce the risk of bone loss. They should also be screened for risks such as family history of osteoporosis, low body weight, prior fractures, excessive alcohol use, smoking, glucocorticoid use, low vitamin D levels, and other medical comorbidities.

Hot Flashes

Hot flashes, a troublesome adverse effect, can impair quality of life for men on ADT. They occur in up to 80% of patients undergoing treatment with GnRH-A [206]. In some studies, megestrol acetate reduced hot flashes in 74% of men on ADT vs. 20% for placebo [207, 208]. Other trials have studied the effectiveness of antidepressants [209, 210], but to date there have been no large-scale placebo-controlled trials of any of these interventions in patients with prostate cancer [211].

Metabolic Syndrome

Recently, male hypogonadism has emerged as an independent risk factor in the development of metabolic syndrome. Men with low testosterone levels have a higher prevalence of metabolic syndrome, after controlling for other risk factors [212]. Serum testosterone levels have a negative correlation with fat mass and a positive correlation with muscle mass. Several prospective studies have compared body composition and metabolism in cohorts of men with prostate cancer before ADT and 6 to 12 months after ADT [213-215], with the following results ($n = 35$): increased body mass index of 1.6% to 2.4%; increased fat body mass of 10% to 20% in 7 (20%) men, 20% to 50% in 8 (22.8%) men, and more than 50% in 5 (14.3%) men; decreased lean body mass of 2% to 5% in 8 (22.8%) men and > 5% in 7 (20%) men [214], as well as increases in total cholesterol and triglycerides, HDL, LDL, and, in one study, fasting glucose. All of these studies were comparisons of the same patient population before and after ADT and therefore lacked a true control group.

A cross-sectional study divided 58 men into 1) an ADT group consisting of 20 patients with prostate cancer undergoing ADT for at least 12 months, 2) a non-ADT group of 18 age-matched men with nonmetastatic prostate cancer who had rising PSA after local treatment, and 3) a control group of 20 age-matched men. Patients on ADT had significantly higher body mass indexes and lower total and free testosterone levels. The prevalence of metabolic syndrome was higher in the ADT group compared with the non-ADT ($p < 0.01$) and control ($p = 0.03$) groups [216]. Among the components of metabolic syndrome, men on ADT had a higher prevalence of abdominal obesity and hyperglycemia. Androgen-deprived men also had elevated triglycerides compared with controls ($p = 0.02$). The prevalence of hypertension and low HDL levels was similar. In a large observational population-based cohort study of 73,196 Medicare enrollees 66 years old or older who had locoregional prostate cancer, GnRH-A use was associated with an increased risk of coronary heart disease (adjusted HR = 1.16; $p = 0.004$), myocardial infarction (adjusted HR = 1.11; $p = 0.03$), sudden cardiac death (adjusted HR = 1.34; $p < 0.001$), and diabetes (adjusted HR = 1.44; $p < 0.001$). Men treated with orchiectomy alone were more likely to develop diabetes (adjusted HR = 1.34; $p < 0.001$) but not coronary heart disease, myocardial infarction, or sudden cardiac death (all $p > 0.20$) [217]. Taken together, these data suggest that metabolic syndrome may promote the development of cardiovascular risk factors. Given the risks and uncertain benefits of ADT for patients with biochemical recurrence, use of this therapy in this patient population should be carefully considered.

Sexual Dysfunction

Testosterone plays an important role in sexual function and the vast majority of men treated with ADT develop some form of sexual dysfunction [218]. Loss of libido usually develops first, followed by erectile dysfunction. An early cross-sectional study examined the effects of at least 12 months of ADT for prostate cancer on different parameters, including sexual function, lean body mass, muscle strength, BMD, and quality of life. On the Watts Sexual Function Questionnaire, patients receiving ADT had lower overall scores than either patients who had not undergone ADT or healthy age-matched controls ($p = 0.0001$), particularly in the areas of arousal, desire, and frequency of spontaneous early morning erections [219]. A study of 431 patients treated with GnRH-A and orchiectomy in the Prostate Cancer Outcomes Study of the SEER program found similar effects on sexual function [220]. Therapeutic efforts to prevent or ameliorate the sexual side effects of ADT have included intermittent ADT and AA monotherapy [95, 97, 98]. Other available options include vacuum devices, carnitine, and intracavernosal injections of prostaglandin [221, 222].

Emotional and Cognitive Side Effects

Men with prostate cancer often experience depression, especially if they have a history of depressive episodes. In men surviving at least 5 years after diagnosis, the incidence of at least one diagnosis of depression or cognitive dysfunction was significantly higher compared to controls (31.3% vs. 23.7%; $p < 0.001$) [223]. However, after adjusting for age, comorbidity, and tumor characteristics, the risks for patients on ADT were substantially reduced or eliminated. There are conflicting reports concerning the effects of ADT on cognitive function. Some data suggest a decline in attention and memory [224], as well as verbal fluency and visual memory [225], even in short-term ADT of 6 to 12 months [226]. Other data suggest a noted improvement in object recall among men undergoing ADT [227].

Systemic Effects

Up to 90% of patients receiving ADT experience normocytic normochromic anemia [228]. Although other etiologies should be ruled out, the anemia is typically temporary and related to androgen blockade. Treatment with erythropoietin is effective, though rarely necessary since the condition usually resolves when ADT is discontinued. Patients may experience fatigue that is independent of either anemia or psychological issues [218]. Gynecomastia resulting from ADT has been treated prophylactically with breast irradiation or with surgery and tamoxifen [100, 101]. Other systemic effects include dry eyes, thinning or loss of body hair, and vertigo [221].

Biology of Castrate-Resistant Prostate Cancer

While clinical studies of various forms of ADT have proven its clinical efficacy in several disease states and select prostate cancer patient populations, there is controversy regarding the use of such strategies in patients with biochemical failure. Current standard clinical practice dictates continued testosterone suppression even for CRPC, based on recent data that suggest that androgens and AR continue to play an important role in the biology of CRPC.

Patients with metastatic prostate cancer typically respond to ADT for an average of 14 to 20 months [83, 87], at which time CRPC develops. Once this occurs, survival ranges from 12 to 46 months [229, 230]. CRPC is sometimes referred to as androgen-independent prostate cancer, but "androgen-independent" is not a fully descriptive term since laboratory evidence suggests that castrate resistance is at least partially caused by sensitization to low (or castrate) levels of androgens. Other terms used in reference to castrate resistance, such as androgen-resistant, androgen-refractory, and hormone-refractory, are indistinct and vague, and are not appropriately descriptive of this disease state [231]. Androgen depletion-independent prostate cancer has been suggested as an alternative term [232] because it reflects the persistence or progression of prostate cancer in the presence of low, but not absent, levels of testosterone. However, castrate-resistant is the preferred term because it accurately describes the biology of the underlying mechanisms.

When ADT is instituted, a majority of prostate cancer cells undergo apoptosis, but some persist in the G1 phase of the cell cycle [233]. Clinical progression occurs with the proliferation of cells resistant to androgen ablation. In the last few years, compelling research has indicated that the biology and survival of CRPC is largely dependent on reactivation of AR, despite castrate levels of testosterone [234, 235]. Evidence suggesting different mechanisms of AR reactivation include the fact that CRPC manifests as progression that is accompanied by a rise in PSA that may still be sensitive to secondary treatments [235], and often responds to second-line hormonal therapy such as AR antagonists and adrenal ablation [236], indicating that CRPC is still dependent on AR. However, lack of response to secondary hormonal therapy does not necessarily rule out AR dependence. In a study of patients with CRPC treated with flutamide, men who previously had responded well to castration responded better to AR antagonists as secondary hormonal therapy. Men who had an incomplete response to castration did not respond as well to secondary hormonal therapy [237]. It may be that the men who responded well to ADT and secondary hormonal therapy had tumors whose biology was more reliant on AR.

Other evidence downstream of AR suggests that AR is reactivated and that the signal is intact. DNA microarray studies of human prostate cancer cell line xenografts that examined initial tumor growth, tumor response in the initial castrate setting, and castrate-resistant tumor growth showed that a subset of AR-responsive genes that are down-regulated upon castration are re-expressed in the castrate-resistant tumor [238]. DNA microarray studies from prostate cancer specimens collected from patients in similar states also suggest AR reactivation in castrate resistance. In fact, the gene expression patterns of castrate-resistant tumors were more similar to androgen-dependent tumors growing with normal levels of testosterone than to androgen-dependent tumors after initial exposure to castration [239].

Reactivation of AR function after castration occurs in part through increased expression of this gene. Gene amplification, or an increase in the genomic copy number of AR, occurs infrequently before ADT. However, AR gene amplification occurs in over 20% of CRPC [240, 241]. The mechanism of increased AR expression may not necessarily be limited to gene amplification. A DNA microarray study of mouse xenograft tumors comparing androgen-dependent and castrate-resistant tumors suggests that an increase in AR mRNA, by whatever mechanism, is common among CRPCs. Of all the genes analyzed in 7 matched sets of isogenic androgen-dependent and castrate-resistant tumors, AR was the only consistent transcript that increased in the transition to CRPC [242].

Several other mechanisms have been postulated for gain-of-function changes in AR signaling that lead to persistent activation despite castration. One mechanism involves changes in coregulatory molecules, such as overexpression of steroid receptor coactivators, which are proteins required for the full function of steroid receptors such as AR. This is perhaps best illustrated by mouse knockout models, such as that of steroid receptor coactivator-1 (SRC-1), in which organs responsive to sex steroids, such as the prostate, uterus, and mammary gland, failed to fully develop [243]. While a loss of steroid receptor coactivator expression may decrease AR function, increased expression may augment androgen signaling and therefore account for AR signaling in the castrate setting. While some findings suggest that this occurs, other studies on steroid receptor coactivator expression changes are not always consistent with this hypothesis [234].

Another mechanism of castrate resistance involves changes in the level of cytokines, growth factors, and membrane receptors in tumor tissue. Investigators have described a growing list of soluble factors that play a role in AR activation. Interleukin-6 (IL-6) is one of the most widely studied of these agents and has been shown to activate AR in a STAT3-dependent manner [244]. Furthermore, administration of an anti-IL-6 antibody inhibits the conversion of androgen-dependent to castrate-resistant phenotype in mice [245]. Insulin-like growth factor-1 has also been shown to activate AR and may be implicated in CRPC [246]. Her2/neu, a member of the epidermal growth factor receptor family, has a prominent role in the biology and treatment of breast cancer [247], but there is evidence that Her2/neu also plays a role in AR activation, in part by stabilizing AR protein and augmenting DNA binding activity [248]. The long list of cytokines and growth factors purported to activate AR is reviewed in detail elsewhere [249, 250]. It may be that these various growth factors all converge on a common signaling intermediary to activate AR, perhaps explaining the wide variety of growth factors on this list [251].

There is also evidence that AR activity may be up-regulated in the CRPC tumor microenvironment by an increase in the synthesis and availability of androgens. One study examined tissue concentrations of testosterone and DHT in benign prostate of men who had no hormonal treatment and compared it to androgen levels in locally recurrent CRPC [252]. Although DHT levels were over 90% lower in locally recurrent CRPC, testosterone levels were not significantly different between the 2 groups, suggesting that there may be local androgen production. This may be explained in part by an increase in genes, such as aldo-keto reductase family 1, member C3, that are responsible for converting adrenal androgens to testosterone in CRPC [253].

Data on the mechanisms involved in the development of castrate resistance suggest that various stimuli converge on AR as a nodal point, perhaps redundantly, and stimulate the activation of a subset of androgen-responsive genes. In addition, the majority of prostate cancers develop a translocation between the upstream, androgen-responsive TMPRSS2 gene and erythroblast transformation-specific (ETS) family oncogenes [254]. AR-mediated ETS activation may further hasten tumor growth upon reactivation of AR in the castrate-resistant state. These new data on this class of translocations further strengthen the argument for developing novel drugs to target AR in CRPC.

Potentially Therapeutic Approaches Targeting AR

There are several potential strategies for directing a novel therapy at AR in CRPC. The first would be to target the growth factors and receptors responsible for activating AR. However, there are several such growth factors and there is likely some redundancy to growth-factor activation of AR. Therefore, targeting only one growth factor may not be sufficient to prevent AR activation. It has been proposed that the intracellular signaling proteins at a point of convergence downstream of these growth factors would serve as a more attractive target [251]. Drugs fitting this description would mainly be kinase inhibitors.

At the level of AR itself, the interaction between AR and a required steroid receptor coactivator could, in principle, be inhibited. The observation that one patient with complete androgen insufficiency syndrome and complete loss of AR function has a wild-type AR and likely a mutation in a steroid receptor coactivator, suggests that at least one coactivator is absolutely required for AR function [255]. However, developing small-molecule inhibitors of protein-protein interactions is problematic. "Clefts" or "pockets" in which small molecules readily bind are typically not as obvious in the interface of 2 proteins as they are in catalytic domains of kinases, although these problems may not be insurmountable. Peptides that bind AR in steroid receptor coactivator binding domains have been developed, along with crystal structures of the interaction between these peptides and AR [256]. Such studies may pave the way to developing small molecules that antagonize coactivator function.

The interaction between the AR zinc-finger DNA binding domain and the androgen response element DNA motif to which it binds may also be interrupted. A compound that antagonizes the interaction between the estrogen receptor zinc-finger domain and the estrogen response element has been developed. This compound inhibits estrogen-induced transcription and cell proliferation. Furthermore, it reduces tumor growth in a mouse xenograft model of breast cancer [257]. In principle, such a strategy is also possible with AR. Since this strategy involves a drug that does not bind the classical steroid receptor ligand binding domain, it should also be effective in cells that have become resistant to classical antagonists.

Heat-shock proteins are required for normal protein folding, processing, and turnover [258]. Normal AR activity and processing are also dependent on heat-shock protein 90 (hsp90). Inhibitors of hsp90, such as geldanamycin and its analogs, disrupt AR activity and AR-mediated transcription [259]. However, inhibitors of hsp90 are not specific for AR and, like conventional cytotoxic chemotherapy, their development for the treatment of CRPC will depend on their therapeutic index [260]. Proteolysis targeting chimeric molecules (PROTACS), a strategy for selectively targeting AR, has been developed. This system uses an androgen ligand linked to a moiety that targets bound proteins to the ubiquitin-proteosome pathway, thereby specifically targeting and degrading AR [261]. Such strategies for developing specific drugs to target AR are promising for the development and treatment of CRPC.

Given the multiple levels of AR activation in CRPC, some have argued for a multifaceted approach to targeting AR for inhibition [262]. Strategies that combine newer targeted agents against AR could be undertaken as early as initiation of ADT to minimize the opportunity for castrate-resistant cells to arise. A similar strategy is being adopted, for instance, in the setting of chronic myelogenous leukemia, for which there are now multiple drugs, such as imatinib and dasatinib, to target a central, critical protein (BCR-ABL) for tumor survival [263].

Finally, there are new data on the existence of prostate cancer stem cells [264, 265]. Cancer stem cells are thought to represent a small subset of the total tumor-cell population, yet they have the potential for continuous replication. If prostate cancer arises from bona fide stem cells, then CRPC must originate from these stem cells as well. However, evidence suggests that neither normal prostate stem cells nor prostate cancer stem cells express AR. The castrate-resistance conundrum is that CRPC leads to gain-of-function changes in AR, yet it arises from AR-negative prostate cancer stem cells, which by definition can neither directly respond to ADT nor undergo selection for changes in AR function [266]. Resolution of the castrate-resistance conundrum will aid in understanding the development of CRPC and identifying new targets for therapy.

Conclusion

ADT is being employed more frequently for prostate cancer patients with symptomatic and asymptomatic metastatic disease, patients with biochemical recurrence, and about 14% of newly diagnosed patients [218]. ADT offers palliation of bone pain and, in some patient populations, a survival benefit. Unfortunately, nearly all men progress to castrate-resistant phenotype within 2 years, and overall survival after the start of ADT is 28 to 63 months [82, 229, 267]. For some disease states and patient populations, the issue of who should receive

ADT, and when and how they should receive it, remains controversial. Data suggest that ADT is most strongly indicated for prostate cancer patients with metastatic disease, as an adjunct to RT for high-risk patients (Gleason score $\geq$ 8, stage $\geq$ T2c), for patients with microscopic lymph node disease after RP, and as primary therapy for patients who are not candidates for local therapy (figure 3). Of the available options for testosterone-lowering therapy, orchiectomy and GnRH-A have similar efficacy and safety. The choice to undergo one or the other should therefore be a matter of patient preference after factors such as comorbidities or side effects of each procedure have been thoroughly discussed. Whether CAB is better than ADT monotherapy is still unclear. Although several trials showed a small survival benefit (1% to 5%) within 5 to 10 years of analysis, the large United States intergroup study (INT-0105), which was negative, is considered by many to be the definitive trial comparing CAB to ADT monotherapy because of its size and prospective evaluation of quality-of-life benefits in men with minimal disease and good performance status. Given the considerable cost, toxicity, and minimal survival benefit, the consensus has not been in favor of routine use of CAB over ADT monotherapy.

The timing of hormonal therapy is also a subject of ongoing debate. The benefits of early treatment—a trend towards survival benefit, reduced disease progression, and lower morbidity from the complications of urethral obstruction, pathologic fractures, spinal cord compression, ureteral obstruction, and extraskeletal metastases—must be weighed against the potential side effects of prolonged ADT. The side effects of continuous ADT treatment have not raised specific concerns for patients with metastatic disease since, on average, these men do not survive long enough for the side effects to become clinically significant. However, because improved diagnostic methods have resulted in earlier diagnosis of prostate cancer and earlier detection of biochemical recurrence, ADT is being instituted in men with earlier stages of disease, whose life expectancy could well be over 10 years. For these men, systemic side effects can be a substantial burden. This is especially true for patients presenting with biochemical recurrence, where no data from prospective trials are currently available to specifically address a possible overall survival benefit. However, given the benefits seen in patients with locally advanced or high-grade disease, and the risk of earlier metastasis in patients with aggressive high-risk features, there is a trend toward initiating ADT earlier in the course of disease. Alternative methods of delivering ADT have been studied, including the use of intermittent ADT as opposed to continuous ADT, and although its survival benefit and impact on disease control have not been fully ascertained, the strategy is gaining favor as a way to improve quality of life and lower health care costs for prostate cancer patients. When disease progresses after first-line ADT, secondary ADT should be considered. In addition, there is a rationale for combining ADT with other therapies, and studies are ongoing to determine the clinical benefit of this approach. Eventually, most patients with metastatic prostate cancer treated with ADT will develop CRPC. Recent insights into the biology of CRPC have led to the search for novel therapies targeting the AR pathway. This may eventually lead to another class of drugs that could lengthen the period when prostate cancer is responsive to hormonal therapy.

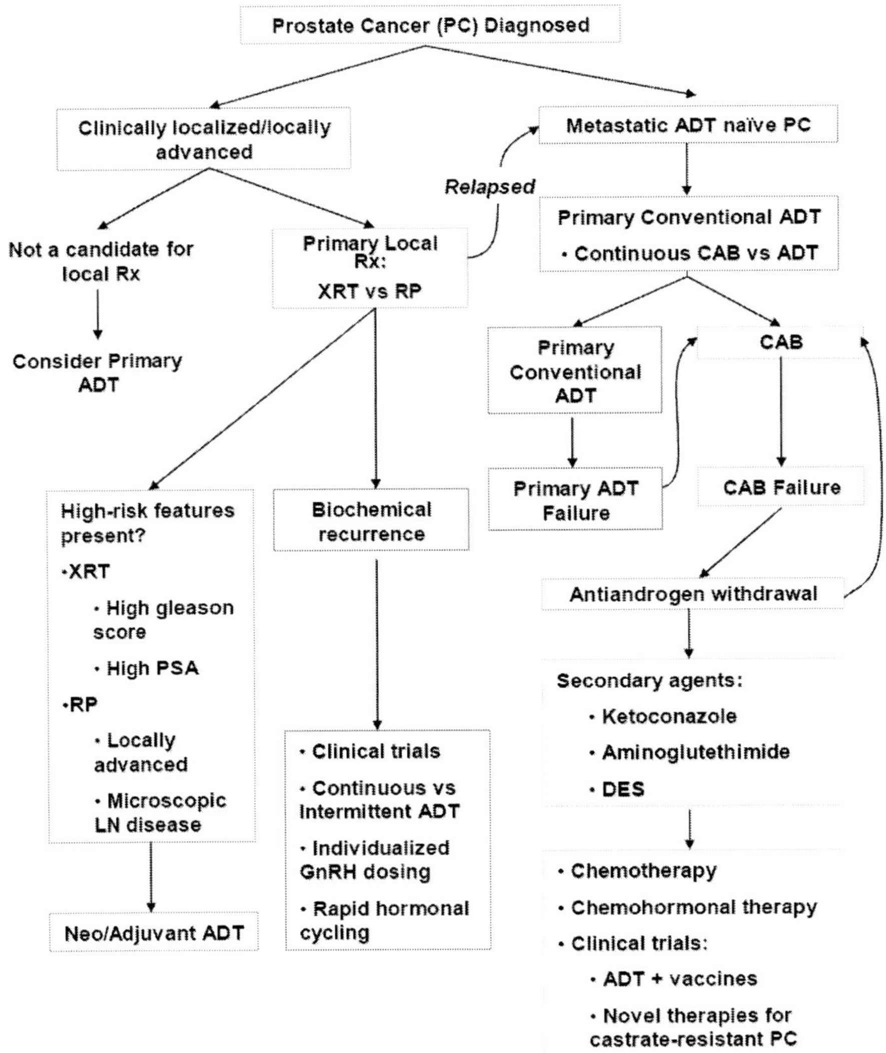

Figure 3. Algorithm for Clinical Application of ADT.

References

[1] Huggins C, Hodges C. Studies on prostatic cancer: I. The effect of estrogen and of androgen injection on serum phosphatases in metastatic carcinoma of the prostate. *Cancer Res.* 1941;1:293-7.

[2] Gelmann EP. Molecular biology of the androgen receptor. *J. Clin. Oncol.* 2002 Jul 1;20(13):3001-15.

[3] Tyagi RK, Lavrovsky Y, Ahn SC, Song CS, Chatterjee B, Roy AK. Dynamics of intracellular movement and nucleocytoplasmic recycling of the ligand-activated androgen receptor in living cells. *Mol. Endocrinol.* 2000 Aug;14(8):1162-74.

[4] DePrimo SE, Diehn M, Nelson JB, Reiter RE, Matese J, Fero M, et al. Transcriptional programs activated by exposure of human prostate cancer cells to androgen. *Genome Biol.* 2002 Jun 14;3(7):RESEARCH0032.

[5] Zhou ZX, Lane MV, Kemppainen JA, French FS, Wilson EM. Specificity of ligand-dependent androgen receptor stabilization: receptor domain interactions influence ligand dissociation and receptor stability. *Mol. Endocrinol.* 1995 Feb;9(2):208-18.

[6] Gottlieb B, Pinsky L, Beitel LK, Trifiro M. Androgen insensitivity. *Am. J. Med. Genet.* 1999 Dec 29;89(4):210-7.

[7] Treatment and survival of patients with cancer of the prostate. The Veterans Administration Co-operative Urological Research Group. *Surg. Gynecol. Obstet.* 1967 May;124(5):1011-7.

[8] Loblaw DA, Mendelson DS, Talcott JA, Virgo KS, Somerfield MR, Ben-Josef E, et al. American Society of Clinical Oncology recommendations for the initial hormonal management of androgen-sensitive metastatic, recurrent, or progressive prostate cancer. *J. Clin. Oncol.* 2004 Jul 15;22(14):2927-41.

[9] McLeod DG. Hormonal therapy: historical perspective to future directions. *Urology.* 2003 Feb;61(2 Suppl 1):3-7.

[10] Grayhack JT, Keeler TC, Kozlowski JM. Carcinoma of the prostate. Hormonal therapy. *Cancer.* 1987 Aug 1;60(3 Suppl):589-601.

[11] de Voogt HJ, Smith PH, Pavone-Macaluso M, de Pauw M, Suciu S. Cardiovascular side effects of diethylstilbestrol, cyproterone acetate, medroxyprogesterone acetate and estramustine phosphate used for the treatment of advanced prostatic cancer: results from European Organization for Research on Treatment of Cancer trials 30761 and 30762. *J. Urol.* 1986 Feb;135(2):303-7.

[12] Matsuo H, Baba Y, Nair RM, Arimura A, Schally AV. Structure of the porcine LH- and FSH-releasing hormone. I. The proposed amino acid sequence. *Biochem. Biophys. Res. Commun.* 1971 Jun 18;43(6):1334-9.

[13] Schally AV, Arimura A, Kastin AJ, Matsuo H, Baba Y, Redding TW, et al. Gonadotropin-releasing hormone: one polypeptide regulates secretion of luteinizing and follicle-stimulating hormones. *Science.* 1971 Sep 10;173(4001):1036-8.

[14] Schally AV. Luteinizing hormone-releasing hormone analogs: their impact on the control of tumorigenesis. *Peptides.* 1999;20(10):1247-62.

[15] Casper RF. Clinical uses of gonadotropin-releasing hormone analogues. *CMAJ.* 1991 Jan 15;144(2):153-8.

[16] Filicori M. Gonadotropin-releasing hormone agonists. A guide to use and selection. *Drugs.* 1994 Jul;48(1):41-58.

[17] Kraus S, Naor Z, Seger R. Gonadotropin-releasing hormone in apoptosis of prostate cancer cells. *Cancer Lett.* 2006 Mar 28;234(2):109-23.

[18] Kuhn JM, Billebaud T, Navratil H, Moulonguet A, Fiet J, Grise P, et al. Prevention of the transient adverse effects of a gonadotropin-releasing hormone analogue (buserelin) in metastatic prostatic carcinoma by administration of an antiandrogen (nilutamide). *N. Engl. J. Med.* 1989 Aug 17;321(7):413-8.

[19] Scardino PT. National Comprehensive Cancer Network (NCCN) Practice Guidelines version 2. 2005 [cited; Available from: http://www.nccn.org

[20] Mongiat-Artus P, Teillac P. Abarelix: the first gonadotrophin-releasing hormone antagonist for the treatment of prostate cancer. Expert Opin Pharmacother. 2004 Oct;5(10):2171-9.

[21] Abarelix package insert. [cited 2006 September 2]; Available from: http://www.fda.gov/CDER/foi/label/2003/021320lbl.pdf

[22] Seidenfeld J, Samson DJ, Hasselblad V, Aronson N, Albertsen PC, Bennett CL, et al. Single-therapy androgen suppression in men with advanced prostate cancer: a systematic review and meta-analysis. *Ann. Intern. Med.* 2000 Apr 4;132(7):566-77.

[23] Cassileth BR, Soloway MS, Vogelzang NJ, Schellhammer PS, Seidmon EJ, Hait HI, et al. Patients' choice of treatment in stage D prostate cancer. *Urology.* 1989 May;33(5 Suppl):57-62.

[24] Thompson IM, Pauler DK, Goodman PJ, Tangen CM, Lucia MS, Parnes HL, et al. Prevalence of prostate cancer among men with a prostate-specific antigen level < or =4.0 ng per milliliter. *N. Engl. J. Med.* 2004 May 27;350(22):2239-46.

[25] Bubley GJ, Carducci M, Dahut W, Dawson N, Daliani D, Eisenberger M, et al. Eligibility and response guidelines for phase II clinical trials in androgen-independent prostate cancer: recommendations from the Prostate-Specific Antigen Working Group. *J. Clin. Oncol.* 1999 Nov;17(11):3461-7.

[26] Oefelein MG, Feng A, Scolieri MJ, Ricchiutti D, Resnick MI. Reassessment of the definition of castrate levels of testosterone: implications for clinical decision making. *Urology.* 2000 Dec 20;56(6):1021-4.

[27] Russell DW, Wilson JD. Steroid 5 alpha-reductase: two genes/two enzymes. *Annu. Rev. Biochem.* 1994;63:25-61.

[28] Titus MA, Gregory CW, Ford OH, 3rd, Schell MJ, Maygarden SJ, Mohler JL. Steroid 5alpha-reductase isozymes I and II in recurrent prostate cancer. *Clin. Cancer Res.* 2005 Jun 15;11(12):4365-71.

[29] McConnell JD, Wilson JD, George FW, Geller J, Pappas F, Stoner E. Finasteride, an inhibitor of 5 alpha-reductase, suppresses prostatic dihydrotestosterone in men with benign prostatic hyperplasia. *J. Clin. Endocrinol. Metab.* 1992 Mar;74(3):505-8.

[30] Thompson IM, Goodman PJ, Tangen CM, Lucia MS, Miller GJ, Ford LG, et al. The influence of finasteride on the development of prostate cancer. *N. Engl. J. Med.* 2003 Jul 17;349(3):215-24.

[31] Thompson IM, Chi C, Ankerst DP, Goodman PJ, Tangen CM, Lippman SM, et al. Effect of finasteride on the sensitivity of PSA for detecting prostate cancer. *J. Natl. Cancer Inst.* 2006 Aug 16;98(16):1128-33.

[32] Bramson HN, Hermann D, Batchelor KW, Lee FW, James MK, Frye SV. Unique preclinical characteristics of GG745, a potent dual inhibitor of 5AR. *J. Pharmacol. Exp. Ther.* 1997 Sep;282(3):1496-502.

[33] Roehrborn CG, Boyle P, Nickel JC, Hoefner K, Andriole G. Efficacy and safety of a dual inhibitor of 5-alpha-reductase types 1 and 2 (dutasteride) in men with benign prostatic hyperplasia. *Urology.* 2002 Sep;60(3):434-41.

[34] Gomella LG. Chemoprevention using dutasteride: the REDUCE trial. *Curr. Opin. Urol.* 2005 Jan;15(1):29-32.

[35] SELECT Trial SWOG page. [cited 2006 September 12]; Available from: http://www.crab.org/select/

[36] Virtamo J, Pietinen P, Huttunen JK, Korhonen P, Malila N, Virtanen MJ, et al. Incidence of cancer and mortality following alpha-tocopherol and beta-carotene supplementation: a postintervention follow-up. *JAMA.* 2003 Jul 23;290(4):476-85.

[37] Duffield-Lillico AJ, Dalkin BL, Reid ME, Turnbull BW, Slate EH, Jacobs ET, et al. Selenium supplementation, baseline plasma selenium status and incidence of prostate cancer: an analysis of the complete treatment period of the Nutritional Prevention of Cancer Trial. *BJU Int.* 2003 May;91(7):608-12.

[38] Pilepich MV, Krall JM, John MJ, Rubin P, Porter AT, Marcial VA, et al. Hormonal cytoreduction in locally advanced carcinoma of the prostate treated with definitive radiotherapy: preliminary results of RTOG 83-07. *Int. J. Radiat. Oncol. Biol. Phys.* 1989 Mar;16(3):813-7.

[39] Bolla M, Gonzalez D, Warde P, Dubois JB, Mirimanoff RO, Storme G, et al. Improved survival in patients with locally advanced prostate cancer treated with radiotherapy and goserelin. *N. Engl. J. Med.* 1997 Jul 31;337(5):295-300.

[40] Bolla M, Collette L, Blank L, Warde P, Dubois JB, Mirimanoff RO, et al. Long-term results with immediate androgen suppression and external irradiation in patients with locally advanced prostate cancer (an EORTC study): a phase III randomised trial. *Lancet.* 2002 Jul 13;360(9327):103-6.

[41] Pilepich MV, Caplan R, Byhardt RW, Lawton CA, Gallagher MJ, Mesic JB, et al. Phase III trial of androgen suppression using goserelin in unfavorable-prognosis carcinoma of the prostate treated with definitive radiotherapy: report of Radiation Therapy Oncology Group Protocol 85-31. *J. Clin. Oncol.* 1997 Mar;15(3):1013-21.

[42] Lawton CA, Winter K, Murray K, Machtay M, Mesic JB, Hanks GE, et al. Updated results of the phase III Radiation Therapy Oncology Group (RTOG) trial 85-31 evaluating the potential benefit of androgen suppression following standard radiation therapy for unfavorable prognosis carcinoma of the prostate. *Int. J. Radiat. Oncol. Biol. Phys.* 2001 Mar 15;49(4):937-46.

[43] Pilepich M, Winter K, Lawton C, Do D, Re R, Mi M, et al. Phase III trial of androgen suppression adjuvant to definitive radiotherapy. Long term results of RTOG 85-31 [abstract]. *Proc. Am. Soc. Clin. Oncol.* 2003;22:A1530.

[44] Pilepich MV, Winter K, Lawton CA, Krisch RE, Wolkov HB, Movsas B, et al. Androgen suppression adjuvant to definitive radiotherapy in prostate carcinoma--long-term results of phase III RTOG 85-31. *Int. J. Radiat. Oncol. Biol. Phys.* 2005 Apr 1;61(5):1285-90.

[45] Lawton CA, Winter K, Grignon D, Pilepich MV. Androgen suppression plus radiation versus radiation alone for patients with stage D1/pathologic node-positive adenocarcinoma of the prostate: updated results based on national prospective randomized trial Radiation Therapy Oncology Group 85-31. *J. Clin. Oncol.* 2005 Feb 1;23(4):800-7.

[46] D'Amico AV, Manola J, Loffredo M, Renshaw AA, DellaCroce A, Kantoff PW. 6-month androgen suppression plus radiation therapy vs radiation therapy alone for

patients with clinically localized prostate cancer: a randomized controlled trial. *JAMA.* 2004 Aug 18;292(7):821-7.

[47] D'Amico AV, Loffredo M, Renshaw AA, Loffredo B, Chen MH. Six-month androgen suppression plus radiation therapy compared with radiation therapy alone for men with prostate cancer and a rapidly increasing pretreatment prostate-specific antigen level. *J. Clin. Oncol.* 2006 Sep 1;24(25):4190-5.

[48] Pilepich MV, Krall JM, al-Sarraf M, John MJ, Doggett RL, Sause WT, et al. Androgen deprivation with radiation therapy compared with radiation therapy alone for locally advanced prostatic carcinoma: a randomized comparative trial of the Radiation Therapy Oncology Group. *Urology.* 1995 Apr;45(4):616-23.

[49] Pilepich MV, Winter K, John MJ, Mesic JB, Sause W, Rubin P, et al. Phase III radiation therapy oncology group (RTOG) trial 86-10 of androgen deprivation adjuvant to definitive radiotherapy in locally advanced carcinoma of the prostate. *Int. J. Radiat. Oncol. Biol. Phys.* 2001 Aug 1;50(5):1243-52.

[50] Shipley WU, Desilvio M, Pilepich MV, Roach M, 3rd, Wolkov HB, Sause WT, et al. Early initiation of salvage hormone therapy influences survival in patients who failed initial radiation for locally advanced prostate cancer: A secondary analysis of RTOG protocol 86-10. *Int. J. Radiat. Oncol. Biol. Phys.* 2006 Mar 15;64(4):1162-7.

[51] Hellerstedt BA, Pienta KJ. The truth is out there: an overall perspective on androgen deprivation. *Urol. Oncol.* 2003 Jul-Aug;21(4):272-81.

[52] Soloway MS, Pareek K, Sharifi R, Wajsman Z, McLeod D, Wood DP, Jr., et al. Neoadjuvant androgen ablation before radical prostatectomy in cT2bNxMo prostate cancer: 5-year results. *J. Urol.* 2002 Jan;167(1):112-6.

[53] Gleave ME, La Bianca SE, Goldenberg SL, Jones EC, Bruchovsky N, Sullivan LD. Long-term neoadjuvant hormone therapy prior to radical prostatectomy: evaluation of risk for biochemical recurrence at 5-year follow-up. *Urology.* 2000 Aug 1;56(2):289-94.

[54] Gleave ME, Goldenberg SL, Chin JL, Warner J, Saad F, Klotz LH, et al. Randomized comparative study of 3 versus 8-month neoadjuvant hormonal therapy before radical prostatectomy: biochemical and pathological effects. *J. Urol.* 2001 Aug;166(2):500-6; discussion 6-7.

[55] Gerber GS, Thisted RA, Chodak GW, Schroder FH, Frohmuller HG, Scardino PT, et al. Results of radical prostatectomy in men with locally advanced prostate cancer: multi-institutional pooled analysis. *Eur. Urol.* 1997;32(4):385-90.

[56] Messing EM, Manola J, Sarosdy M, Wilding G, Crawford ED, Trump D. Immediate hormonal therapy compared with observation after radical prostatectomy and pelvic lymphadenectomy in men with node-positive prostate cancer. *N. Engl. J. Med.* 1999 Dec 9;341(24):1781-8.

[57] Cheng L, Zincke H, Blute ML, Bergstralh EJ, Scherer B, Bostwick DG. Risk of prostate carcinoma death in patients with lymph node metastasis. *Cancer.* 2001 Jan 1;91(1):66-73.

[58] Studer UE, Hauri D, Hanselmann S, Chollet D, Leisinger HJ, Gasser T, et al. Immediate versus deferred hormonal treatment for patients with prostate cancer who

are not suitable for curative local treatment: results of the randomized trial SAKK 08/88. *J. Clin. Oncol.* 2004 Oct 15;22(20):4109-18.

[59] Studer UE, Whelan P, Albrecht W, Casselman J, de Reijke T, Hauri D, et al. Immediate or deferred androgen deprivation for patients with prostate cancer not suitable for local treatment with curative intent: European Organisation for Research and Treatment of Cancer (EORTC) Trial 30891. *J. Clin. Oncol.* 2006 Apr 20;24(12):1868-76.

[60] Sorensen HT, Mellemkjaer L, Steffensen FH, Olsen JH, Nielsen GL. The risk of a diagnosis of cancer after primary deep venous thrombosis or pulmonary embolism. *N. Engl. J. Med.* 1998 Apr 23;338(17):1169-73.

[61] Gulley J, Parnes H, Wright J, Dahut W. Early treatment gets the benefit [letter]. *J. Clin. Oncol.* 2006;24(32):in press.

[62] Ravery V. The significance of recurrent PSA after radical prostatectomy: benign versus malignant sources. *Semin. Urol. Oncol.* 1999 Aug;17(3):127-9.

[63] Ciezki JP, Reddy CA, Garcia J, Angermeier K, Ulchaker J, Mahadevan A, et al. PSA kinetics after prostate brachytherapy: PSA bounce phenomenon and its implications for PSA doubling time. *Int. J. Radiat. Oncol. Biol. Phys.* 2006 Feb 1;64(2):512-7.

[64] Jhaveri FM, Zippe CD, Klein EA, Kupelian PA. Biochemical failure does not predict overall survival after radical prostatectomy for localized prostate cancer: 10-year results. *Urology.* 1999 Nov;54(5):884-90.

[65] Pound CR, Partin AW, Eisenberger MA, Chan DW, Pearson JD, Walsh PC. Natural history of progression after PSA elevation following radical prostatectomy. *Jama.* 1999 May 5;281(17):1591-7.

[66] Freedland SJ, Humphreys EB, Mangold LA, Eisenberger M, Dorey FJ, Walsh PC, et al. Risk of prostate cancer-specific mortality following biochemical recurrence after radical prostatectomy. *Jama.* 2005 Jul 27;294(4):433-9.

[67] Cannon GM, Jr., Walsh PC, Partin AW, Pound CR. Prostate-specific antigen doubling time in the identification of patients at risk for progression after treatment and biochemical recurrence for prostate cancer. *Urology.* 2003 Dec 29;62 Suppl 1:2-8.

[68] Partin AW, Pearson JD, Landis PK, Carter HB, Pound CR, Clemens JQ, et al. Evaluation of serum prostate-specific antigen velocity after radical prostatectomy to distinguish local recurrence from distant metastases. *Urology.* 1994 May;43(5):649-59.

[69] Zhou P, Chen MH, McLeod D, Carroll PR, Moul JW, D'Amico AV. Predictors of prostate cancer-specific mortality after radical prostatectomy or radiation therapy. *J. Clin. Oncol.* 2005 Oct 1;23(28):6992-8.

[70] D'Amico AV, Moul JW, Carroll PR, Sun L, Lubeck D, Chen MH. Surrogate end point for prostate cancer-specific mortality after radical prostatectomy or radiation therapy. *J. Natl. Cancer Inst.* 2003 Sep 17;95(18):1376-83.

[71] Isaacs JT, Coffey DS. Adaptation versus selection as the mechanism responsible for the relapse of prostatic cancer to androgen ablation therapy as studied in the Dunning R-3327-H adenocarcinoma. *Cancer Res.* 1981 Dec;41(12 Pt 1):5070-5.

[72] Zincke H, Lau W, Bergstralh E, Blute ML. Role of early adjuvant hormonal therapy after radical prostatectomy for prostate cancer. *J. Urol.* 2001 Dec;166(6):2208-15.

[73] Moul JW, Wu H, Sun L, McLeod DG, Amling C, Donahue T, et al. Early versus delayed hormonal therapy for prostate specific antigen only recurrence of prostate cancer after radical prostatectomy. *J. Urol.* 2004 Mar;171(3):1141-7.

[74] [74] Immediate versus deferred treatment for advanced prostatic cancer: initial results of the Medical Research Council Trial. The Medical Research Council Prostate Cancer Working Party Investigators Group. *Br. J. Urol.* 1997 Feb;79(2):235-46.

[75] Kirk D. Immediate vs deferred hormone treatment for prostate cancer. How safe is androgen deprivation? *Br. J. Urol.* 2000;86(Suppl 3):S220.

[76] Nair B, Wilt T, MacDonald R, Rutks I. Early versus deferred androgen suppression in the treatment of advanced prostatic cancer. *Cochrane Database Syst. Rev.* 2002(1):CD003506.

[77] Picus J, Halabi S, Small E, Do D, Re R, Mi M, et al. Long term efficacy of peripheral androgen blockade on prostate cancer: CALGB 9782 [abstract]. *J. Clin. Oncol.* 2006;24(18S Pt 1):A4573.

[78] Huggins C, Stevens R, Hodges C. Studies in prostatic cancer. II. The effects of castration on advanced cancer of the prostate gland. *Arch. Surg.* 1941;43:209-23.

[79] Ferrari P, Castagnetti G, Ferrari G, Pollastri CA, Tavoni F, Dotti A. Combination treatment in M1 prostate cancer. *Cancer.* 1993 Dec 15;72(12 Suppl):3880-5.

[80] Robinson MR, Smith PH, Richards B, Newling DW, de Pauw M, Sylvester R. The final analysis of the EORTC Genito-Urinary Tract Cancer Co-Operative Group phase III clinical trial (protocol 30805) comparing orchidectomy, orchidectomy plus cyproterone acetate and low dose stilboestrol in the management of metastatic carcinoma of the prostate. *Eur. Urol.* 1995;28(4):273-83.

[81] Labrie F, Dupont A, Belanger A, Lacoursiere Y, Raynaud JP, Husson JM, et al. New approach in the treatment of prostate cancer: complete instead of partial withdrawal of androgens. *Prostate.* 1983;4(6):579-94.

[82] Denis L, Murphy GP. Overview of phase III trials on combined androgen treatment in patients with metastatic prostate cancer. *Cancer.* 1993 Dec 15;72(12 Suppl):3888-95.

[83] Crawford ED, Eisenberger MA, McLeod DG, Spaulding JT, Benson R, Dorr FA, et al. A controlled trial of leuprolide with and without flutamide in prostatic carcinoma. *N. Engl. J. Med.* 1989 Aug 17;321(7):419-24.

[84] Denis LJ, Carneiro de Moura JL, Bono A, Sylvester R, Whelan P, Newling D, et al. Goserelin acetate and flutamide versus bilateral orchiectomy: a phase III EORTC trial (30853). EORTC GU Group and EORTC Data Center. *Urology.* 1993 Aug;42(2):119-29; discussion 29-30.

[85] Janknegt RA, Abbou CC, Bartoletti R, Bernstein-Hahn L, Bracken B, Brisset JM, et al. Orchiectomy and nilutamide or placebo as treatment of metastatic prostatic cancer in a multinational double-blind randomized trial. *J. Urol.* 1993 Jan;149(1):77-82; discussion 3.

[86] Dijkman GA, Janknegt RA, De Reijke TM, Debruyne FM. Long-term efficacy and safety of nilutamide plus castration in advanced prostate cancer, and the significance of early prostate specific antigen normalization. International Anandron Study Group. *J. Urol.* 1997 Jul;158(1):160-3.

[87] Eisenberger MA, Blumenstein BA, Crawford ED, Miller G, McLeod DG, Loehrer PJ, et al. Bilateral orchiectomy with or without flutamide for metastatic prostate cancer. *N. Engl. J. Med.* 1998 Oct 8;339(15):1036-42.

[88] Maximum androgen blockade in advanced prostate cancer: an overview of 22 randomised trials with 3283 deaths in 5710 patients. Prostate Cancer Trialists' Collaborative Group. *Lancet.* 1995 Jul 29;346(8970):265-9.

[89] Samson DJ, Seidenfeld J, Schmitt B, Hasselblad V, Albertsen PC, Bennett CL, et al. Systematic review and meta-analysis of monotherapy compared with combined androgen blockade for patients with advanced prostate carcinoma. *Cancer.* 2002 Jul 15;95(2):361-76.

[90] Verhelst J, Denis L, Van Vliet P, Van Poppel H, Braeckman J, Van Cangh P, et al. Endocrine profiles during administration of the new non-steroidal anti-androgen Casodex in prostate cancer. *Clin. Endocrinol.* (Oxf). 1994 Oct;41(4):525-30.

[91] Boccon-Gibod L, Fournier G, Bottet P, Marechal JM, Guiter J, Rischman P, et al. Flutamide versus orchidectomy in the treatment of metastatic prostate carcinoma. *Eur. Urol.* 1997;32(4):391-5; discussion 5-6.

[92] Pavone-Macaluso M. Flutamide monotherapy versus combined androgen blockade in advanced prostate cancer. Interim report of an Italian multicenter randomized study [abstract]. Proceedings of the 23rd Congress of the Societe Internationale d'Urologie, Sydney, Australia. 1994:A354.

[93] Boccardo F, Rubagotti A, Barichello M, Battaglia M, Carmignani G, Comeri G, et al. Bicalutamide monotherapy versus flutamide plus goserelin in prostate cancer patients: results of an Italian Prostate Cancer Project study. *J. Clin. Oncol.* 1999 Jul;17(7):2027-38.

[94] Kolvenbag GJ, Nash A. Bicalutamide dosages used in the treatment of prostate cancer. *Prostate.* 1999 Apr 1;39(1):47-53.

[95] Tyrrell CJ, Kaisary AV, Iversen P, Anderson JB, Baert L, Tammela T, et al. A randomised comparison of 'Casodex' (bicalutamide) 150 mg monotherapy versus castration in the treatment of metastatic and locally advanced prostate cancer. *Eur. Urol.* 1998;33(5):447-56.

[96] Kaisary AV, Iversen P, Tyrrell CJ, Carroll K, Morris T. Is there a role for antiandrogen monotherapy in patients with metastatic prostate cancer? *Prostate Cancer Prostatic Dis.* 2001;4(4):196-203.

[97] Iversen P, Tyrrell CJ, Kaisary AV, Anderson JB, Van Poppel H, Tammela TL, et al. Bicalutamide monotherapy compared with castration in patients with nonmetastatic locally advanced prostate cancer: 6.3 years of followup. *J. Urol.* 2000 Nov;164(5):1579-82.

[98] Kolvenbag GJ, Iversen P, Newling DW. Antiandrogen monotherapy: a new form of treatment for patients with prostate cancer. *Urology.* 2001 Aug;58(2 Suppl 1):16-23.

[99] McLeod DG, Iversen P, See WA, Morris T, Armstrong J, Wirth MP. Bicalutamide 150 mg plus standard care vs standard care alone for early prostate cancer. *BJU Int.* 2006 Feb;97(2):247-54.

[100] Widmark A, Damber L, Fossa S, Do D, Re R, Mi M, et al. Does prophylactic radiotherapy prevent antiandrogen induced gynecomastia? Evaluation of patients in

the randomized Scandinavian trial SPCG7/SFUO-3. *Int. J. Radiat. Oncol. Biol. Phys.* 1999;45(Suppl):262-3.

[101] McLeod DG, Iversen P. Gynecomastia in patients with prostate cancer: a review of treatment options. *Urology*. 2000 Nov 1;56(5):713-20.

[102] See WA, Wirth MP, McLeod DG, Iversen P, Klimberg I, Gleason D, et al. Bicalutamide as immediate therapy either alone or as adjuvant to standard care of patients with localized or locally advanced prostate cancer: first analysis of the early prostate cancer program. *J. Urol.* 2002 Aug;168(2):429-35.

[103] Wirth MP, See WA, McLeod DG, Iversen P, Morris T, Carroll K. Bicalutamide 150 mg in addition to standard care in patients with localized or locally advanced prostate cancer: results from the second analysis of the early prostate cancer program at median followup of 5.4 years. *J. Urol.* 2004 Nov;172(5 Pt 1):1865-70.

[104] McLeod DG, See WA, Klimberg I, Gleason D, Chodak G, Montie J, et al. The bicalutamide 150 mg early prostate cancer program: findings of the North American trial at 7.7-year median followup. *J. Urol.* 2006 Jul;176(1):75-80.

[105] EORTC Protocol 30991. 2003 [cited September 11, 2006]; Available from: http://www.eortc.be/protoc/Details.asp?Protocol=30991

[106] Kelly WK, Scher HI. Prostate specific antigen decline after antiandrogen withdrawal: the flutamide withdrawal syndrome. *J. Urol.* 1993 Mar;149(3):607-9.

[107] Gleave M, Small E. Androgen deprivation therapy for prostate cancer. In: Carroll P, Nelson W, eds. *Report to the Nation on Prostate Cancer 2004*. Elmwood Park: Medscape 2004:27-36.

[108] Dupont A, Gomez JL, Cusan L, Koutsilieris M, Labrie F. Response to flutamide withdrawal in advanced prostate cancer in progression under combination therapy. *J. Urol.* 1993 Sep;150(3):908-13.

[109] Scher HI, Kelly WK. Flutamide withdrawal syndrome: its impact on clinical trials in hormone-refractory prostate cancer. *J. Clin. Oncol.* 1993 Aug;11(8):1566-72.

[110] Veldscholte J, Ris-Stalpers C, Kuiper GG, Jenster G, Berrevoets C, Claassen E, et al. A mutation in the ligand binding domain of the androgen receptor of human LNCaP cells affects steroid binding characteristics and response to anti-androgens. *Biochem. Biophys. Res. Commun.* 1990 Dec 14;173(2):534-40.

[111] Young CY, Montgomery BT, Andrews PE, Qui SD, Bilhartz DL, Tindall DJ. Hormonal regulation of prostate-specific antigen messenger RNA in human prostatic adenocarcinoma cell line LNCaP. *Cancer Res.* 1991 Jul 15;51(14):3748-52.

[112] Schuurmans AL, Bolt J, Voorhorst MM, Blankenstein RA, Mulder E. Regulation of growth and epidermal growth factor receptor levels of LNCaP prostate tumor cells by different steroids. *Int. J. Cancer.* 1988 Dec 15;42(6):917-22.

[113] Nieh PT. Withdrawal phenomenon with the antiandrogen casodex. *J. Urol.* 1995 Mar;153(3 Pt 2):1070-2; discussion 2-3.

[114] Feldman BJ, Feldman D. The development of androgen-independent prostate cancer. *Nat. Rev. Cancer.* 2001 Oct;1(1):34-45.

[115] Akakura K, Bruchovsky N, Goldenberg SL, Rennie PS, Buckley AR, Sullivan LD. Effects of intermittent androgen suppression on androgen-dependent tumors. Apoptosis and serum prostate-specific antigen. *Cancer.* 1993 May 1;71(9):2782-90.

[116] Gleave M, Miyake H, Chi K. Beyond simple castration: targeting the molecular basis of treatment resistance in advanced prostate cancer. *Cancer Chemother. Pharmacol.* 2005 Nov;56 Suppl 1:47-57.

[117] Gulley J, Figg W, Dahut W. Even more cost savings? Letter to the Editor. *J. Oncol. Pract.* 2006;2(4):202.

[118] Tunn U, Kurek R, Kienle E, Do D, Re R, Mi M, et al. Intermittent is as effective as continuous androgen deprivation in patients with PSA relapse after radical prostatectomy. *J. Urol.* 2004;171:A1458.

[119] Gulley JL, Figg WD, Steinberg SM, Carter J, Sartor O, Higano CS, et al. A prospective analysis of the time to normalization of serum androgens following 6 months of androgen deprivation therapy in patients on a randomized phase III clinical trial using limited hormonal therapy. *J. Urol.* 2005 May;173(5):1567-71.

[120] Bruchovsky N, Klotz L, Crook J, Malone S, Ludgate C, Morris WJ, et al. Final results of the Canadian prospective phase II trial of intermittent androgen suppression for men in biochemical recurrence after radiotherapy for locally advanced prostate cancer: clinical parameters. *Cancer.* 2006 Jul 15;107(2):389-95.

[121] Klotz LH, Herr HW, Morse MJ, Whitmore WF, Jr. Intermittent endocrine therapy for advanced prostate cancer. *Cancer.* 1986 Dec 1;58(11):2546-50.

[122] Goldenberg SL, Bruchovsky N, Gleave ME, Sullivan LD, Akakura K. Intermittent androgen suppression in the treatment of prostate cancer: a preliminary report. *Urology.* 1995 May;45(5):839-44; discussion 44-5.

[123] Strum SB, Scholz MC, McDermed JE. Intermittent androgen deprivation in prostate cancer patients: factors predictive of prolonged time off therapy. *Oncologist.* 2000;5(1):45-52.

[124] Calais Da Silva F, Calais Da Silva F, Bono A, Do D, Re R, Mi M, et al. Phase III intermittent MAB vs continuous MAB [abstract]. *J. Clin. Oncol.* 2006;24(18S Pt 1):A4513.

[125] Bruchovsky N, Klotz L, Crook J, Do D, Re R, Mi M, et al. A phase II study of intermittent androgen suppression (IAS) in men with a rising serum PSA after radiation for localized prostate cancer. *J. Urol.* 1998;159(5):1287.

[126] Higano CS, Ellis W, Russell K, Lange PH. Intermittent androgen suppression with leuprolide and flutamide for prostate cancer: a pilot study. *Urology.* 1996 Nov;48(5):800-4.

[127] Rashid MH, Chaudhary UB. Intermittent androgen deprivation therapy for prostate cancer. *Oncologist.* 2004;9(3):295-301.

[128] Salonen A, Viitanen J, Ala-Opas M, Do D, Re R, Mi M, et al. Finnish multicenter study to compare intermittent and continuous androgen deprivation in patients with advanced prostate cancer [abstract]. *J. Urol.* 2006;175(4 Suppl):1198.

[129] Bhandari MS, Crook J, Hussain M. Should intermittent androgen deprivation be used in routine clinical practice? *J. Clin. Oncol.* 2005 Nov 10;23(32):8212-8.

[130] Hussain M, Tangen CM, Higano C, Schelhammer PF, Faulkner J, Crawford ED, et al. Absolute prostate-specific antigen value after androgen deprivation is a strong independent predictor of survival in new metastatic prostate cancer: data from

Southwest Oncology Group Trial 9346 (INT-0162). *J. Clin. Oncol.* 2006 Aug 20;24(24):3984-90.

[131] Wagmiller J, Griggs J, Dick A, Sahasrabudhe D. Individualized strategy for dosing luteinizing hormone-releasing hormone agonists for androgen-independent prostate cancer: identification of outcomes and costs. *J. Oncol. Pract.* 2006;2(2):57-66.

[132] Oefelein MG. Health related quality of life using serum testosterone as the trigger to re-dose long acting depot luteinizing hormone-releasing hormone agonists in patients with prostate cancer. *J. Urol.* 2003 Jan;169(1):251-5.

[133] Pedraza R, Kwart AM. Hormonal therapy for patients with advanced adenocarcinoma of the prostate: is there a role for discontinuing treatment after prolonged androgen suppression? *Urology.* 2003 Apr;61(4):770-3.

[134] Oefelein MG. Serum testosterone-based luteinizing hormone-releasing hormone agonist redosing schedule for chronic androgen ablation: a phase I assessment. *Urology.* 1999 Oct;54(4):694-9.

[135] Nordquist L, Morris M, Sauter N, Do D, Re R, Mi M, et al. Rapid hormone cycling for prostate cancer (PC) patients: the MENS cycle [abstract]. *Proc. Am. Soc. Clin. Oncol.* 2003;22:A1669.

[136] Nordquist L, Sauter N, Morris M, Do D, Re R, Mi M, et al. Hormonal induction followed by rapid hormonal cycling for prostate cancer (PC): the MENS cycle [abstract]. *Proc. Am. Soc. Clin. Oncol.* 2004;22(14S):A4609.

[137] Beekman K, Kelly W, Carducci M, Do D, Re R, Mi M, et al. Rapid hormonal cycling with docetaxel for patients with rising PSA after definitive local therapy for prostate cancer [abstract]. Multidisciplinary Prostate Cancer Symposium: Current Status and Future Directions for Prevention and Management Orlando, FL. 2005:A145.

[138] Clinical Trials Webpage. [cited 2006 September 27]; Available from: http://clinicaltrials.gov/show/NCT00070369

[139] Trachtenberg J, Halpern N, Pont A. Ketoconazole: a novel and rapid treatment for advanced prostatic cancer. *J. Urol.* 1983 Jul;130(1):152-3.

[140] Trachtenberg J. High-dose ketoconazole in the treatment of metastatic prostatic cancer. *Prostate.* 1985;6(4):455.

[141] Harris KA, Weinberg V, Bok RA, Kakefuda M, Small EJ. Low dose ketoconazole with replacement doses of hydrocortisone in patients with progressive androgen independent prostate cancer. *J. Urol.* 2002 Aug;168(2):542-5.

[142] Eichenberger T, Trachtenberg J, Toor P, Keating A. Ketoconazole: a possible direct cytotoxic effect on prostate carcinoma cells. *J. Urol.* 1989 Jan;141(1):190-1.

[143] Small EJ, Baron A, Bok R. Simultaneous antiandrogen withdrawal and treatment with ketoconazole and hydrocortisone in patients with advanced prostate carcinoma. *Cancer.* 1997 Nov 1;80(9):1755-9.

[144] Lowe FC, Somers WJ. The use of ketoconazole in the emergency management of disseminated intravascular coagulation due to metastatic prostatic cancer. *J. Urol.* 1987 May;137(5):1000-2.

[145] Litt MR, Bell WR, Lepor HA. Disseminated intravascular coagulation in prostatic carcinoma reversed by ketoconazole. *JAMA.* 1987 Sep 11;258(10):1361-2.

[146] Johnson DE, Babaian RJ, von Eschenbach AC, Wishnow KI, Tenney D. Ketoconazole therapy for hormonally refractive metastatic prostate cancer. *Urology.* 1988 Feb;31(2):132-4.
[147] Kruit WH, Stoter G, Klijn JG. Effect of combination therapy with aminoglutethimide and hydrocortisone on prostate-specific antigen response in metastatic prostate cancer refractory to standard endocrine therapy. *Anticancer Drugs.* 2004 Oct;15(9):843-7.
[148] Elomaa I, Taube T, Blomqvist C, Rissanen P, Rannikko S, Alfthan O. Aminoglutethimide for advanced prostatic cancer resistant to conventional hormonal therapy. *Eur. Urol.* 1988;14(2):104-6.
[149] Chang AY, Bennett JM, Pandya KJ, Asbury R, McCune C. A study of aminoglutethemide and hydrocortisone in patients with advanced and refractory prostate carcinoma. *Am. J. Clin. Oncol.* 1989 Aug;12(4):358-60.
[150] Lam JS, Leppert JT, Vemulapalli SN, Shvarts O, Belldegrun AS. Secondary hormonal therapy for advanced prostate cancer. *J. Urol.* 2006 Jan;175(1):27-34.
[151] O'Donnell A, Judson I, Dowsett M, Raynaud F, Dearnaley D, Mason M, et al. Hormonal impact of the 17alpha-hydroxylase/C(17,20)-lyase inhibitor abiraterone acetate (CB7630) in patients with prostate cancer. *Br. J. Cancer.* 2004 Jun 14;90(12):2317-25.
[152] de Bono J, O'Donnell A, Attard G, Do D, Re R, Mi M, et al. Clinical and endocrine evaluation of abiraterone acetate (AA), a rationally designed small molecule inhibitor of androgen synthesis targeting 17a hydroxylase (17OH)/17,20 lyase, in patients with hormone refractory prostate cancer [abstract]. *ASCO 2005 Prostate Cancer Symposium.* 2005:A290.
[153] Gulley J, Dahut WL. Chemotherapy for prostate cancer: finally an advance! *Am. J. Ther.* 2004 Jul-Aug;11(4):288-94.
[154] Isaacs JT, Heston WD, Weissman RM, Coffey DS. Animal models of the hormone-sensitive and -insensitive prostatic adenocarcinomas, Dunning R-3327-H, R-3327-HI, and R-3327-AT. *Cancer Res.* 1978 Nov;38(11 Pt 2):4353-9.
[155] Murphy GP, Beckley S, Brady MF, Chu TM, deKernion JB, Dhabuwala C, et al. Treatment of newly diagnosed metastatic prostate cancer patients with chemotherapy agents in combination with hormones versus hormones alone. *Cancer.* 1983 Apr 1;51(7):1264-72.
[156] Murphy GP, Huben RP, Priore R. Results of another trial of chemotherapy with and without hormones in patients with newly diagnosed metastatic prostate cancer. *Urology.* 1986 Jul;28(1):36-40.
[157] Wang J, Halford S, Rigg A, Roylance R, Lynch M, Waxman J. Adjuvant mitozantrone chemotherapy in advanced prostate cancer. *BJU Int.* 2000 Oct;86(6):675-80.
[158] Hudes G. Estramustine-based chemotherapy. *Semin. Urol. Oncol.* 1997 Feb;15(1):13-9.
[159] Benson R, Hartley-Asp B. Mechanisms of action and clinical uses of estramustine. *Cancer Invest.* 1990;8(3-4):375-80.

[160] Clark PE, Peereboom DM, Dreicer R, Levin HS, Clark SB, Klein EA. Phase II trial of neoadjuvant estramustine and etoposide plus radical prostatectomy for locally advanced prostate cancer. *Urology.* 2001 Feb;57(2):281-5.

[161] Zelefsky MJ, Kelly WK, Scher HI, Lee H, Smart T, Metz E, et al. Results of a phase II study using estramustine phosphate and vinblastine in combination with high-dose three-dimensional conformal radiotherapy for patients with locally advanced prostate cancer. *J. Clin. Oncol.* 2000 May;18(9):1936-41.

[162] Khil MS, Kim JH, Bricker LJ, Cerny JC. Tumor control of locally advanced prostate cancer following combined estramustine, vinblastine, and radiation therapy. *Cancer J. Sci. Am.* 1997 Sep-Oct;3(5):289-96.

[163] Ben-Josef E, Porter AT, Han S, Mertens W, Chuba P, Fontana J, et al. Neoadjuvant estramustine and etoposide followed by concurrent estramustine and definitive radiotherapy for locally advanced prostate cancer: feasibility and preliminary results. *Int. J. Radiat. Oncol. Biol. Phys.* 2001 Mar 1;49(3):699-703.

[164] Pettaway CA, Pisters LL, Troncoso P, Slaton J, Finn L, Kamoi K, et al. Neoadjuvant chemotherapy and hormonal therapy followed by radical prostatectomy: feasibility and preliminary results. *J. Clin. Oncol.* 2000 Mar;18(5):1050-7.

[165] Hussain M, Smith DC, El-Rayes BF, Du W, Vaishampayan U, Fontana J, et al. Neoadjuvant docetaxel and estramustine chemotherapy in high-risk/locallyadvanced prostate cancer. *Urology.* 2003 Apr;61(4):774-80.

[166] Petrylak D, Shelton G, England-Owen C, Do D, Re R, Mi M, et al. Response and preliminary survival results of a phase II study of docetaxel (D) + estramustine (E) in patients with androgen-independent prostate cancer (AIPC) [abstract]. *Proc. Am. Soc. Clin. Oncol.* 2000;19:A334.

[167] Kent EC, Hussain MH. The rationale for adjuvant chemotherapy for high-risk prostate cancer. *Curr. Opin. Urol.* 2003 Mar;13(2):123-31.

[168] Hudes G, Einhorn L, Ross E, Balsham A, Loehrer P, Ramsey H, et al. Vinblastine versus vinblastine plus oral estramustine phosphate for patients with hormone-refractory prostate cancer: a Hoosier Oncology Group and Fox Chase Network phase III trial. *J. Clin. Oncol.* 1999 Oct;17(10):3160-6.

[169] Petrylak DP, Tangen CM, Hussain MH, Lara PN, Jr., Jones JA, Taplin ME, et al. Docetaxel and estramustine compared with mitoxantrone and prednisone for advanced refractory prostate cancer. *N. Engl. J. Med.* 2004 Oct 7;351(15):1513-20.

[170] Berry DL, Moinpour CM, Jiang CS, Ankerst DP, Petrylak DP, Vinson LV, et al. Quality of life and pain in advanced stage prostate cancer: results of a Southwest Oncology Group randomized trial comparing docetaxel and estramustine to mitoxantrone and prednisone. *J. Clin. Oncol.* 2006 Jun 20;24(18):2828-35.

[171] Tannock IF, de Wit R, Berry WR, Horti J, Pluzanska A, Chi KN, et al. Docetaxel plus prednisone or mitoxantrone plus prednisone for advanced prostate cancer. *N. Engl. J. Med.* 2004 Oct 7;351(15):1502-12.

[172] Tang Y, Khan MA, Goloubeva O, Lee DI, Jelovac D, Brodie AM, et al. Docetaxel followed by castration improves outcomes in LNCaP prostate cancer-bearing severe combined immunodeficient mice. *Clin. Cancer Res.* 2006 Jan 1;12(1):169-74.

[173] Perlman H, Zhang X, Chen MW, Walsh K, Buttyan R. An elevated bax/bcl-2 ratio corresponds with the onset of prostate epithelial cell apoptosis. *Cell Death Differ.* 1999 Jan;6(1):48-54.

[174] Hussain A, Dawson N, Amin P, Engstrom C, Dorsey B, Siegel E, et al. Docetaxel followed by hormone therapy in men experiencing increasing prostate-specific antigen after primary local treatments for prostate cancer. *J. Clin. Oncol.* 2005 Apr 20;23(12):2789-96.

[175] Olsen NJ, Zhou P, Ong H, Kovacs WJ. Testosterone induces expression of transforming growth factor-beta 1 in the murine thymus. *J. Steroid Biochem. Mol. Biol.* 1993 May;45(5):327-32.

[176] Kim IY, Kim JH, Zelner DJ, Ahn HJ, Sensibar JA, Lee C. Transforming growth factor-beta1 is a mediator of androgen-regulated growth arrest in an androgen-responsive prostatic cancer cell line, LNCaP. *Endocrinology.* 1996 Mar;137(3):991-9.

[177] Zatelli MC, Rossi R, degli Uberti EC. Androgen influences transforming growth factor-beta1 gene expression in human adrenocortical cells. *J. Clin. Endocrinol. Metab.* 2000 Feb;85(2):847-52.

[178] Zatelli MC, Rossi R, del Senno L, degli Uberti EC. Role of transforming growth factor beta 1 (TGF beta 1) in mediating androgen-induced growth inhibition in human adrenal cortex in vitro. *Steroids.* 1998 May-Jun;63(5-6):243-5.

[179] Salm SN, Koikawa Y, Ogilvie V, Tsujimura A, Coetzee S, Moscatelli D, et al. Transforming growth factor-beta is an autocrine mitogen for a novel androgen-responsive murine prostatic smooth muscle cell line, PSMC1. *J. Cell Physiol.* 2000 Dec;185(3):416-24.

[180] Dammann CE, Ramadurai SM, McCants DD, Pham LD, Nielsen HC. Androgen regulation of signaling pathways in late fetal mouse lung development. *Endocrinology.* 2000 Aug;141(8):2923-9.

[181] Inui S, Fukuzato Y, Nakajima T, Yoshikawa K, Itami S. Androgen-inducible TGF-beta1 from balding dermal papilla cells inhibits epithelial cell growth: a clue to understand paradoxical effects of androgen on human hair growth. *FASEB J.* 2002 Dec;16(14):1967-9.

[182] Roden AC, Moser MT, Tri SD, Mercader M, Kuntz SM, Dong H, et al. Augmentation of T cell levels and responses induced by androgen deprivation. *J. Immunol.* 2004 Nov 15;173(10):6098-108.

[183] Hsueh EC, Gupta RK, Lefor A, Reyzin G, Ye W, Morton DL. Androgen blockade enhances response to melanoma vaccine. *J. Surg. Res.* 2003 Apr;110(2):393-8.

[184] Drake CG, Doody AD, Mihalyo MA, Huang CT, Kelleher E, Ravi S, et al. Androgen ablation mitigates tolerance to a prostate/prostate cancer-restricted antigen. *Cancer Cell.* 2005 Mar;7(3):239-49.

[185] Olsen NJ, Kovacs WJ. Gonadal steroids and immunity. *Endocr. Rev.* 1996 Aug;17(4):369-84.

[186] Mercader M, Bodner BK, Moser MT, Kwon PS, Park ES, Manecke RG, et al. T cell infiltration of the prostate induced by androgen withdrawal in patients with prostate cancer. *Proc. Natl. Acad. Sci. U. S. A.* 2001 Dec 4;98(25):14565-70.

[187] Sutherland JS, Goldberg GL, Hammett MV, Uldrich AP, Berzins SP, Heng TS, et al. Activation of thymic regeneration in mice and humans following androgen blockade. *J. Immunol.* 2005 Aug 15;175(4):2741-53.

[188] Schwarer A, Sutherland J, Muirhead J, Prince H. Sex steroid suppression with luteinizing hormone-releasing hormone agonist (LHRH-A) allows thymic reactivation and improved immunological recovery after allogeneic hematopoietic stem cell transplantation (alloHSCT). American Society of Hematology Annual Meeting [abstract]. *Blood.* 2003;102(11):A260.

[189] Sanda MG, Smith DC, Charles LG, Hwang C, Pienta KJ, Schlom J, et al. Recombinant vaccinia-PSA (PROSTVAC) can induce a prostate-specific immune response in androgen-modulated human prostate cancer. *Urology.* 1999 Feb;53(2):260-6.

[190] Eder JP, Kantoff PW, Roper K, Xu GX, Bubley GJ, Boyden J, et al. A phase I trial of a recombinant vaccinia virus expressing prostate-specific antigen in advanced prostate cancer. *Clin. Cancer Res.* 2000 May;6(5):1632-8.

[191] Gulley J, Chen AP, Dahut W, Arlen PM, Bastian A, Steinberg SM, et al. Phase I study of a vaccine using recombinant vaccinia virus expressing PSA (rV-PSA) in patients with metastatic androgen-independent prostate cancer. *Prostate.* 2002 Oct 1;53(2):109-17.

[192] Arlen PM, Gulley JL, Todd N, Lieberman R, Steinberg SM, Morin S, et al. Antiandrogen, vaccine and combination therapy in patients with nonmetastatic hormone refractory prostate cancer. *J. Urol.* 2005 Aug;174(2):539-46.

[193] Kassouf W, Tanguay S, Aprikian AG. Nilutamide as second line hormone therapy for prostate cancer after androgen ablation fails. *J. Urol.* 2003 May;169(5):1742-4.

[194] Desai A, Stadler WM, Vogelzang NJ. Nilutamide: possible utility as a second-line hormonal agent. *Urology.* 2001 Dec;58(6):1016-20.

[195] Daniell HW, Dunn SR, Ferguson DW, Lomas G, Niazi Z, Stratte PT. Progressive osteoporosis during androgen deprivation therapy for prostate cancer. *J. Urol.* 2000 Jan;163(1):181-6.

[196] Stoch SA, Parker RA, Chen L, Bubley G, Ko YJ, Vincelette A, et al. Bone loss in men with prostate cancer treated with gonadotropin-releasing hormone agonists. *J. Clin. Endocrinol.* Metab. 2001 Jun;86(6):2787-91.

[197] Preston DM, Torrens JI, Harding P, Howard RS, Duncan WE, McLeod DG. Androgen deprivation in men with prostate cancer is associated with an increased rate of bone loss. *Prostate Cancer Prostatic Dis.* 2002;5(4):304-10.

[198] Oefelein MG, Ricchuiti V, Conrad W, Seftel A, Bodner D, Goldman H, et al. Skeletal fracture associated with androgen suppression induced osteoporosis: the clinical incidence and risk factors for patients with prostate cancer. *J. Urol.* 2001 Nov;166(5):1724-8.

[199] Diamond TH, Bucci J, Kersley JH, Aslan P, Lynch WB, Bryant C. Osteoporosis and spinal fractures in men with prostate cancer: risk factors and effects of androgen deprivation therapy. *J. Urol.* 2004 Aug;172(2):529-32.

[200] Shahinian VB, Kuo YF, Freeman JL, Goodwin JS. Risk of fracture after androgen deprivation for prostate cancer. *N. Engl. J. Med.* 2005 Jan 13;352(2):154-64.

[201] Smith MR, McGovern FJ, Zietman AL, Fallon MA, Hayden DL, Schoenfeld DA, et al. Pamidronate to prevent bone loss during androgen-deprivation therapy for prostate cancer. *N. Engl. J. Med.* 2001 Sep 27;345(13):948-55.
[202] Smith MR, Eastham J, Gleason DM, Shasha D, Tchekmedyian S, Zinner N. Randomized controlled trial of zoledronic acid to prevent bone loss in men receiving androgen deprivation therapy for nonmetastatic prostate cancer. *J. Urol.* 2003 Jun;169(6):2008-12.
[203] Michaelson M, Lee H, Kaufman D, Kantoff P, Finkelstein J, Smith M. Annual zoledronic acid to prevent gonadotropin-releasing hormone agonist-induced bone loss in men with prostate cancer: a randomized placebo-controlled trial [abstract]. *J. Clin. Oncol.* 2006;24(18S Pt I):4515.
[204] Alibhai SM, Rahman S, Warde PR, Jewett MA, Jaffer T, Cheung AM. Prevention and management of osteoporosis in men receiving androgen deprivation therapy: a survey of urologists and radiation oncologists. *Urology.* 2006 Jul;68(1):126-31.
[205] Higano CS. Management of bone loss in men with prostate cancer. *J. Urol.* 2003 Dec;170(6 Pt 2):S59-63; discussion S4.
[206] Holzbeierlein JM, McLaughlin MD, Thrasher JB. Complications of androgen deprivation therapy for prostate cancer. *Curr. Opin. Urol.* 2004 May;14(3):177-83.
[207] Loprinzi CL, Michalak JC, Quella SK, O'Fallon JR, Hatfield AK, Nelimark RA, et al. Megestrol acetate for the prevention of hot flashes. *N. Engl. J. Med.* 1994 Aug 11;331(6):347-52.
[208] Sartor O, Eastham JA. Progressive prostate cancer associated with use of megestrol acetate administered for control of hot flashes. *South Med. J.* 1999 Apr;92(4):415-6.
[209] Quella SK, Loprinzi CL, Sloan J, Novotny P, Perez EA, Burch PA, et al. Pilot evaluation of venlafaxine for the treatment of hot flashes in men undergoing androgen ablation therapy for prostate cancer. *J. Urol.* 1999 Jul;162(1):98-102.
[210] Loprinzi CL, Barton DL, Carpenter LA, Sloan JA, Novotny PJ, Gettman MT, et al. Pilot evaluation of paroxetine for treating hot flashes in men. *Mayo Clin. Proc.* 2004 Oct;79(10):1247-51.
[211] Sharifi N, Gulley JL, Dahut WL. Androgen deprivation therapy for prostate cancer. *JAMA.* 2005 Jul 13;294(2):238-44.
[212] Muller M, Grobbee DE, den Tonkelaar I, Lamberts SW, van der Schouw YT. Endogenous sex hormones and metabolic syndrome in aging men. *J. Clin. Endocrinol. Metab.* 2005 May;90(5):2618-23.
[213] Smith MR, Finkelstein JS, McGovern FJ, Zietman AL, Fallon MA, Schoenfeld DA, et al. Changes in body composition during androgen deprivation therapy for prostate cancer. *J. Clin. Endocrinol. Metab.* 2002 Feb;87(2):599-603.
[214] Berruti A, Dogliotti L, Terrone C, Cerutti S, Isaia G, Tarabuzzi R, et al. Changes in bone mineral density, lean body mass and fat content as measured by dual energy x-ray absorptiometry in patients with prostate cancer without apparent bone metastases given androgen deprivation therapy. *J. Urol.* 2002 Jun;167(6):2361-7; discussion 7.
[215] Nishiyama T, Ishizaki F, Anraku T, Shimura H, Takahashi K. The influence of androgen deprivation therapy on metabolism in patients with prostate cancer. *J. Clin. Endocrinol. Metab.* 2005 Feb;90(2):657-60.

[216] Braga-Basaria M, Dobs AS, Muller DC, Carducci MA, John M, Egan J, et al. Metabolic syndrome in men with prostate cancer undergoing long-term androgen-deprivation therapy. *J. Clin. Oncol.* 2006 Aug 20;24(24):3979-83.
[217] Keating NL, O'Malley AJ, Smith MR. Diabetes and cardiovascular disease during androgen deprivation therapy for prostate cancer. *J. Clin. Oncol.* 2006 Sep 20;24(27):4448-56.
[218] Managing the side effects of androgen deprivation therapy. *J. Support Oncol.* 2006 Feb;4(2):97-8.
[219] Basaria S, Lieb J, 2nd, Tang AM, DeWeese T, Carducci M, Eisenberger M, et al. Long-term effects of androgen deprivation therapy in prostate cancer patients. *Clin. Endocrinol.* (Oxf). 2002 Jun;56(6):779-86.
[220] Potosky AL, Knopf K, Clegg LX, Albertsen PC, Stanford JL, Hamilton AS, et al. Quality-of-life outcomes after primary androgen deprivation therapy: results from the Prostate Cancer Outcomes Study. *J. Clin. Oncol.* 2001 Sep 1;19(17):3750-7.
[221] Chen AC, Petrylak DP. Complications of androgen deprivation therapy in men with prostate cancer. *Curr. Oncol. Rep.* 2004 May;6(3):209-15.
[222] Cavallini G, Caracciolo S, Vitali G, Modenini F, Biagiotti G. Carnitine versus androgen administration in the treatment of sexual dysfunction, depressed mood, and fatigue associated with male aging. *Urology.* 2004 Apr;63(4):641-6.
[223] Shahinian VB, Kuo YF, Freeman JL, Goodwin JS. Risk of the "androgen deprivation syndrome" in men receiving androgen deprivation for prostate cancer. *Arch. Intern. Med.* 2006 Feb 27;166(4):465-71.
[224] Green HJ, Pakenham KI, Headley BC, Yaxley J, Nicol DL, Mactaggart PN, et al. Altered cognitive function in men treated for prostate cancer with luteinizing hormone-releasing hormone analogues and cyproterone acetate: a randomized controlled trial. *BJU Int.* 2002 Sep;90(4):427-32.
[225] Salminen EK, Portin RI, Koskinen AI, Helenius HY, Nurmi MJ. Estradiol and cognition during androgen deprivation in men with prostate carcinoma. *Cancer.* 2005 Apr 1;103(7):1381-7.
[226] Jenkins VA, Bloomfield DJ, Shilling VM, Edginton TL. Does neoadjuvant hormone therapy for early prostate cancer affect cognition? Results from a pilot study. *BJU Int.* 2005 Jul;96(1):48-53.
[227] Salminen E, Portin R, Korpela J, Backman H, Parvinen LM, Helenius H, et al. Androgen deprivation and cognition in prostate cancer. *Br. J. Cancer.* 2003 Sep 15;89(6):971-6.
[228] Strum SB, McDermed JE, Scholz MC, Johnson H, Tisman G. Anaemia associated with androgen deprivation in patients with prostate cancer receiving combined hormone blockade. *Br. J. Urol.* 1997 Jun;79(6):933-41.
[229] Sharifi N, Dahut WL, Steinberg SM, Figg WD, Tarassoff C, Arlen P, et al. A retrospective study of the time to clinical endpoints for advanced prostate cancer. *BJU Int.* 2005 Nov;96(7):985-9.
[230] Oefelein MG, Agarwal PK, Resnick MI. Survival of patients with hormone refractory prostate cancer in the prostate specific antigen era. *J. Urol.* 2004 Apr;171(4):1525-8.

[231] Gregory CW, Johnson RT, Jr., Mohler JL, French FS, Wilson EM. Androgen receptor stabilization in recurrent prostate cancer is associated with hypersensitivity to low androgen. *Cancer Res.* 2001 Apr 1;61(7):2892-8.

[232] Roy-Burman P, Tindall DJ, Robins DM, Greenberg NM, Hendrix MJ, Mohla S, et al. Androgens and prostate cancer: are the descriptors valid? *Cancer Biol. Ther.* 2005 Jan;4(1):4-5.

[233] Agus DB, Cordon-Cardo C, Fox W, Drobnjak M, Koff A, Golde DW, et al. Prostate cancer cell cycle regulators: response to androgen withdrawal and development of androgen independence. *J. Natl. Cancer Inst.* 1999 Nov 3;91(21):1869-76.

[234] Sharifi N, Farrar WL. Androgen receptor as a therapeutic target for androgen independent prostate cancer. *Am. J. Ther.* 2006 Mar-Apr;13(2):166-70.

[235] Scher HI, Sawyers CL. Biology of progressive, castration-resistant prostate cancer: directed therapies targeting the androgen-receptor signaling axis. *J. Clin. Oncol.* 2005 Nov 10;23(32):8253-61.

[236] Figg WD, Liu Y, Arlen P, Gulley J, Steinberg SM, Liewehr DJ, et al. A randomized, phase II trial of ketoconazole plus alendronate versus ketoconazole alone in patients with androgen independent prostate cancer and bone metastases. *J. Urol.* 2005 Mar;173(3):790-6.

[237] Fujikawa K, Matsui Y, Fukuzawa S, Takeuchi H. Prostate-specific antigen levels and clinical response to flutamide as the second hormone therapy for hormone-refractory prostate carcinoma. *Eur. Urol.* 2000 Feb;37(2):218-22.

[238] Mousses S, Wagner U, Chen Y, Kim JW, Bubendorf L, Bittner M, et al. Failure of hormone therapy in prostate cancer involves systematic restoration of androgen responsive genes and activation of rapamycin sensitive signaling. *Oncogene.* 2001 Oct 11;20(46):6718-23.

[239] Holzbeierlein J, Lal P, LaTulippe E, Smith A, Satagopan J, Zhang L, et al. Gene expression analysis of human prostate carcinoma during hormonal therapy identifies androgen-responsive genes and mechanisms of therapy resistance. *Am. J. Pathol.* 2004 Jan;164(1):217-27.

[240] Edwards J, Krishna NS, Grigor KM, Bartlett JM. Androgen receptor gene amplification and protein expression in hormone refractory prostate cancer. *Br. J. Cancer.* 2003 Aug 4;89(3):552-6.

[241] Bubendorf L, Kononen J, Koivisto P, Schraml P, Moch H, Gasser TC, et al. Survey of gene amplifications during prostate cancer progression by high-throughput fluorescence in situ hybridization on tissue microarrays. *Cancer Res.* 1999 Feb 15;59(4):803-6.

[242] Chen CD, Welsbie DS, Tran C, Baek SH, Chen R, Vessella R, et al. Molecular determinants of resistance to antiandrogen therapy. *Nat. Med.* 2004 Jan;10(1):33-9.

[243] Xu J, Qiu Y, DeMayo FJ, Tsai SY, Tsai MJ, O'Malley BW. Partial hormone resistance in mice with disruption of the steroid receptor coactivator-1 (SRC-1) gene. *Science.* 1998 Mar 20;279(5358):1922-5.

[244] Chen T, Wang LH, Farrar WL. Interleukin 6 activates androgen receptor-mediated gene expression through a signal transducer and activator of transcription 3-dependent pathway in LNCaP prostate cancer cells. *Cancer Res.* 2000 Apr 15;60(8):2132-5.

[245] Wallner L, Dai J, Escara-Wilke J, Zhang J, Yao Z, Lu Y, et al. Inhibition of interleukin-6 with CNTO328, an anti-interleukin-6 monoclonal antibody, inhibits conversion of androgen-dependent prostate cancer to an androgen-independent phenotype in orchiectomized mice. *Cancer Res.* 2006 Mar 15;66(6):3087-95.

[246] Papatsoris AG, Karamouzis MV, Papavassiliou AG. Novel insights into the implication of the IGF-1 network in prostate cancer. *Trends Mol. Med.* 2005 Feb;11(2):52-5.

[247] Finn RS, Slamon DJ. Monoclonal antibody therapy for breast cancer: herceptin. *Cancer Chemother. Biol. Response Modif.* 2003;21:223-33.

[248] Mellinghoff IK, Vivanco I, Kwon A, Tran C, Wongvipat J, Sawyers CL. HER2/neu kinase-dependent modulation of androgen receptor function through effects on DNA binding and stability. *Cancer Cell.* 2004 Nov;6(5):517-27.

[249] Gioeli D. Signal transduction in prostate cancer progression. *Clin. Sci.* (Lond). 2005 Apr;108(4):293-308.

[250] Heinlein CA, Chang C. Androgen receptor in prostate cancer. *Endocr. Rev.* 2004 Apr;25(2):276-308.

[251] Weber MJ, Gioeli D. Ras signaling in prostate cancer progression. *J. Cell Biochem.* 2004 Jan 1;91(1):13-25.

[252] Titus MA, Schell MJ, Lih FB, Tomer KB, Mohler JL. Testosterone and dihydrotestosterone tissue levels in recurrent prostate cancer. *Clin. Cancer Res.* 2005 Jul 1;11(13):4653-7.

[253] Stanbrough M, Bubley GJ, Ross K, Golub TR, Rubin MA, Penning TM, et al. Increased expression of genes converting adrenal androgens to testosterone in androgen-independent prostate cancer. *Cancer Res.* 2006 Mar 1;66(5):2815-25.

[254] Tomlins SA, Rhodes DR, Perner S, Dhanasekaran SM, Mehra R, Sun XW, et al. Recurrent fusion of TMPRSS2 and ETS transcription factor genes in prostate cancer. *Science.* 2005 Oct 28;310(5748):644-8.

[255] Adachi M, Takayanagi R, Tomura A, Imasaki K, Kato S, Goto K, et al. Androgen-insensitivity syndrome as a possible coactivator disease. N Engl J Med. 2000 Sep 21;343(12):856-62.

[256] Hur E, Pfaff SJ, Payne ES, Gron H, Buehrer BM, Fletterick RJ. Recognition and accommodation at the androgen receptor coactivator binding interface. *PLoS Biol.* 2004 Sep;2(9):E274.

[257] Wang LH, Yang XY, Zhang X, Mihalic K, Fan YX, Xiao W, et al. Suppression of breast cancer by chemical modulation of vulnerable zinc fingers in estrogen receptor. *Nat. Med.* 2004 Jan;10(1):40-7.

[258] Whitesell L, Lindquist SL. HSP90 and the chaperoning of cancer. *Nat. Rev. Cancer.* 2005 Oct;5(10):761-72.

[259] Georget V, Terouanne B, Nicolas JC, Sultan C. Mechanism of antiandrogen action: key role of hsp90 in conformational change and transcriptional activity of the androgen receptor. *Biochemistry.* 2002 Oct 1;41(39):11824-31.

[260] Drysdale MJ, Brough PA, Massey A, Jensen MR, Schoepfer J. Targeting Hsp90 for the treatment of cancer. *Curr. Opin. Drug Discov. Devel.* 2006 Jul;9(4):483-95.

[261] Schneekloth JS, Jr., Fonseca FN, Koldobskiy M, Mandal A, Deshaies R, Sakamoto K, et al. Chemical genetic control of protein levels: selective in vivo targeted degradation. *J. Am. Chem. Soc.* 2004 Mar 31;126(12):3748-54.

[262] Singh P, Uzgare A, Litvinov I, Denmeade SR, Isaacs JT. Combinatorial androgen receptor targeted therapy for prostate cancer. *Endocr. Relat. Cancer.* 2006 Sep;13(3):653-66.

[263] Talpaz M, Shah NP, Kantarjian H, Donato N, Nicoll J, Paquette R, et al. Dasatinib in imatinib-resistant Philadelphia chromosome-positive leukemias. *N. Engl. J. Med.* 2006 Jun 15;354(24):2531-41.

[264] Collins AT, Berry PA, Hyde C, Stower MJ, Maitland NJ. Prospective identification of tumorigenic prostate cancer stem cells. *Cancer Res.* 2005 Dec 1;65(23):10946-51.

[265] Patrawala L, Calhoun T, Schneider-Broussard R, Li H, Bhatia B, Tang S, et al. Highly purified CD44+ prostate cancer cells from xenograft human tumors are enriched in tumorigenic and metastatic progenitor cells. *Oncogene.* 2006 Mar 16;25(12):1696-708.

[266] Sharifi N, Kawasaki BT, Hurt EM, Farrar WL. Stem cells in prostate cancer: resolving the castrate-resistant conundrum and implications for hormonal therapy. *Cancer Biol. Ther.* 2006 Aug 28;5(8):[Epub ahead of print].

[267] Smaletz O, Scher HI, Small EJ, Verbel DA, McMillan A, Regan K, et al. Nomogram for overall survival of patients with progressive metastatic prostate cancer after castration. *J. Clin. Oncol.* 2002 Oct 1;20(19):3972-82.

[268] Hanks G, Lu J, Machtay M, Do D, Re R, Mi M, et al. RTOG Protocol 92-02: a phase III trial of the use of long term androgen suppression following neoadjuvant hormonal cytoreduction and radiotherapy in locally advanced carcinoma of the prostate [abstract]. *Proc. Am. Soc. Clin. Oncol.* 2000;19:1264.

[269] D'Amico AV, Schultz D, Loffredo M, Dugal R, Hurwitz M, Kaplan I, et al. Biochemical outcome following external beam radiation therapy with or without androgen suppression therapy for clinically localized prostate cancer. *Jama.* 2000 Sep 13;284(10):1280-3.

[270] Schulman CC, Debruyne FM, Forster G, Selvaggi FP, Zlotta AR, Witjes WP. 4-Year follow-up results of a European prospective randomized study on neoadjuvant hormonal therapy prior to radical prostatectomy in T2-3N0M0 prostate cancer. European Study Group on Neoadjuvant Treatment of Prostate Cancer. *Eur Urol.* 2000 Dec;38(6):706-13.

[271] Aus G, Abrahamsson PA, Ahlgren G, Hugosson J, Lundberg S, Schain M, et al. Three-month neoadjuvant hormonal therapy before radical prostatectomy: a 7-year follow-up of a randomized controlled trial. *BJU Int.* 2002 Oct;90(6):561-6.

[272] Denis LJ, Keuppens F, Smith PH, Whelan P, de Moura JL, Newling D, et al. Maximal androgen blockade: final analysis of EORTC phase III trial 30853. EORTC Genito-Urinary Tract Cancer Cooperative Group and the EORTC Data Center. *Eur Urol.* 1998;33(2):144-51.

[273] Tyrrell CJ, Altwein JE, Klippel F, Varenhorst E, Lunglmayr G, Boccardo F, et al. Multicenter randomized trial comparing Zoladex with Zoladex plus flutamide in the

treatment of advanced prostate cancer. Survival update. International Prostate Cancer Study Group. *Cancer.* 1993 Dec 15;72(12 Suppl):3878-9.

[274] Iversen P, Rasmussen F, Klarskov P, Christensen IJ. Long-term results of Danish Prostatic Cancer Group trial 86. Goserelin acetate plus flutamide versus orchiectomy in advanced prostate cancer. *Cancer.* 1993 Dec 15;72(12 Suppl):3851-4.

[275] Boccardo F, Decensi A, Guarneri D, Rubagotti A, Oneto F, Martorana G, et al. Zoladex with or without flutamide in the treatment of locally advanced or metastatic prostate cancer: interim analysis of an ongoing PONCAP study. Italian Prostatic Cancer Project (PONCAP). *Eur. Urol.* 1990;18 Suppl 3:48-53.

[276] Bracarda S, Rosi P, Pizzirusso G, Do D, Re R, Mi M, et al. Intermittent androgen suppression (IAS) in advanced or inoperable prostate cancer. Ann Oncol. 1998;9:272O.

[277] Theyer G, Hamilton G. Current status of intermittent androgen suppression in the treatment of prostate cancer. *Urology.* 1998 Sep;52(3):353-9.

[278] Gleave M, Bruchovsky N, Goldenberg SL, Rennie P. Intermittent androgen suppression for prostate cancer: rationale and clinical experience. *Eur. Urol.* 1998;34 Suppl 3:37-41.

[279] Crook JM, Szumacher E, Malone S, Huan S, Segal R. Intermittent androgen suppression in the management of prostate cancer. *Urology.* 1999 Mar;53(3):530-4.

[280] Grossfeld GD, Chaudhary UB, Reese DM, Carroll PR, Small EJ. Intermittent androgen deprivation: update of cycling characteristics in patients without clinically apparent metastatic prostate cancer. *Urology.* 2001 Aug;58(2):240-5.

[281] Prapotnich D, Fizazi K, Escudier B, Mombet A, Cathala N, Vallancien G. A 10-year clinical experience with intermittent hormonal therapy for prostate cancer. *Eur. Urol.* 2003 Mar;43(3):233-39; discussion 9-40.

[282] Tangen C, Hussain M, Wilding G, Do D, Re R, Mi M, et al. Determinants of prostate specific antigen normalization in prostate cancer patients treated with androgen deprivation on Southwest Oncology Group Study 9346 (INT-0162) [abstract]. *Proc. Am. Soc. Clin. Oncol.* 2003;22:A1591.

In: Trends in Testosterone Research
Editor: Raymund E. Veritos
ISBN: 978-1-60456-127-2

Chapter II

Testosterone or Gonadotropin Lowering Treatment for Alzheimer's Disease: Predicting Risk or Benefit

Stephan Bandelow and Eef Hogervorst*
Department of Human Sciences, Loughborough University, United Kingdom

Abstract

This review investigates whether lowering gonadotropin levels using leuprolide acetate would be preferable to testosterone (T) treatment for men with Alzheimer's disease (AD). There is considerable evidence from animal and cell culture studies that high gonodatropin and low T levels may have detrimental effects on the brain. Several observational studies have also reported low levels of T and high levels of gonadotropins in men with AD. Chemical castration using leuprolide acetate in men with prostate cancer has shown some improvements, but also significant decline in memory functions. Limited data suggest that this effect may be worse in older men. However, we only found high gonadotropin levels in older (80+ years), but not younger AD cases. Possibly, increased gonadotropin levels may be an adequate, if failed, response to earlier lowered levels of T in the disease. As T treatment also decreases gonadotropin levels, is neuroprotective and has shown positive effects on cognition in AD, it might be a more suitable alternative than leuprolide acetate. Age, genetics, prior levels of T and estrogens may all play a role in determining optimal levels of T to improve cognition in AD.

Keywords: Alzheimer, testosterone, leuprolide, gonadotropin, cognition, memory, castration.

* Correspondence should be addressed to: Prof. E. Hogervorst; Department of Human Sciences; Loughborough University; LE11 3TU; United Kingdom; tel + 1509 223020; fax + 1509 223940; email:e.hogervorst@lboro.ac.uk

1. Introduction

1.1. Biological Plausibility of the Association between High Gonadotropin Levels and AD Pathology

A flurry of research papers has been published over the last years, which all convincingly argue that high gonadotropin, such as Luteinising hormone (LH) levels are associated with Alzheimer's disease (AD). Studies into biological plausible mechanisms have been reviewed and can be summed up as follows[1]. LH was found to be significantly increased in serum, but also in pyramidal neurons and neurofibrillary tangles in AD cases compared to controls. LH is known to be mitogenic, and could therefore initiate the cell cycle abnormalities seen in AD, affecting neurons particularly in those regions (e.g. the hippocampus) where LH receptors are abundant and which are vulnerable to AD pathological processes. Using genetically modified mice, LH did not alter amyloid-β precursor protein (AβPP) expression, but did alter AβPP processing toward the amyloidogenic pathway, as evidenced by increased secretion and insolubility of amyloid β. Amyloid β is neurotoxic and is a major constituent of the plaques seen in AD. Treatment to lower LH levels using leuprolide acetate, a prostate cancer agent, was successful in improving cognitive performance and decreasing amyloid-β deposition in transgenic mice.

This work lead to a large multi-center clinical trial (ALADDIN), which aimed to include more than 500 AD patients to test the effect of lowering LH levels through leuprolide acetate. Leuprolide is a GnRH analogue, which initially increases LH and testosterone (T) levels, but lowers both after a couple of weeks. Leuprolide thus also leads to chemical castration, by indirectly lowering T activity. While results of this trial presented at the Alzheimer's Association conference in Madrid in 2006 were positive for women with AD, results for men with AD were withheld.

As the literature reviewed suggests that T has neuroprotective properties, either directly or through its conversion into estradiol (E2)[2], evidence is further reviewed to scrutinize the theory that leuprolide acetate would be beneficial for cognitive function in men with AD or that it might actually have negative effects and that T treatment would be preferable.

1. 2. Are Levels of Gonadotropins Really Lowered in AD Cases when Compared to Age-Matched Controls ? Why Would this Be the Case ?

An initial study reported that levels of gonadotropins were increased in men with dementia compared to controls[3]. Investigating different cohorts, we found, however, that this was age-dependent. For instance, data from another cohort indicated that levels of gonadotropins were not different between AD cases and controls when analyses were adjusted for age[4]. Results did remain significant for women with AD not using hormone treatment. While some [5] found no differences in gonadotropin levels in women with AD compared to a group of somewhat younger controls, we [6], in contrast, found lower levels of LH in women with AD compared to controls of the Oxford Project To Investigate Memory and Ageing (OPTIMA).

This was consistent with the finding of higher estrogen levels in women with AD. Data from OPTIMA did show higher levels of gonadotropins in men with AD, but only in the older (average age 85 years) and not in the younger (average age 66 years) cases [7]. This was hypothesized to tie in with findings of lower T levels in men with AD.

2. Lowering Testosterone Levels through Lowering LH Levels, Is that a Good Idea ?

2.1. Levels of Testosterone in Men with AD Compared to Controls

Several research groups, including our own in Oxford which is led by Professor David Smith (Oxford project To Investigate Memory and Ageing or OPTIMA), found that men with both clinical and post-mortem confirmed AD had lower levels of T [7-9], even when controlled for a wide variety of potential confounds. Most convincing were the data from the Baltimore Longitudinal Study of Aging [10] (BLSA) which showed that levels of free or bioavailable T (FT) were lowered years before the actual onset of AD. Increased LH levels in the older cases with AD might thus be an appropriate response to their lowered T levels. In OPTIMA, we found that in younger men with AD, of a similar age as those investigated in the BLSA, levels of FT and sex hormone binding globulin (SHBG) were more pronouncedly different from controls, while in older cases of OPTIMA, total T and gonadotropin levels were more pronouncedly and significantly different from age-matched controls [7].

2.1. The Chicken or the Egg: Is Lowered T a Result of Brain Degeneration ?

So why would FT levels be lower in cases with AD early in the disease process? Data suggest an acceleration of a pattern of endocrinological change seen in normal aging, possibly related to genetic factors or DNA damage. For instance, we also found lowered thyroid stimulating hormone (TSH) levels in cases with AD early in the disease [11]. Lowered TSH levels lead to increased sex hormone binding globulin (SHBG) levels, which then lead to a decrease in FT levels [7].

The BLSA data suggest that total T is initially not significantly lower in those at risk for AD, also indicating a low probability of primary hypogonadism as a causal factor in AD. The subsequent later adequate, but failed, response with an increase in gonadotropin levels, when total T levels are also decreased in cases, may be an attempt to normalize T levels. This suggests that the hypothalamic-pituitary-gonadal (HPG) axis is still intact in AD and that low FT levels are not just a consequence of the degeneration of lower brain areas. Rosario et al. [12] also concluded that T depletion is a contributor rather than a result from the development of AD. In an autopsy study of subjects with definite AD, Rosario et al. reported that brain levels of T (but not of E2) were significantly lower in men with AD (also in those with very mild early pathological and non clinical signs) compared to controls [12].

However, as low T levels can lead to higher levels of gonadotropins, which, as described, could be neurotoxic, there may still be a good rational for lowering levels of LH medically.

3. Proof of the Pudding: Does Chemical Castration Improve AD Pathology or Cognitive Function?

3.1. Effects of Chemical Castration on Neuropeptides Related to AD

Men with prostate cancer, who underwent chemical castration with leuprolide acetate (leuprorelin) and flutamide, showed increased plasma amyloid β levels which corresponded to the decrease seen in T levels [13]. Others [14] also reported an inverse correlation between total T, FT and plasma amyloid β peptide 40 (Aβ40) levels in men with dementia or with memory impairment. No association was seen with LH or E2 levels and amyloid β levels. Animal studies, as reviewed by Pike [15], indicated that androgens (such as T), but not E2, decrease amyloid β in castrated animals. As E2, similar to T, reverses LH elevation after castration, this reduces the likelihood of LH being an important regulatory factor in AD-related neuropathology. Rather, subclinical androgen deficiency, whether or not induced biochemically by using leuprolide, may promote AD related peptides.

3.2. The Effect of Chemical Castration on Cognitive Function

Several controlled studies indicated that women who undergo surgical (reviewed in [16]) or chemical [17-18] menopause (using leuprolide acetate) have a subsequent and significant drop in cognitive functions, of which a decline in episodic verbal memory functions is often the most apparent and the most susceptible to treatment with E2.

For men, however, contrasting results were seen after leuprolide acetate induced castration (table 1). Memory deficits are the most prominent and early signs of AD and are hypothesized to be most sensitive to effects of sex steroids. Two studies [19,20] of relatively younger men (in their mid sixties) showed an improvement in memory recall 12 months after chemical castration using leuprolide acetate. However, two studies of older men (average age mid seventies) showed negative effects of leuprolide on memory function. One study [21] showed worse memory in patients who had received leuprolide after 6 months, while another [13] showed improvements in verbal memory and global cognitive function but only *after* leuprolide acetate in patients was discontinued. Other cognitive functions showed inconsistent results after leuprolide treatment, with no change or a decline in visuospatial performance [19] or visuomotor speed [20,21]. Differences between studies could not be attributed to differences in treatment regimens (e.g. intermittent or continuous treatment, see table 1).

Table 1. Studies investigating lowered and increased testosterone levels and cognitive function

Author/yr	n	treatment	duration	outcome	age
Chemical castration in men with prostate cancer					
Almeida 2004	n=40 prostate cancer	flutamide for 1 week then leuprolide acetate every 3 months (intermittent treatment)	36 wks, + 18 wks follow-up	decline T and E2, increased depression and anxiety symptoms, global cognition and verbal recall improved only AFTER therapy was stopped, no effect visuospatial function	72 years of age on average (44-83 yrs)
Green 2004	n=62 prostate cancer and n=15 community controls	random allocation to leuprolide (LEU), goserelin (GOS), cyproterone acetate (CPA) or close monitoring (MON)	12 months	sexual difficulty LEU, GOS and CPA; distress after CPA (less in MON): also attention (Stroop) worse after CPA ; digit symbol (visuomotor speed): MON+CON > LEU, GOS, CPA; verbal memory: at 6 mnth GOS<LEU, at 1yr :CON>MON> LEU=CPA=GOS (T lowering)	patients 74+/-6yrs, controls 69+/-6yrs)
Salminen 2004	n=26 prostate cancer	flutamide for 4 wks, leuprolide after 2 wks for 12 months	12 months	decline T by 6 months, at 6 months decline concentration, at 12 months: associations decline T and decrease visuomotor speed, vigilance, RT attention BUT delayed recall objects improved. No effect visuospatial memory or function or word list recall	mean age 65 years
Cherrier 2003	n=19 prostate cancer and n=19 healthy community controls	leuprolide acetate and flutamide (intermittent treatment)	9 months + 3 months follow-up	decline T, no change measures verbal, spatal memory, executive function, language. Decline spatial rotation BUT improved verbal memory into follow-up	52 to 76 years old
Testosterone treatment in patients with AD					
Li 2003	n=9 SDAT	oral T, 120 mg	6 wks	7 improved, 2 declined CGI	
Tan 2003	n=10 AD (hypogonadal)	IM T 200 mg 2 wks (TT from 4 to 10 nmol/L) or placebo	12 mnths	MMSE 19->23, placebo declined, specifically visuospatial skills	
Lu 2006	n=16 AD, n=22 healthy controls	testogel 75 mg orr placebo	24 wks	Quality of life better (ns improvement visuospatial function in AD cases)	
Cherrier 2005	n=15 AD, n=17 MCI	IM T 100 mg or saline	6 wks	verbal and spatial memory, constructional functions improved	

However, these limited data may suggest that older (average age 73 years) men perform worse after leuprolide treatment than slightly younger (in their mid sixties) men. This would be line with Muller's et al. findings [22] who found optimal endogenous T levels for cognitive function in older, but not younger (middle-aged) men, who, she argued, were less susceptible to loss of androgen function.

A caveat of the above studies is only men with cancer were included for whom leuprolide acetate would be indicated. It is not clear how results translate to men with AD. Green et al. [21] showed that controls overall had better performance than cancer patients. This is in line with findings by Shahinian et al 2006 [23], who analyzed data of 50,613 men who had undergone androgen deprivation therapy and 50,476 men without cancer. They found that the risk for cognitive impairment in men who had undergone androgen deprivation treatment, was explained by age, co-morbid conditions and having been diagnosed with cancer itself. Cancer may thus have confounded the above studies as these often only had performance of healthy controls as comparisons rather than placebo treatment which would have been unethical. Effects of cancers on cognition depend on location, type and spread of tumors, but may also be mediated by psychological effects of being diagnosed with a life threatening disease.

However, these data taken together seem to indicate that a drop in T levels or decrease in T function by using leuprolide acetate does not necessarily induce overall cognitive decline in men, but also does not lead to overall improvement of cognitive function.

In sum, limited data suggest that age may be an important factor. Older participants seemed to fare worse with leuprolide treatment and (as AD cases are usually older men) we would thus predict that male AD participants would have worse performance on memory tests after leuprolide acetate treatment. In ALLADIN, however, men were also given testosterone treatment alongside and it is unclear how this would have affected the overall picture, as data were not released.

Some might argue that sufficient damage to the brain needs to be present for leuprolide to show its positive effects on cognition. However, similarly was argued for hormone treatment in women. This lead inclusion of an older population in the largest study of hormone treatment to date: the Women's Health Initiative Memory Study (WHIMS) [16]. This study showed that estrogen treatment in women over 65 years of age increased the risk for dementia. The argument thus may not be valid.

4. Treatment Studies Using T in Men with Dementia

The effects of testosterone treatment in men with dementia have shown mainly positive results (table 1), which are reviewed in more detail elsewhere [6]. However, these results may mirror the earlier positive hormone treatment trials, which had methodological issues (size, statistical analyses etc.), and which were later disputed by results of larger well controlled randomised trials (see [16]).

5. Conclusion

At present we cannot conclude whether effects of leuprolide acetate are most likely to be negative in men with AD, but there are a number of arguments to suggest that this may be the case. An increase of amyloid β levels and worsening of memory function (particularly in older men who are, perhaps, more susceptible to loss of androgen function) in some of the previous studies of leuprolide acetate, could suggest this. From our earlier review [6], it seems likely that age, genetics (e.g. having at least one APOE ε4 allele) and prior T, but also E2 levels (see below) may modify the optimal T level required for optimal cognitive function. The role of age is not entirely clear as one of our observational studies suggested detrimental effects of high T levels on verbal memory in older men, while curvilinear associations were seen for middle-aged men with optimal levels around the normal physiological range of T [24]. This may indicate that different optimal T levels are needed for men of different ages to optimize cognitive function.

In addition, the elegant work by Cherrier and her group [25] suggested that improvement of verbal memory with T treatment was dependent on E2 levels. Others [26] found that E2 administration could reverse verbal memory impairment in men with prostate cancer undergoing androgen deprivation [26].

Whether bioavailable sex hormones, determined by SHBG, are more important than total levels, also remains to be determined. While T treatment lowers SHBG, lowering T through leuprolide will most likely raise SHBG levels paradoxically, resulting in even less FT, which we saw earlier, was a risk factor for cognitive decline in other studies. Results of the leuprolide trial for men with AD as well as large controlled trials of testosterone treatment in men with AD and healthy elderly men are eagerly awaited.

Acknowledgements

We are indebted to the OPTIMA team, nurses and participants. Mrs. A. Yesufu and Dr S. Bandelow from Loughborough University are thanked for their help writing this review. Funding for the work described in this article was gratefully received from the Alzheimer's Association, Dutch Brain Foundation (Nederlandse Hersenstichting), Bristol-Myers Squibb, the MRC, the Blaschko fellowship, Somerville College, RIA/Help the Aged.

Financial Disclosure

Richard Bowen (Voyager Pharm) paid for the LH and FSH assays done in OPTIMA in 2002. In 2003/2004 Prof. Hogervorst acted as consultant for Wyett (WHIMS study) and Solvay Pharmaceuticals (QALY data) and the Androgen Deficiency Society. We have no other conflicts of interest.

References

[1] Casadesus G, Atwood CS, Zhu X, et al. Evidence for the role of gonadotropin hormones in the development of Alzheimer disease. *Cell Mol. Life Sci.* 2005;Feb;62(3):293-298.

[2] Janowsky JS. The role of androgens in cognition and brain aging in men. *Neuroscience.* 2006;138(3):1015-1020.

[3] Bowen RL, Isley JP, Atkinson RL. An association of elevated serum gonadotropin concentrations and Alzheimer Disease ? *J. Neuroendocrinol.* 2000;Apr;12(4):351-354.

[4] Short RA, Bowen RL, O'Brien PC, Graff Radford NR. Elevated gonadotropin levels in patients with Alzheimer disease. *Mayo Clin. Proc.* 2001;76(9):906-909.

[5] Tsolaki M, Grammaticos P, Karanasou C, et al. Serum estradiol, progesterone, testosterone, FSH and LH levels in postmenopausal women with Alzheimer's dementia. *Hell J. Nucl. Med.* 2005;Jan-Apr;8(1):39-42.

[6] Hogervorst E, Bandelow S, Moffat SD. Increasing testosterone levels and effects on cognitive functions in elderly men and women: a review. *Curr. Drug Targets CNS Neurol. Disord.* 2005;Oct;4(5):531-540.

[7] Hogervorst E, Bandelow S, Combrinck M, Smith AD. Low free testosterone is an independent risk factor for Alzheimer's disease. *Exp. Gerontol.* 2004;39(11-12):1633-1639.

[8] Watanabe T, Koba S, Kawamura M, et al. Small dense low-density lipoprotein and carotid atherosclerosis in relation to vascular dementia. *Metabolism.* 2004;53(4):476-482.

[9] Paoletti AM, Congia S, Lello S, et al. Low androgenization index in elderly women and elderly men with Alzheimer's disease. *Neurology.* 2004;62(2):301-303.

[10] Moffat SD, Zonderman AB, Metter EJ, et al. Free testosterone and risk for Alzheimer disease in older men. *Neurology.* 2004;62(2):188-193.

[11] van Osch LA, Hogervorst E, Combrinck M, Smith A, D. Low thyroid-stimulating hormone as an independent risk factor for Alzheimer disease. *Neurology.* 2004;62(11):1967-1971.

[12] Rosario ER, Chang L, Stanczyk FZ, Pike CJ. Age-related testosterone depletion and the development of Alzheimer disease. *JAMA.* 2004;Sep 22;292(12):1431-1432.

[13] Almeida OP, Waterreus A, Spry N, Flicker L, Martins RN. One year follow-up study of the association between chemical castration, sex hormones, beta-amyloid, memory and depression in men. *Psychoneuroendocrinology.* 2004;29(8):1071-1081.

[14] Gillett MJ, Martins RN, Clarnette RM, Chubb SA, Bruce DG, Yeap BB. Relationship between testosterone, sex hormone binding globulin and plasma amyloid beta peptide 40 in older men with subjective memory loss or dementia. *J. Alzheimers Dis.* 2003;5(4):267-269.

[15] Pike CJ. Reply to R. Bowen re. Dementia and Testosterone levels in men. *JAMA.* 2005;Feb 2; 293(5):551-552.

[16] Hogervorst E. The short-lived effect of HRT on cognitive function. In: N.Rasgon, ed. *The Effects of Estrogen on Brain Function.* Baltimore: The Johns Hopkins University Press; 2006.

[17] Sherwin BB, Tulandi T. "Add-back" estrogen reverses cognitive deficits induced by a gonadotropin-releasing hormone agonist in women with leiomyomata uteri. *J. Clin. Endocrinol. Metab.* 1996;81(7):2545-2549.
[18] Varney NR, Syrop C, Kubu CS, Struchen M, Hahn S, Franzen K. Neuropsychologic dysfunction in women following leuprolide acetate induction of hypoestrogenism. *J. Assist. Reprod. Genet.* 1993;10(1):53-57.
[19] Cherrier MM, Rose AL, Higano C. The effects of combined androgen blockade on cognitive function during the first cycle of intermittent androgen suppression in patients with prostate cancer. *J. Urol.* 2003;170(5):1808-1811.
[20] Salminen EK, Portin RI, Koskinen A, Helenius H, Nurmi M. Associations between serum testosterone fall and cognitive function in prostate cancer patients. *Clin. Cancer Res.* 2004;10(22):7575-7582.
[21] Green HJ, Pakenham KI, Headley BC, et al. Quality of life compared during pharmacological treatments and clinical monitoring for non-localized prostate cancer: a randomized controlled trial. *BJU Int.* 2004;May;93(7):975-979.
[22] Muller M, Aleman A, Grobbee DE, de Haan EH, van der Schouw YT. Endogenous sex hormone levels and cognitive function in aging men: is there an optimal level? *Neurology.* 2005;64(5):866-871.
[23] Shahinian VB, Kuo YF, Freeman JL, Goodwin JS. Risk of the "androgen deprivation syndrome" in men receiving androgen deprivation for prostate cancer. *Arch. Intern. Med.* 2006;166(4):465-471.
[24] Hogervorst E, De Jager C, Budge M, Smith AD. Serum levels of estradiol and testosterone and performance in different cognitive domains in healthy elderly men and women. *Psychoneuroendocrinology.* 2004;29(3):405-421.
[25] Cherrier MM, Matsumoto AM, Amory JK, et al. The role of aromatization in testosterone supplementation: effects on cognition in older men. *Neurology.* 2005;64(2):290-296.
[26] Beer TM, Bland LB, Bussiere JR, et al. Androgen deprivation impairs memory in older men. *Behav. Neurosci.* 2006;119(6):1429-1437.

In: Trends in Testosterone Research
Editor: Raymund E. Veritos
ISBN: 978-1-60456-127-2

Chapter III

Stress, Testosterone Suppression and Nitric Oxide

Ben Avi Weissman1 **and Matthew P. Hardy**2*

[1] Department of Pharmacology, Israel Institute for Biological Research, P.O> Box 19, Ness Ziona 70450, Israel, and
[2] Center for Biomedical Research, Population Council, The Rockefeller University, New York, NY, 10021, USA

Abstract

Stress that can be exerted in various ways, including immobilization (IMO), induces a rapid increase in glucocorticoid secretion (in rodents, corticosterone, CORT) and a parallel decrease in circulating testosterone (T) levels. At the same time, nitric oxide (NO), a reactive free radical and fast acting neurotransmitter that is thought to be produced at higher rates in some tissues during stress, has been shown to suppress the biosynthesis of T by Leydig cells. Assessment of the respective roles of CORT and/or NO in acute stress-mediated reduction of T production is an ongoing area of research. The pharmacokinetics and pharmacodynamics of CORT have been studied in IMO-stressed wild type (WT) and inducible nitric oxide synthase knockout (iNOS-/-) mice. Notably, similar basal plasma and testicular T levels are present in both genotypes and their exposure to 3 h of IMO results in a marked elevation in plasma CORT and a dramatic reduction in T concentrations. In addition, testicular T levels exhibit the same pattern while the concentrations of nitrite and nitrate, the stable metabolites of NO in testicular extracts did not differ. Studies performed using WT mice have shown that the changes in CORT and T levels are very rapid. Together, these findings raise the issue of what role, if any, NO has as a mediator of stress in mammals. This question has additional relevance in that the presence of the NO synthase (NOS) enzyme family members in Leydig cells, which has also been reported, is subject to doubt. We will show in the present chapter that testicular expression of NO synthase (NOS) isoforms that

* Send correspondence to: Ben Avi Weissman, Ph.D. Dept. of Pharmacology; IIBR; P.O. Box 19; Ness Ziona 74100; Israel; Tel: +972-8-938-1753; Fax: +972-8-938-15590; Email: baw@iibr.gov.il

catalyze synthesis of NO is not linked to stress physiology. In tissues such as brain or adrenal glands, NOS isoforms may act as mediators of enzymatic activity and hormone release, thereby modulating the response of the testis to stress.

Keywords: Stress; Testosterone; Nitric oxide; Steroidogenesis; Glucocorticoids; Infertility.

Introduction

Stress is a widespread condition, and stressors are increasingly present in modern society - among them noise, over-crowding, and pollution – leading to health problems that all trace back to stress as a contributing cause (Munck and Guyre, 1986; Chrousos and Gold, 1992). In humans, the severe psychological stress brought on by the death of a relative or spouse consistently lowers the sperm count (Fenster et al., 1997). Stress is recognized by clinicians as a contributing factor to human infertility and couples needing assisted reproduction are now counseled in measures to reduce stress (Hjollund *et al.*, 2004b; Hjollund *et al.*, 2004a; Eskiocak *et al.*, 2005). Physiologically, the stress response is comprised of the adjustments made by the body to compensate for the stressor while preserving balance of its internal milieu (Selye, 1946). An over abundance of glucocorticoid activity, perhaps even locally, is the hallmark of stress (Chrousos and Gold, 1992; Sapolsky et al., 2000). Some of the earliest studies of gonadal and sexual dysfunction associated with elevated circulating cortisol (the glucocorticoid in humans) were made on men with Cushing's syndrome. These patients already had low plasma T concentrations, which were further suppressed during the administration of dexamethasone (a synthetic glucocorticoid that further increased the level of glucocorticoid action) given for diagnostic or treatment reasons (Smals et al., 1977). Other causes of stress, including anesthesia, surgery, anticipation of battle, or training show the same glucocorticoid-induced suppression of androgen levels, with a inverse reciprocal glucocorticoid rise and T decrease (Nakashima et al., 1975).

The Role of Glucocorticoid Action in Stress

Although glucocorticoids are referred to as stress hormones and are extensively studied for their actions resulting in pathology, basal glucocorticoid signaling is essential for normal developmental events including lung maturation and for maintenance of homeostatic metabolism as typified by gluconeogenesis in the liver (Schmid et al., 1995). Though it has now been established that Leydig cells express glucocorticoid receptors (Stalker *et al.*, 1989; Stalker *et al.*, 1991), the biochemical consequences of basal levels of glucocorticoid stimulation in Leydig cells remain unclear. In contrast, elevated glucocorticoid concentrations (five-fold and higher above the basal 80 – 100 nM) have been shown to act directly on Leydig cells to inhibit T biosynthesis (Bambino and Hsueh, 1981; Welsh *et al.*, 1982; Hales and Payne, 1989). Elevations in circulating corticosteroid in response to stress are associated with testicular involution and a significant drop in T secretion. These changes are accompanied by diminished libido and fertility. A similar pattern is observed in rats subjected to immobilization (or restraint) stress (Monder et al., 1994). In males, this potential reduction in fertility in response to stress is most likely caused by the stress-induced decline in testosterone, although direct effects of stress on the seminiferous epithelium have also been reported (Yazawa et al., 1999). A number of *in vitro* studies have shown that increased glucocorticoid directly inhibits T production by Leydig cells (Orr et al., 1994).

Recent studies have shown that excessive glucocorticoid exposures not only inhibit androgen synthesis but may also decrease serum T levels by inducing Leydig cell apoptosis, reducing the numbers of Leydig cells per testis (Gao et al., 2002; Gao et al., 2003). Additionally, a number of *in vitro* studies demonstrated that increased glucocorticoid directly inhibits T production by Leydig cells (Hales and Payne, 1989; Orr et al., 1994). Moreover, it is now known that glucocorticoid directly inhibits the transcription of genes encoding T biosynthetic enzymes (Bambino and Hsueh, 1981; Hales and Payne, 1989; Bain *et al.*, 1991; Agular *et al.*, 1992; Orr *et al.*, 1994; Agular and Vind, 1995), and these same genes are positively induced by luteinizing hormone (LH) (Ge et al., 2005). In this respect, the stress-mediated action of glucocorticoid stands as a counterpoint to the stimulatory effect of LH on Leydig cell steroidogenesis.

The Role of NO in Stress

Despite the large body of evidence positioning CORT as the major agent responsible for the reduced circulating T levels that ensues stress, other candidate mediators have also been proposed. One endogenously-produced compound, NO appears to be similar to glucocorticoid in that it has been seen to suppress Leydig cell steroidogenesis *in vitro*. The possibility that NO modulates Leydig cell T biosynthesis, is inferred from experiments in which NO donors reduce testicular T production when administered *in vivo* (Adams et al., 1994) as well as *in vitro* (Del Punta et al., 1996). In addition, a short period of restraint stress causes a marked decline of serum T levels and blocks LH-stimulated increases in T production by hemi-testis preparations *in vitro*, an effect attributed to NO (Kostic et al., 1998). Inhibitors of NOSs, the family of enzymes that catalyze NO synthesis from L-Arginine, prevent a similar blockade of Leydig cell function. In the present article, we will focus on the classic stress response and, in particular, the role of NO as a potential mediator. The observations discussed herein derive from several species although the main emphasis is on the rat, reflecting the number of studies. Careful examination of the available information leads to the conclusion that under conditions of acute stress, the testicular NO pathway is not directly involved in the rapidly-occurring regulation of T biosynthesis. There remains the probability of functional roles for NO and NOSs in the testis despite the uncertainty of a connection to stress. These include suppression of T production during the inflammatory response and vascular smooth tone in the control of testicular blood flow. In addition, NO action in response to acute IMO stress has been documented in the brain and adrenal gland, and may lead to atrophic changes in the reproductive system.

Nitric Oxide and T Biosynthesis: General Considerations

As noted above, T, the predominant hormone that promotes the development and maintenance of male sexual characteristics, is produced by Leydig cells. Only recently has NO received attention as a potential mediator of testicular function. This reactive free radical is generated by NOSs, a family of enzymes that oxidize the amino acid L-Arginine into both L-Citrulline and NO. The NOS family consists of the constitutive, Ca^{2+}-dependent neuronal and endothelial isoforms (n- and eNOS, respectively), and the Ca^{2+}-independent, inducible enzyme iNOS. Nitric oxide can be generated from numerous synthetic donors and the administration of NO donors *in vivo* has been shown to decrease testicular T production (Adams et al., 1994). While a direct T-suppressing action of NO on Leydig cells can be inferred from studies of Leydig cells *in vitro* (Del Punta et al., 1996; Weissman et al., 2005), the results of *in vivo* experiments indicate that indirect effects may also occur. One possibility is that NO action lowers LH secretion by the pituitary. When delivered intraperitoneally or intratesticularly, L-Arginine methyl ester (L-AME), an exogenous substrate of NOS, decreases serum T concentrations, but LH declines as well (Gaytan et al., 1997). It is clear that Leydig cells are sensitive to NO, even if it is uncertain whether Leydig cells are exposed directly to NO generated locally during stress. However, intratesticular application of the NO donor sodium nitroprusside (SNP) induces a decrease in serum and interstitial fluid T concentrations without a significant change in LH concentrations (Gaytan et al., 1997). Furthermore, the response of Leydig cells to directly introduced NO was recently demonstrated by exposing isolated rat Leydig cells to S-nitrosoglutathione (GSNO) that acts as a 'natural' source for NO and inhibits T secretion at low micromolar concentrations (Weissman et al., 2005) (figure 1). Interestingly, these *in vitro* effects of NO on Leydig cell T production are mirrored in animal and human experiments with NO generators (see below).

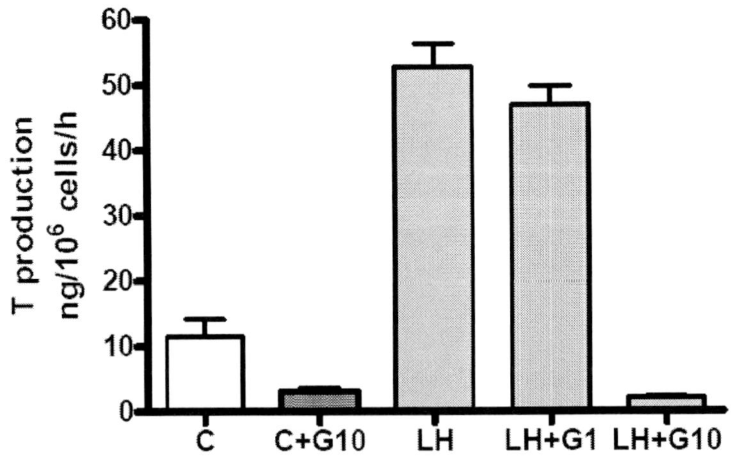

Figure 1. S-nitrosoglutathione (GSNO) potently inhibits T production by Leydig cells. Purified rat Leydig cells were incubated for 1 h in LCM in the absence (C, control; LH, 0.5 ng/ml) or presence of 1 or 10 μM of GSNO (G1 or G10, respectively). The production of T was estimated by T RIA and is expressed as ng of T per 10^6 cells.

A number of reports point to decrements in male reproductive function subsequent to treatment with NO donors, but the sites of NO action remain unresolved. Injections of the NO precursors isosorbide dinitrite (ISDN) or L-AME decrease plasma T levels without affecting LH secretion (Adams et al., 1993; Kostic et al., 1998; Kostic et al., 2000). Additionally, an intratesticular injection of the endogenous substrate of NOS, the amino acid L-Arginine, lowers serum T concentrations (Kostic et al., 1998). Similarly, SNP, a potent NO donor and a clinically used antihypertensive drug, as well as L-AME both lower T levels (Pinilla et al., 2001). Consistent with these declines, SNP has also been shown to cause decrements in sexual competence that can be attributed to diminished androgen action (Ratnasooriya et al., 2004). Although these results would appear to support the concept that NO is an endogenous negative regulator of T production in the testis, data in humans have failed to demonstrate a functional linkage. For example, when three groups of human males, divided according to semen analysis, i.e., normozoospermic, oligozoospermic and azoospermic, were submitted to T and nitrite/nitrate (NOx) analyses, NOx, but not T, levels varied according to spermatogenic status, being elevated in subjects with defective spermatogenesis (Battaglia et al., 2000). Surprisingly, the NOx content in seminal plasma of normozoospermic men was considerably higher compared to the other two groups. These findings indicate that the cellular source of NO must first be identified before its regulatory role can be understood. Thus, Leydig cells, which are sensitive to the suppressive effects of NO, may be under the control of NO diffusing from cells in close proximity. In the interstitium, Leydig cells are close to other Leydig cells, testicular macrophages, blood vessel and lymphatic endothelial cells and peritubular myoid cells. Of these interstitial cell types, testicular macrophages are best candidates for T suppression because these cells are able to express iNOS and generate substantial quantities of NO (Weissman et al., 2005).

Pathological states such as inflammation caused by endotoxemia, i.e., following the administration of lipopolysaccharide (LPS), are characterized by a large outpouring of NO that is followed by a sharp drop in plasma T concentrations (Bosmann et al., 1996; Sharma et al., 1998). This decline could be brought about by several agents other than NO such as TNF-α or IL-1β, but, given that LPS-stimulated J774 cells (Di Rosa et al., 1990) and testicular macrophages (Weissman et al., 2005) both express inducible NOS and release large amounts of NO, this agent becomes a likely contender for the observed effects. Testicular macrophages typically located adjacent to and in close contact with Leydig cells in the interstitial tissue (Hutson, 1992), have been hypothesized to act as a source of NO under conditions of inflammation or intoxication. Indeed, NO released from stimulated macrophages (Sun *et al.*, 1993; Pomerantz and Pitelka, 1998), under *in vitro* conditions that mimic the immune-activated state, causes depressed androgen biosynthesis. The suppression of T production is reversible upon addition of the non selective NOS inhibitor L-N^G-nitro-arginine methyl ester (L-NAME) or the NO scavenger hemoglobin. In another set of experiments, aluminum has been shown to induce reproductive toxicity in male mice, associated with a marked decrease in serum and testicular T concentrations. These alterations are accompanied by a considerable expression of iNOS and are ensued by significant increases in serum and testicular NOx content (Guo et al., 2001). However, NO is only one candidate in a lengthy list of potential mediators of T suppression under inflammatory conditions. Examination of wild type and iNOS null mice (Laubach et al., 1998) shows that while basal levels of T are similar between WT and KO saline-treated mice, LPS administration decreases T to nearly undetectable levels in both WT and KO male mice. This is consistent with studies showing reduced T content in male sepsis patients (Christeff et al., 1992) and in endotoxemic mice (Sharma et al., 1998). Thus, while the literature is compatible with the hypothesis that NO can be an inflammatory mediator, it is not essential in the reduction of T secretion. Notably, macrophages from various origins, including the rat testis, respond to the presentation of LPS with a massive secretion of NO (Weissman et al., 2005). Nevertheless, a firm conclusion on the importance of NO signaling under inflammatory conditions will have to await further clarification of which testicular cell types are expressing NOS isoforms.

Despite reports of NOS expression in Leydig cells, as detected by immunohistochemical staining of the cells, *in situ* analyses of mRNA expression levels show that NOS isoforms are present below the detection sensitivity in Leydig cells and iNOS mRNA is abundant in testicular macrophages. Indeed, purified Leydig cells are resistant to the stimulatory effect of the bacterial toxin LPS and fail to produce NO even after 24 h incubation period in the presence of a substantial concentration of this agent (figure 2). It is unlikely that isolated rat Leydig cells lose their ability to express NOS isoforms *in vitro* because they maintain their ability to produce T (figure 3) and exhibit a typical pattern of sensitivity to a NO donor (figure 1).

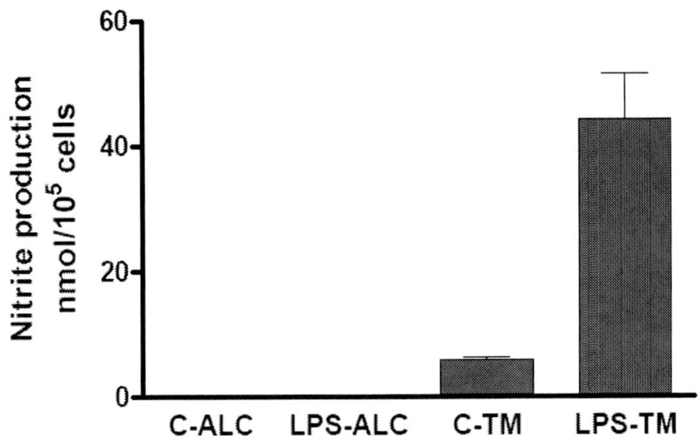

Figure 2. Nitrite accumulation in Lipopolysaccharide (LPS) treated adult rat Leydig cells and testicular macrophages. Purified rat Leydig cells (ALC) and isolated testicular macrophages (TM) were incubated for 24 h in the absence (C-) or presence of LPS (LPS-, 10 µg/ml). The concentration of nitrite in the incubation medium was assessed by a modified Griess assay.

Stress, Nitric Oxide and T

Administration of a 2 h immobilization stress in rats decreases serum T levels and attenuates the hCG-induced T production in hemitestis preparations (Kostic *et al.*, 1998; Kostic *et al.*, 1999; Kostic *et al.*, 2000). Results obtained in this *ex vivo* model, consisting of a 3 h incubation *in vitro* following the decapitation of control and stressed animals, indicate that the process is associated with the accumulation of NO stable metabolites, namely, nitrite and nitrate in the testis. Moreover, bilateral, dual intratesticular injections of either L-NAME (Kostic et al., 1998) or aminoguanidine (AG) (Kostic et al., 1999) prevent the stress-mediated reduction of T content in the incubation medium. These findings were interpreted to implicate NO in the stress-evoked decline of testicular steroidogenesis. In this instance, however, the *ex vivo* conditions could promote the expression of iNOS and thus, create a higher background under which it then becomes possible to detect the activity of an iNOS inhibitor. More importantly, when the influence of AG on a 2 h IMO-induced suppression of plasma T concentration was examined, no reversal could be detected (Kostic et al., 1999). Small IMO-evoked increases in NOx concentration that were not sensitive to the iNOS inhibitor and may not be physiologically relevant. When assessing the involvement of iNOS in stress, it is important to address whether iNOS could have been expressed and activated in the tissue during the *in vitro* incubation period, as seems possible in several previous studies (Kostic *et al.*, 1998; Kostic *et al.*, 1999; Kostic *et al.*, 2000), The release of cytokines such as TNF-α or IL-1β resulting from the killing of animals and preparing the tissues (Fassbender et al., 2000), could cause a rapid NO production, thus leading to the suppression of T formation (Tatsumi et al., 1997).

Recent research on neural regulation of testicular steroidogenesis casts doubt on the involvement of the NO pathway in the observed decline in Leydig cell function (Herman and Rivier, 2006). In this model of stress, intracerebroventricular (icv) applications of compounds such as isoproterenol or ethanol cause a rapid and dramatic decrease in plasma T concentration concurrent with elevated levels of NOx and a testis-specific nNOS (TnNOS) expression in the rat testis. However, pretreatment with L-NAME, which blocked the isoproterenol-induced increase in TnNOS protein expression, did not restore the steroidogenic response to hCG. One may infer, therefore, that other factors are responsible for T suppression in this paradigm.

Based on the suggestion that testicular iNOS and NO are involved in the decline of T production that accompany stress (Kostic *et al.*, 1998; Kostic *et al.*, 1999; Kostic *et al.*, 2000), it follows that iNOS deficient animals should exhibit either little or no response to IMO. However, WT and iNOS-/- mice subjected to 3 h of IMO have the same concentrations of CORT, T and NOx (Weissman *et al.*, 2007). The results show that following restraint, both groups of mice exhibit identical patterns of reduced plasma T content associated with increased plasma CORT concentrations. Furthermore, while testicular T concentration sharply declined in stressed WT and mutant mice, the concentration of NOx remained unchanged (table 1). These data suggest that, in contrast to CORT, signaling by testicular NO is unlikely to be involved in the suppression of T biosynthesis mediated by IMO stress.

Table 1. Testicular NOx levels in WT and iNOS-/- mice

Genotype	Control	Stress
Wild type	19.8 ± 3.1 (n=21)	22.1 ± 4.6 (n=17)
iNOS-/-	19.2 ± 3.5 (n=12)	24.1 ± 4.5 (n=13)

Table 1 WT and iNOS-/- mice were exposed to 3 h IMO and the content of nitrite/nitrate (NOx) was estimated in testicular extracts using a modified Griess assay immediately thereafter. Data are expressed as nmol/g tissue with the number of mice evaluated in parentheses.

Nitric Oxide in Leydig Cells

The neuronal NOS (nNOS) (Davidoff et al., 1995) and TnNOS (Wang et al., 1997) protein have been immunolocalized to human Leydig cells. In addition, nNOS (Lissbrant et al., 1997) and constitutively expressed iNOS mRNA and protein were identified in rat Leydig cells by immunocytochemistry (Koksal et al., 2003) and immunohistochemistry (O'Bryan et al., 2000), respectively. Using similar approaches, eNOS has been detected in rat Sertoli, Leydig, and germ cells (Zini et al., 1996). As expected, eNOS is found in testicular blood vessels which are devoid of any immunoreactivity for iNOS (Moon et al., 2005). Reports of testicular iNOS expression are particularly difficult to categorize. Whereas some investigators have reported iNOS expression in Leydig cells, other laboratories have not observed iNOS anywhere in the testis, at least under normal conditions (Shiraishi et al., 2001). Notably, none of the studies referred to above measured NOS enzyme activity in Leydig cells. The absence of nicotinamide adenine dinucleotide phosphate-diaphorase (NADPH-d) histochemical activity in Leydig cells may indicate the existence of an inactive form of NOS (Lissbrant et al., 1997). Other reports, however, show the presence of NADPH-d activity in Leydig cells (Giannessi et al., 1998; Ruffoli et al., 2001). In summary, these accounts exhibit the profound lack of consensus in the literature concerning the issue of whether NOS enzyme family members are present in Leydig cells.

An extensive effort to detect NOS activity in purified rat Leydig cells has shown that they have the capacity to generate NO although whether the amounts of NO generated locally in the testis are sufficient to inhibit T production remains unsettled (Weissman et al., 2005). Isolated Leydig cells express the complete battery of steroidogenic enzymes, but only a marginal level of eNOS, i.e., twice the background value.

In humans, while nNOS is reportedly present in Leydig cells (Davidoff et al., 1995), evidence for production and functional activity of NO only exists for other testicular cells types, i.e., seminiferous tubules and blood vessels (Middendorff et al., 1997). Likewise, whereas results from CHO-K1 cells stably transfected with the TnNOS cDNA indicate that this protein is a Ca^{2+}-dependent NOS with a substantial catalytic activity comparable to that of full-length nNOS, generation of NO in primary human Leydig cells has not been established (Wang et al., 1997). Furthermore, despite reports that iNOS is expressed constitutively in rat Leydig cells, implying an incessant NO generation and inhibition of T biosynthesis, administration of the nonspecific NOS inhibitor L-NAME reduced T production rather than increasing it (O'Bryan et al., 2000). Subsequently, the distribution of iNOS was investigated by both immunofluorescent and immunoenzyme methods and the protein was detected in the perinuclear cytoplasm of Sertoli cells throughout the spermatogenic stages (Kon et al., 2002). While this study also employed additional analytical methods such as reverse transcriptase-polymerase chain reaction amplification of mRNA signals (RT-PCR), iNOS was not detected in the Leydig cell.

Direct measurements of NOS activity (i.e., NO formation) in testes and Leydig cells reveal either residual or insignificant levels. When NOS activity was estimated by the conversion of L-[^{14}C]Arginine to L-[^{14}C]Citrulline (and NO) in the human genital tract, the testis and epididymis lacked Ca^{2+}-dependent NOS activity. In addition, no Ca^{2+}-independent NOS activity (i.e., iNOS) was obtained in the urogenital tract (Ehren et al., 1994). This report implies none of the forms of NOS is present in Leydig cells. In general, low levels of NO formation occur in the rat testis and seminal vesicles (i.e., $<$ 0.5 fmol L-[^{3}H]Citrulline formed/min/mg protein) (Burnett et al., 1995). More specifically, purified rat Leydig cells have miniscule amounts of NOS activity when quantified by conversion of L-[^{14}C]Arginine to L-[^{14}C]Citrulline and the Griess assay for NO stable metabolites (nitrite and nitrate) (Weissman et al., 2005). Moreover, neither calcium chelation, nor the application of a calcium ionophore to reduce or increase intracellular Ca^{2+} concentrations, respectively, has an effect on the Leydig cell rate of NO generation. Constitutively expressed NOS isoforms e-, n- or TnNOS, are sensitive to intracellular Ca^{2+} and respond to elevated levels by activation and rapid NO production; the opposite is true for reduced calcium levels. Also, addition of a high concentration of the endogenous NOS substrate L-Arginine does not modulate NO generation or androgen biosynthesis. Under the same conditions in which Leydig cells were seen to be inactive in the generation of NO, they were highly responsive to exogenous LH (Weissman et al., 2005).

The function of NOS isoform expression in the testis cannot be definitively linked to stress, but intriguing patterns have emerged in the literature that may point to an involvement in important housekeeping functions related to spermatogenesis. For example, NOS activity in testes of mice has a circadian rhythm, ranging from 0.5 to about 2 pmol of Citrulline per mg protein/min (Tunctan et al., 2002). Testicular NOS activity has also been measured in the aging Brown-Norway rat model (Hikim et al., 2005). Testes of young rats produce 0.66 pmol/mg protein/min and the rate increases by 90% in old males. Recently, the real-time release of NO was monitored using an NO-selective electrode, and nitrite and nitrate concentrations were measured in the rat testis (Kono et al., 2006). The NOx concentrations in normal rat tissues are in the range of 1 to 3 nmol/mg protein. These observations are in agreement with a recent study on the influence of 3 h IMO on mice lacking the gene for iNOS (iNOS-/- mice), where the same NO metabolites content in testicular extracts from wild type (WT) and mutant animals are detected (Weissman *et al.*, 2007). Nitrite and nitrate concentrations in the testis of the two genotypes were essentially equal under control and immobilization stress conditions (table 1).

NOS Inhibitors and Leydig Cell T Production *In Vitro*

In vitro studies of NOS inhibition using L-NAME or L-N^{G}-Methyl Arginine (L-NMMA) in testicular cell preparations that contained macrophages, Sertoli cells and endothelial cells in addition to Leydig cells, showed that these agents increase basal and hCG-stimulated T secretion (Welch et al., 1995). Whether the small increases were obtained due to the presence of cells other than Leydig cells is unknown. Adding to the uncertainty, high concentrations of L-NAME (10 mM) do not affect basal T production, but inhibit hCG-stimulated T secretion (Pinilla et al., 1995). In preparations of Leydig cells that are enriched to 95%, NOS inhibitors such as L-NAME or L-NMMA, fail to alter either basal or LH-stimulated T production (figure 3). These results gain additional importance when compared to observations made on isolated adreno-cortical cells where the selective nNOS inhibitor L-N^G-nitro-arginine (L-NA) significantly increased CORT secretion (Cymeryng et al., 1998).

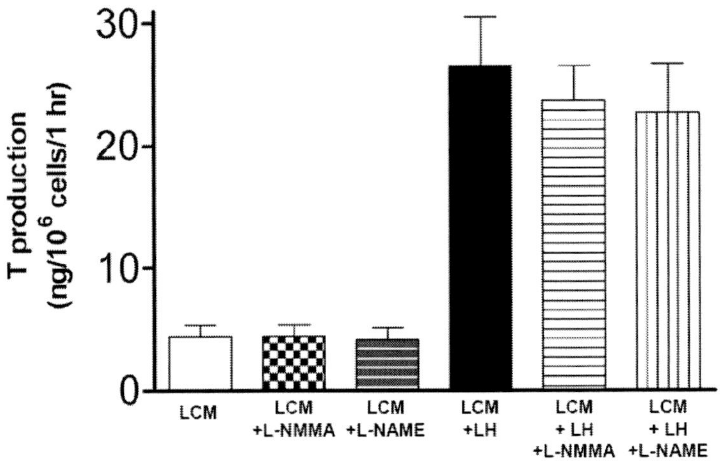

Figure 3. Effects of NOS blockers on Leydig cells T secretion. Purified rat Leydig cells were incubated for 1 h in LCM in the presence of LH (0.5 ng/ml) and L-NMMA or L-NAME (1 mM). The production of T was estimated by T RIA.

NOS Inhibitors and Leydig Cell T Production *In Vivo*

Results obtained from experiments where NOS inhibitors were administered *in vivo* have been invoked to argue for the involvement of NO in physiological modulation of Leydig cells steroidogenesis. In this regard, systemic delivery of L-NAME increases T secretion in a dose dependent fashion without affecting LH concentration (Adams *et al.*, 1992; Adams *et al.*, 1993; Adams *et al.*, 1996). An intraperitoneal injection of a high dose of L-NAME (100 mg/kg) slightly decreases serum LH while doubling testosterone concentrations (Shi et al., 1998). Under similar experimental conditions, the parent acid of L-NAME, specifically, L-NA, (30 mg/kg), has no effect on either T or LH values. These responses to L-NA are comparable to those seen following the administration of single or repeated L-NAME injections (30 mg/kg) to control mice (Budziszewska *et al.*, 1998; Budziszewska *et al.*, 1999). Similarly, parenteral injections of L-NAME (Kostic et al. 1998) or AG, an iNOS specific inhibitor (Kostic et al., 1999), did not change serum T levels in control male rats. In this context, it is important to note that an *in vivo* electron paramagnetic resonance (EPR, a free radical monitoring technique) study demonstrated that AG was unable to affect NO levels in naïve subjects whereas an inhibition of NO formation is evident in animals after stimulation with LPS (Dambrova et al., 2003). In fact, AG had no impact on basal NOx levels in all organs examined including the testis. These results imply that iNOS is not induced or/active in testis of control animals. In addition, dual injections of L-NAME (40 mg/kg x2) to control male rats induced a highly significant rise in LH secretion (Pinilla et al., 2001). Additional experiments reported in this study show that a single administration of L-NAME did not change plasma T content whereas it blocked the T-suppression induced by the NO donor SNP or the NOS substrate L-AME. While the inhibitory activity of L-NAME on the action of L-AME is very well understood, the blocking effect of SNP is unclear. Moreover, increases in secretagogue-induced adrenocorticotropin hormone (ACTH) and CORT, which are known to decrease T secretion, were unaffected by this NOS inhibitor L-NAME in control rats (Rivier and Shen, 1994), indicating the questionable involvement of central NO pathways in this process.

The problematic nature of interpreting data obtained from experiments utilizing NOS inhibitors such as L-NAME could be a consequence of the finding that a 50 mg/kg dose of this blocker differentially reduced plasma nitrate concentrations, ranging from a 14% decline in brain to an 83% decrease in lung (Tuncel et al., 2001). Furthermore, while an intravenous injection of L-NAME (50 mg/kg) induced no change in plasma NO metabolites and only a small and insignificant increase of testicular blood flow, a considerable elevation in circulating T concentrations was measured in LPS treated rats (Sharma et al., 1998). Whereas a low dose of L-NAME (i.e., 10 mg/kg) increased blood pressure and consequently elevated testicular blood flow (Lissbrant et al., 1997), real-time monitoring of blood flow with a laser Doppler flowmeter showed a sharp decrease in testicular blood flow associated with elevated NOx concentrations (Kono et al., 2006). Research on neural regulation of testicular steroidogenesis has questioned the importance of testicular blood flow in the decrease in plasma T content (Selvage et al., 2004). In this model of stress, icv applications of compounds such as ethanol (EtOH) caused a rapid and dramatic decline in plasma T concentration. Concomitant evaluation of testicular blood flow and changes in androgen secretion following an icv administration of EtOH clearly shows their independence.

These results portray the *in vivo* effects of NOS inhibition on T levels in an ambiguous light and indicate that under basal conditions, endogenous NO may have a limited role in modulating rates of Leydig cell steroidogenesis. This conclusion differs from results obtained with NO donors or NOS precursors. In spite of the fact that elevated endogenous NO levels may interact with a large number of physiological systems, increasing NO content uniformly decreased T secretion. It is important to note that NOS inhibitors could affect tissues other than the hypothalamic-pituitary-gonadal axis or the gonads. Thus, the changes could be secondary to alterations in CORT secretion and/or blood circulation, due to a reduction in eNOS activity in blood vessels (Adams et al., 1992; 1993).

Stress and the Nitric Oxide Pathway in the Central Nervous System

Previous investigations have shown that NOS is present in the CNS in general and the perikarya of the hypothalamus, specifically in nuclei closely associated with the regulation of pituitary activity (cf. Rivier and Shen, 1994). This suggests that NO may have a physiological role in the regulation of neuroendocrine functions. These might include the control of ACTH release and consequently, the regulation of CORT and T homeostasis. Therefore, it is notable that a direct association between acute immobilization stress and expression and/or activation of NOS isoforms in the CNS has been demonstrated. For example, in rats restrained for 2 h, the density of neurons exhibiting NADPH-d activity and nNOS expression in the amygdaloid nuclei are increased (Echeverry et al., 2004). Neuronal NOS expression also appeared to be increased in the dentate gyrus of the hippocampus and piriform cortex during stress. These results are reminiscent to earlier studies showing that a single stress episode causes immediate changes in nitric oxide system in the HPA axis (Kishimoto et al., 1996). In this context, it is interesting to note that 2 h of restraint stress induces an increase in nNOS mRNA in the paraventricular nucleus (PVN), medial parvocellular part, dorsolateral periaqueductal grey and medial amygdaloid nucleus, but not in the hippocampal formation (de Oliveira et al., 2000). Modifications in the expression of nNOS mRNA could be detected in the anterior pituitary and in the PVN following 2 or 6 h of stress, respectively. Furthermore, a 50% elevation in the activity of nNOS in the anterior pituitary is evident after 6 h of stress. This substantial change is apparent only at the termination of stress and it rapidly declines thereafter (Kishimoto et al., 1996). In old rats a 3-fold increase in NOS mRNA occurs in the PVN immediately following 3 h of stress, whereas in young rats the increase reaches significance when animals were killed 3 h after the end of the stress procedure (Calza et al., 1993). The differences observed in NOS mRNA between young and old rats could be related to an age-dependent different responsiveness to stressful stimuli. Short (30 and 60 min) restraint periods resulted in distinct trends in the expression of nNOS mRNA in the hypothalamus and PVN (Hori et al., 2005). Following 30 min of isolation, nNOS mRNA quantities increase in both tissues while 30 min later they returned to control values in the former while showing an additional increase in the PVN. A recent publication reporting on the histological localization of NADPH-d extended this phenomenon to the raphe nucleus (Okere and Waterhouse, 2006). In general, these findings support the view that stress produces a transient increase in nNOS expression in the CNS.

The L-Arginine-NO pathway evoked by stress may be monitored by measuring NO stable metabolites. Nitrite concentrations in brain dialysate are elevated to more than 150% after 30 min of restraint stress compared with its level before stress (Shirakawa et al., 2004). This increase was sensitive to L-NAME and declined rapidly (30 to 60 min) to pre-stress level. Exposure of rats to a short (1 h) isolation stress evoked a sharp (i.e., 57%) decrease in brain NOx content (Masood et al., 2004). A study concerning the effects of acute stress on extra-cellular total antioxidant capacity measured as plasma ferric reducing antioxidant power and plasma nitric oxide production (NOx), revealed an imbalance as oxidant generation was increased and non-enzymatic antioxidants were depleted. Augmentation of antioxidant defenses might be beneficial in long-term stress. It is notable, however, that this pattern was not mirrored in plasma NOx values, in that the levels of NOx remained unchanged during stress (Nadeem et al., 2006). Thus, three independent studies that were aimed at the same goal yielded conflicting results which might be attributed to different methodologies and sample origin.

In mice, a higher NOx content in brain is evoked by social isolation (Huong et al., 2005). This effect was detected at a single time point (6 h), and was absent after 2 or 4 h of stress; NOx concentrations returned to control values following 8 h of IMO. When measured immediately after a 4 h stress exposure, the total NOx level in the brain was significantly higher in psychologically stressed animals than in unstressed control mice (Matsumoto et al., 1999). No significant difference in the level of this parameter between the two groups of mice could be observed at 30 min after termination of stress session. Notably, the reported stress-mediated changes in brain NOx levels are generally small in magnitude and of short duration (i.e., < 30 min.).

It was reported that acute restraint stress for 6 h increases the activity and expression of the calcium-independent NOS isoform in brain cortex in adult male rats (Madrigal et al., 2001). However, it is important to remember that iNOS activity in the rat cortex increased from an almost undetectable conversion of L-Arginine in controls to a level of ca. 1.5 pmol/mg protein/min in rats subjected to 6 h of IMO (Madrigal et al., 2002). Compared to the robust production of L-Citrulline and NO by the constitutive nNOS, namely, ~200 pmol/mg protein/min, the functional significance of iNOS activity must be considered questionable.

Acute restraint stress has differential effects on i- and nNOS thereby controlling the NO pathway in a regionally-specific pattern within the CNS. The role of neural iNOS expression appears to be marginal, but nNOS is likely to be a significant mediator of stress. It is apparent that in most cases NO signaling in various brain structures is characterized by its low amplitude and short duration.

Stress and the Nitric Oxide Pathway in the Adrenal Gland

Western blots and RT-PCR analyses with nNOS, eNOS and iNOS-specific antibodies and primers, respectively, identify nNOS and eNOS in several brain regions and the adrenal gland, whereas iNOS is under the detection limit in these tissues (Hauser et al., 2005). This confirms that iNOS is not expressed in the adrenals of normal rats (Rettori et al., 2003). The presence of nNOS mRNAs in the adrenal zona fasciculata is seen by RT-PCR, immunohistochemistry, and immunoblot analysis, as well as biochemical characterization of nNOS enzymatic activity (Cymeryng et al., 2002). Data from *in vitro* investigations reveal that NO potently changes adrenal gland CORT and aldosterone biosynthesis (Cymeryng et al., 1998). Thus, the possible recruitment of the NO pathway in this organ during stress is a relevant and principal issue to be addressed.

Exposure of rats to a single restraint episode lasting 6 h yields a remarkable increase in nNOS mRNA in the adrenal cortex (Kishimoto et al., 1996). Elevated nNOS activity, as assessed by either L-Arginine conversion or NADPH-d histology, could be observed in the rat adrenal medulla and cortex after a stress session of the same length (Tsuchiya et al.,

1996). These alterations in NOS expression and NO formation in the rat adrenal glands persist for up to 12 h after the termination of IMO. When rats are exposed to a 2 h immobilization stress, a rapid and long-lasting (> 4 h) increase of NOS activity in the adrenal cortex is evident (Tsuchiya et al., 1997). This effect is accompanied by changes in CORT plasma levels and is sensitive to the NOS inhibitor L-NAME.

Taken together, these results show that acute stress may augments nNOS expression in various brain structures. While the consensus regarding nNOS status in the CNS is incomplete, there is a wide agreement that marked elevations in nNOS expression and activity are associated with the stress response of the NO pathway in the adrenal gland.

Conclusion

Data from animal and human studies have been shown that acute stress induces a marked reduction in plasma and testicular T concentrations. Short periods of social isolation are also associated with a sharp increase in CORT secretion and elevations in NOS activity and NO formation in some tissues (e.g., adrenal gland). Given that NO has been demonstrated to potently suppress Leydig cell T production, it was hypothesized that NO could participate in this process. However, no concurrent alterations in plasma or testicular NO stable metabolites level could be monitored in restrained animals. In addition, the observation that IMO induces robust decline in plasma T content in both WT and iNOS knockout mice, concurrent with similar testicular NOx concentrations, cast a large shadow over the putative role of testicular NO pathways in the stress response. Some consideration should be given to possible localized actions of NO in the testis during stress, but additional evidence will be required before these functions can be accurately assessed. These observations point our attention toward candidates other than NO pathways in the testis (such as glucocorticoid synthesized by the adrenal gland), as critical players in the control of T homeostasis.

References

Adams, M. L., Forman, J. B., Kalicki, J. M., Meyer, E. R., Sewing, B., and Cicero, T. J. (1993). Antagonism of alcohol-induced suppression of rat testosterone secretion by an inhibitor of nitric oxide synthase. *Alcohol Clin Exp Res* 17, 660-664.

Adams, M. L., Meyer, E. R., and Cicero, T. J. (1996). Effects of nitric oxide-related agents on opioid regulation of rat testicular steroidogenesis. *Biol Reprod* 54, 1128-1134.

Adams, M. L., Meyer, E. R., Sewing, B. N., and Cicero, T. J. (1994). Effects of nitric oxide-related agents on rat testicular function. *J Pharmacol Exp Ther* 269, 230-237.

Adams, M. L., Nock, B., Truong, R., and Cicero, T. J. (1992). Nitric oxide control of steroidogenesis: endocrine effects of NG-nitro-L-arginine and comparisons to alcohol. *Life Sci* 50, PL35-40.

Agular, B. M., and Vind, C. (1995). Effects of dexamethasone on steroidogenesis in Leydig cells from rats of different ages. *J Steroid Biochem Mol Biol* 54, 75-81.

Agular, B. M., Vinggaard, A. M., and Vind, C. (1992). Regulation by dexamethasone of the 3β-hydroxysteroid dehydrogenase activity in adult rat Leydig cells. *J. Steroid Biochem. Mol. Biol.* 43, 565-571.

Bain, P. A., Yoo, M., Clarke, T., Hammond, S. H., and Payne, A. H. (1991). Multiple forms of mouse 3β-hydroxysteroid dehydrogenase/delta 5-δ 4 isomerase and differential expression in gonads, adrenal glands, liver, and kidneys of both sexes. *Proc Natl Acad Sci U S A* 88, 8870-8874.

Bambino, T., and Hsueh, A. (1981). Direct inhibitory effect of glucocorticoids upon testicular luteinizing hormone receptor and steroidogenesis *in vivo* and *in vitro*. *Endocrinology* 108, 2142-2148.

Battaglia, C., Giulini, S., Regnani, G., Di Girolamo, R., Paganelli, S., Facchinetti, F., and Volpe, A. (2000). Seminal plasma nitrite/nitrate and intratesticular Doppler flow in fertile and infertile subjects. *Hum Reprod* 15, 2554-2558.

Bosmann, H. B., Hales, K. H., Li, X., Liu, Z., Stocco, D. M., and Hales, D. B. (1996). Acute in vivo inhibition of testosterone by endotoxin parallels loss of steroidogenic acute regulatory (StAR) protein in Leydig cells. *Endocrinology* 137, 4522-4525.

Budziszewska, B., Leskiewicz, M., Jaworska-Feil, L., and Lason, W. (1998). The effect of N-nitro-L-arginine methyl ester on cocaine-induced hormonal changes in mice. *Exp Clin Endocrinol Diabetes* 106, 340-345.

Budziszewska, B., Leskiewicz, M., Jaworska-Feil, L., and Lason, W. (1999). The effect of N-nitro-L-arginine methyl ester on morphine-induced changes in the plasma corticosterone and testosterone levels in mice. *Exp Clin Endocrinol Diabetes* 107, 75-79.

Burnett, A. L., Ricker, D. D., Chamness, S. L., Maguire, M. P., Crone, J. K., Bredt, D. S., Snyder, S. H., and Chang, T. S. (1995). Localization of nitric oxide synthase in the reproductive organs of the male rat. *Biology of Reproduction* 52, 1-7.

Calza, L., Giardino, L., and Ceccatelli, S. (1993). NOS mRNA in the paraventricular nucleus of young and old rats after immobilization stress. *Neuroreport* 4, 627-630.

Christeff, N., Carli, A., Benassayag, C., Bleichner, G., Vaxelaire, J. F., and Nunez, E. A. (1992). Relationship between changes in serum estrone levels and outcome in human males with septic shock. *Circ Shock* 36, 249-255.

Chrousos, G. P., and Gold, P. W. (1992). The concepts of stress and stress system disorders. Overview of physical and behavioral homeostasis. *JAMA* 267, 1244-1252.

Cymeryng, C. B., Dada, L. A., and Podesta, E. J. (1998). Effect of nitric oxide on rat adrenal zona fasciculata steroidogenesis. *J Endocrinol* 158, 197-203.

Cymeryng, C. B., Lotito, S. P., Colonna, C., Finkielstein, C., Pomeraniec, Y., Grion, N., Gadda, L., Maloberti, P., and Podesta, E. J. (2002). Expression of nitric oxide synthases in rat adrenal zona fasciculata cells. *Endocrinology* 143, 1235-1242.

Dambrova, M., Kirjanova, O., Baumane, L., Liepinsh, E., Zvejniece, L., Muceniece, R., Kalvinsh, I., and Wikberg, J. E. (2003). EPR investigation of in vivo inhibitory effect of guanidine compounds on nitric oxide production in rat tissues. *J Physiol Pharmacol* 54, 339-347.

Davidoff, M. S., Middendorff, R., Mayer, B., and Holstein, A. F. (1995). Nitric oxide synthase (NOS-I) in Leydig cells of the human testis. *Arch Histol Cytol* 58, 17-30.

de Oliveira, R. M., Aparecida Del Bel, E., Mamede-Rosa, M. L., Padovan, C. M., Deakin, J. F., and Guimaraes, F. S. (2000). Expression of neuronal nitric oxide synthase mRNA in stress-related brain areas after restraint in rats. *Neurosci Lett* 289, 123-126.

Del Punta, K., Charreau, E. H., and Pignataro, O. P. (1996). Nitric oxide inhibits Leydig cell steroidogenesis. *Endocrinology* 137, 5337-5343.

Di Rosa, M., Radomski, M., Carnuccio, R., and Moncada, S. (1990). Glucocorticoids inhibit the induction of nitric oxide synthase in macrophages. *Biochemical & Biophysical Research Communications* 172, 1246-1252.

Echeverry, M. B., Guimaraes, F. S., and Del Bel, E. A. (2004). Acute and delayed restraint stress-induced changes in nitric oxide producing neurons in limbic regions. *Neuroscience* 125, 981-993.

Ehren, I., Adolfsson, J., and Wiklund, N. P. (1994). Nitric oxide synthase activity in the human urogenital tract. *Urol Res* 22, 287-290.

Eskiocak, S., Gozen, A. S., Yapar, S. B., Tavas, F., Kilic, A. S., and Eskiocak, M. (2005). Glutathione and free sulphydryl content of seminal plasma in healthy medical students during and after exam stress. *Hum Reprod* 20, 2595-2600.

Fassbender, K., Schneider, S., Bertsch, T., Schlueter, D., Fatar, M., Ragoschke, A., Kuhl, S., Kischka, U., and Hennerici, M. (2000). Temporal profile of release of interleukin-1beta in neurotrauma. *Neurosci Lett* 284, 135-138.

Fenster, L., Katz, D. F., Wyrobek, A. J., Pieper, C., Rempel, D. M., Oman, D., and Swan, S. H. (1997). Effects of psychological stress on human semen quality. *J Androl* 18, 194-202.

Gao, H. B., Tong, M. H., Hu, Y. Q., Guo, Q. S., Ge, R., and Hardy, M. P. (2002). Glucocorticoid induces apoptosis in rat Leydig cells. *Endocrinology* 143, 130-138.

Gao, H. B., Tong, M. H., Hu, Y. Q., You, H. Y., Guo, Q. S., Ge, R. S., and Hardy, M. P. (2003). Mechanisms of glucocorticoid-induced Leydig cell apoptosis. *Molecular & Cellular Endocrinology* 199, 153-163.

Gaytan, F., Bellido, C., Aguilar, R., Morales, C., van Rooijen, N., and Aguilar, E. (1997). Role of the testis in the response of the pituitary-testicular axis to nitric oxide-related agents. *Eur J Endocrinol* 137, 301-308.

Ge, R.-S., Dong, Q., Sottas, C. M., Chen, H., Zirkin, B. R., and Hardy, M. P. (2005). Gene Expression in Rat Leydig Cells During Development from the Progenitor to Adult Stage: A Cluster Analysis. *Biol Reprod* 72, 1405-1415.

Giannessi, F., Ruffoli, R., Giambelluca, M. A., Morelli, G., and Menchini Fabris, F. (1998). Cytochemical localisation of the NADPH diaphorase activity in the Leydig cells of the mouse. *Histochem Cell Biol* 109, 241-248.

Guo, C., Huang, C., Chen, S., and Wang Hsu, G. (2001). Serum and testicular testosterone and nitric oxide products in aluminum-treated mice. *Environ. Toxicol. Pharmacol.* 10, 53-60.

Hales, D. B., and Payne, A. H. (1989). Glucocorticoid-mediated repression of P450scc mRNA and de novo synthesis in cultured Leydig cells. *Endocrinology* 124, 2099-2104.

Hauser, W., Sassmann, A., Qadri, F., Johren, O., and Dominiak, P. (2005). Expression of nitric oxide synthase isoforms in hypothalamo-pituitary-adrenal axis during the development of spontaneous hypertension in rats. *Brain Res Mol Brain Res* 138, 198-204.

Herman, M., and Rivier, C. (2006). Activation of a Neural Brain-Testicular Pathway Rapidly Lowers Leydig Cell Levels of the Steroidogenic Acute Regulatory Protein and the Peripheral-Type Benzodiazepine Receptor while Increasing Levels of Neuronal Nitric Oxide Synthase. *Endocrinology* 147, 624-633.

Hikim, A. P., Vera, Y., Vernet, D., Castanares, M., Diaz-Romero, M., Ferrini, M., Swerdloff, R. S., Gonzalez-Cadavid, N. F., and Wang, C. (2005). Involvement of nitric oxide-mediated intrinsic pathway signaling in age-related increase in germ cell apoptosis in male Brown-Norway rats. *J Gerontol A Biol Sci Med Sci* 60, 702-708.

Hjollund, N. H., Bonde, J. P., Henriksen, T. B., Giwercman, A., and Olsen, J. (2004a). Job strain and male fertility. *Epidemiology* 15, 114-117.

Hjollund, N. H., Bonde, J. P., Henriksen, T. B., Giwercman, A., and Olsen, J. (2004b). Reproductive effects of male psychologic stress. *Epidemiology* 15, 21-27.

Hori, N., Lee, M. C., Sasaguri, K., Ishii, H., Kamei, M., Kimoto, K., Toyoda, M., and Sato, S. (2005). Suppression of stress-induced nNOS expression in the rat hypothalamus by biting. *J Dent Res* 84, 624-628.

Huong, N. T., Murakami, Y., Tohda, M., Watanabe, H., and Matsumoto, K. (2005). Social isolation stress-induced oxidative damage in mouse brain and its modulation by majonoside-R2, a Vietnamese ginseng saponin. *Biol Pharm Bull* 28, 1389-1393.

Hutson, J. C. (1992). Development of cytoplasmic digitations between Leydig cells and testicular macrophages of the rat. *Cell Tissue Res* 267, 385-389.

Kishimoto, J., Tsuchiya, T., Emson, P. C., and Nakayama, Y. (1996). Immobilization-induced stress activates neuronal nitric oxide synthase (nNOS) mRNA and protein in hypothalamic-pituitary-adrenal axis in rats. *Brain Res* 720, 159-171.

Koksal, I. T., Usta, M. F., Akkoyunlu, G., Toptas, B., Gulkesen, K. H., Erdogru, T., Tuncer, M., Baykal, A., Ersoy, F., Demir, R., and Baykara, M. (2003). The potential role of advanced glycation end product and iNOS in chronic renal failure-related testicular dysfunction. An experimental study. *Am J Nephrol* 23, 361-368.

Kon, Y., Namiki, Y., and Endoh, D. (2002). Expression and distribution of inducible nitric oxide synthase in mouse testis. *Jpn J Vet Res* 50, 115-123.

Kono, T., Saito, M., Kinoshita, Y., Satoh, I., Shinbori, C., and Satoh, K. (2006). Real-time monitoring of nitric oxide and blood flow during ischemia-reperfusion in the rat testis. *Mol Cell Biochem* 286, 139-145.

Kostic, T., Andric, S., Kovacevic, R., and Maric, D. (1998). The involvement of nitric oxide in stress-impaired testicular steroidogenesis. *Eur. J. Pharmacol.* 346, 267-273.

Kostic, T. S., Andric, S. A., Maric, D., and Kovacevic, R. Z. (2000). Inhibitory effects of stress-activated nitric oxide on antioxidant enzymes and testicular steroidogenesis. *J Steroid Biochem Mol Biol* 75, 299-306.

Kostic, T. S., Andric, S. A., Maric, D., Stojilkovic, S. S., and Kovacevic, R. (1999). Involvement of inducible nitric oxide synthase in stress-impaired testicular steroidogenesis. *J Endocrinol* 163, 409-416.

Laubach, V. E., Foley, P. L., Shockey, K. S., Tribble, C. G., and Kron, I. L. (1998). Protective roles of nitric oxide and testosterone in endotoxemia: evidence from NOS-2-deficient mice. *Am J Physiol* 275, H2211-2218.

Lissbrant, E., Lofmark, U., Collin, O., and Bergh, A. (1997). Is nitric oxide involved in the regulation of the rat testicular vasculature? *Biology of Reproduction* 56, 1221-1227.

Madrigal, J. L., Moro, M. A., Lizasoain, I., Lorenzo, P., Castrillo, A., Bosca, L., and Leza, J. C. (2001). Inducible nitric oxide synthase expression in brain cortex after acute restraint stress is regulated by nuclear factor kappaB-mediated mechanisms. *J Neurochem* 76, 532-538.

Madrigal, J. L., Moro, M. A., Lizasoain, I., Lorenzo, P., and Leza, J. C. (2002). Stress-induced increase in extracellular sucrose space in rats is mediated by nitric oxide. *Brain Res* 938, 87-91.

Masood, A., Banerji, B., Vijayan, V. K., and Ray, A. (2004). Pharmacological and biochemical studies on the possible role of nitric oxide in stress adaptation in rats. *Eur J Pharmacol* 493, 111-115.

Matsumoto, K., Yobimoto, K., Huong, N. T., Abdel-Fattah, M., Van Hien, T., and Watanabe, H. (1999). Psychological stress-induced enhancement of brain lipid peroxidation via nitric oxide systems and its modulation by anxiolytic and anxiogenic drugs in mice. *Brain Res* 839, 74-84.

Middendorff, R., Muller, D., Wichers, S., Holstein, A. F., and Davidoff, M. S. (1997). Evidence for production and functional activity of nitric oxide in seminiferous tubules and blood vessels of the human testis. *J Clin Endocrinol Metab* 82, 4154-4161.

Monder, C., Sakai, R. R., Miroff, Y., Blanchard, D. C., and Blanchard, R. J. (1994). Reciprocal changes in plasma corticosterone and testosterone in stressed male rats maintained in a visible burrow system: evidence for a mediating role of testicular beta-hydroxysteroid
dehydrogenase. *Endocrinology* 134, 1193-1198.

Moon, C., Ahn, M., Kim, S., Yasuzumi, F., and Shin, T. (2005). Increased expression of both constitutive and inducible forms of nitric oxide synthase in the delayed phase of acute experimental testicular torsion. *J Vet Med Sci* 67, 453-456.

Munck, A., and Guyre, P. M. (1986). Glucocorticoid physiology, pharmacology and stress. *Adv. Exp. Med. Biol.* 196, 81-96.

Nadeem, A., Masood, A., Masood, N., Gilani, R. A., and Shah, Z. A. (2006). Immobilization stress causes extra-cellular oxidant-antioxidant imbalance in rats: restoration by L-NAME and vitamin E. *Eur Neuropsychopharmacol* 16, 260-267.

Nakashima, A., Koshiyama, K., Uozumi, T., Monden, Y., Hamanaka, Y., Kurachi, K., Aono, T., Mizutani, S., and Matsumoto, K. (1975). Effects of general anesthesia and severity of surgical stress on serum LH and testosterone in males. *Acta Endocrinol* 78, 258-269.

O'Bryan, M. K., Schlatt, S., Gerdprasert, O., Phillips, D. J., de Kretser, D. M., and Hedger, M. P. (2000). Inducible nitric oxide synthase in the rat testis: evidence for potential roles in both normal function and inflammation-mediated infertility. *Biology of Reproduction* 63, 1285-1293.

Okere, C. O., and Waterhouse, B. D. (2006). Acute restraint increases NADPH-diaphorase staining in distinct subregions of the rat dorsal raphe nucleus: implications for raphe serotonergic and nitrergic transmission. *Brain Res* 1119, 174-181.

Orr, T. E., Taylor, M. F., Bhattacharyya, A. K., Collins, D. C., and Mann, D. R. (1994). Acute immobilization stress disrupts testicular steroidogenesis in adult male rats by inhibiting the activities of 17α-hydroxylase and 17,20-lyase without affecting the binding of LH/hCG receptors. *J Androl* 15, 302-308.

Pinilla, L., Gonzalez, L. C., Tena-Sempere, M., Bellido, C., and Aguilar, E. (2001). Effects of systemic blockade of nitric oxide synthases on pulsatile LH, prolactin, and GH secretion in adult male rats. *Horm Res* 55, 229-235.

Pinilla, L., Tena-Sempere, M., Gonzalez, D., and Aguilar, E. (1995). Mechanisms of altered LH secretion in neonatally oestrogenized male rats. *J Endocrinol* 147, 43-50.

Pomerantz, D. K., and Pitelka, V. (1998). Nitric oxide is a mediator of the inhibitory effect of activated macrophages on production of androgen by the Leydig cell of the mouse. *Endocrinology* 139, 922-931.

Ratnasooriya, W. D., Jayakody, J. R., and Dharmasiri, M. G. (2004). Sodium nitroprusside impairs sexual competence of male rats. *Hum Exp Toxicol* 23, 187-192.

Rettori, V., Mohn, C., Scorticati, C., Vissio, P., Cella, M., Farina, M., Franchi, A., and McCann, S. M. (2003). Effect of neurogenic stress and ethanol on nitric oxide synthase and cyclooxygenase activities in rat adrenals. *Ann N Y Acad Sci* 992, 86-98.

Rivier, C., and Shen, G. H. (1994). In the rat, endogenous nitric oxide modulates the response of the hypothalamic-pituitary-adrenal axis to interleukin-1 beta, vasopressin, and oxytocin. *J Neurosci* 14, 1985-1993.

Ruffoli, R., Giambelluca, M. A., Giannessi, F., Soldani, P., Grasso, L., Gasperi, M., and Giannessi, F. (2001). Ultrastructural localization of the NADPH-diaphorase activity in the Leydig cells of aging mice. *Anat Embryol (Berl)* 203, 383-391.

Sapolsky, R. M., Romero, L. M., and Munck, A. U. (2000). How do glucocorticoids influence stress responses? Integrating permissive, suppressive, stimulatory, and preparative actions. *Endocr Rev* 21, 55-89.

Schmid, W., Cole, T. J., Blendy, J. A., and Schutz, G. (1995). Molecular genetic analysis of glucocorticoid signaling in development. *J Steroid Biochem Mol Biol* 53, 33-35.

Selvage, D. J., Lee, S. Y., Parsons, L. H., Seo, D. O., and Rivier, C. L. (2004). A hypothalamic-testicular neural pathway is influenced by brain catecholamines, but not testicular blood flow. *Endocrinology* 145, 1750-1759.

Selye, H. (1946). The general adaptation syndrome and the disease of adaptation. *J. Clin. Endocrinol.* 6, 117-230.

Sharma, A. C., Sam, A. D., 2nd, Lee, L. Y., Hales, D. B., Law, W. R., Ferguson, J. L., and Bosmann, H. B. (1998). Effect of NG-nitro-L-arginine methyl ester on testicular blood flow and serum steroid hormones during sepsis. *Shock* 9, 416-421.

Shi, Q., Emanuele, N. V., and Emanuele, M. A. (1998). Effect of nitric oxide synthase inhibitors on preventing ethanol-induced suppression of the hypothalamic-pituitary-gonadal axis in the male rat. *Alcohol Clin Exp Res* 22, 1763-1770.

Shiraishi, K., Naito, K., and Yoshida, K. (2001). Nitric oxide promotes germ cell necrosis in the delayed phase after experimental testicular torsion of rat. *Biol Reprod* 65, 514-521.

Shirakawa, T., Mitome, M., Kikuiri, T., Nakamura, W., Oshima, S., Hasegawa, T., Shindoh, M., and Oguchi, H. (2004). Immobilization induces acute nitric oxide production in the rat hypothalamus: a role of ionotropic glutamate receptors in the paraventricular nucleus. *Endocrinology* 145, 3603-3607.

Smals, A. G., Kloppenborg, P. W., and Benraad, T. J. (1977). Plasma testosterone profiles in Cushing's syndrome. *J. Clin. Endocrinol. Metab.* 45, 240-245.

Stalker, A., Hermo, L., and Antakly, T. (1989). Covalent affinity labeling, radioautography, and immunocytochemistry localize the glucocorticoid receptor in rat testicular Leydig cells. *Am J Anat* 186, 369-377.

Stalker, A., Hermo, L., and Antakly, T. (1991). Subcellular distribution of 3H-dexamethasone mesylate binding sites in Leydig cells using electron microscope radioautography. *Am J Anat* 190, 19-30.

Sun, X. R., Hedger, M. P., and Risbridger, G. P. (1993). The effect of testicular macrophages and interleukin-1 on testosterone production by purified adult rat Leydig cells cultured under in vitro maintenance conditions. *Endocrinology* 132, 186-192.

Tatsumi, N., Fujisawa, M., Kanzaki, M., Okuda, Y., Okada, H., Arakawa, S., and Kamidono, S. (1997). Nitric oxide production by cultured rat Leydig cells. *Endocrinology* 138, 994-998.

Tsuchiya, T., Kishimoto, J., Koyama, J., and Ozawa, T. (1997). Modulatory effect of L-NAME, a specific nitric oxide synthase (NOS) inhibitor, on stress-induced changes in plasma adrenocorticotropic hormone (ACTH) and corticosterone levels in rats: physiological significance of stress-induced NOS activation in hypothalamic-pituitary-adrenal axis. *Brain Res* 776, 68-74.

Tsuchiya, T., Kishimoto, J., and Nakayama, Y. (1996). Marked increases in neuronal nitric oxide synthase (nNOS) mRNA and NADPH-diaphorase histostaining in adrenal cortex after immobilization stress in rats. *Psychoneuroendocrinology* 21, 287-293.

Tuncel, M., Dogrukol-Ak, D., and Erkasap, N. (2001). Modified method for the determination of capillary electrophoresis nitric oxide-correlated nitrate in tissue homogenates. *J Chromatogr B Biomed Sci Appl* 751, 257-263.

Tunctan, B., Weigl, Y., Dotan, A., Peleg, L., Zengil, H., Ashkenazi, I., and Abacioglu, N. (2002). Circadian variation of nitric oxide synthase activity in mouse tissue. *Chronobiol Int* 19, 393-404.

Wang, Y., Goligorsky, M. S., Lin, M., Wilcox, J. N., and Marsden, P. A. (1997). A novel, testis-specific mRNA transcript encoding an NH2-terminal truncated nitric-oxide synthase. *Journal of Biological Chemistry* 272, 11392-11401.

Weissman, B. A., Niu, E., Ge, R., Sottas, C. M., Holmes, M., Hutson, J. C., and Hardy, M. P. (2005). Paracrine modulation of androgen synthesis in rat leydig cells by nitric oxide. *J Androl* 26, 369-378.

Weissman, B. A., Sottas, C. M., Zhou, P., Iadecola, C., and Hardy, M. P. (2007). Testosterone production in mice lacking inducible nitric oxide synthase expression is sensitive to restraint stress. *Am J Physiol Endocrinol Metab* 292, E615-620.

Welch, C., Watson, M. E., Poth, M., Hong, T., and Francis, G. L. (1995). Evidence to suggest nitric oxide is an interstitial regulator of Leydig cell steroidogenesis. *Metabolism* 44, 234-238.

Welsh, T. H., Bambino, T. H., and Hsueh, A. J. W. (1982). Mechanism of glucocorticoid-induced suppression of testicular androgen biosynthesis *in vitro*. *Biol Reprod* 27, 1138-1146.

Yazawa, H., Sasagawa, I., Ishigooka, M., and Nakada, T. (1999). Effect of immobilization stress on testicular germ cell apoptosis in rats. *Human Reproduction* 14, 1806-1810.

Zini, A., O'Bryan, M. K., Magid, M. S., and Schlegel, P. N. (1996). Immunohistochemical localization of endothelial nitric oxide synthase in human testis, epididymis, and vas deferens suggests a possible role for nitric oxide in spermatogenesis, sperm maturation, and programmed cell death. *Biology of Reproduction* 55, 935-941.

In: Trends in Testosterone Research
Editor: Raymund E. Veritos

ISBN: 978-1-60456-127-2

Chapter IV

Role of FSH and Testosterone in Male Germ Cell Differentiation

Andrés Aragón Martínez
Laboratorio de Biología de la Reproducción, Facultad de Medicina Veterinaria y Zootecnia, Universidad Autónoma del Estado de México, México;

Abstract

Follicle stimulating hormone (FSH) and testosterone have been described as necessary factors for proliferation of Sertoli and germ cells, as well as having a role in apoptosis. However, their role in germ cell differentiation has not been studied in detail. FSH is a proteic hormone produced in the anterior hypophysis and has receptors located in Sertoli cells, which in turn function as nurse cells for germ cells in the seminiferous epithelium. The expression of FSH receptors changes during the cycle of seminiferous epithelium. Germ cells in consecutive steps of differentiation are located in each progressive stage of the seminiferous epithelium, indicating a role for FSH signaling in the differentiation of germ cells. CREB (CRE-protein binding) is a transcription factor involved in differentiation of germ cells and it is modulated by FSH. Some CREM-regulated products have been shown to participate in germ cell differentiation. Recent studies have focused on the intracellular signaling after FSH joins with its receptor, and how it influences germ cell differentiation. Testosterone-stimulated germ cell development occurs via paracrine communication with Sertoli cells. The androgen receptor is expressed in a stage-specific manner during the seminiferous epithelium cycle. Recent studies on gene expression show a number of genes modulated by testosterone, many of which do not follow the traditional pathway of androgen/receptor/gene expression, but are activated by another signalization pathway. This chapter begins with the background necessary to understand the general role of FSH and testosterone in seminiferous epithelium and then addresses the molecular signaling initiated by these chemical messengers.

Introduction

Cell differentiation occurs as a response to the signals of neighbor cells. This interaction permits the differentiating cell to express its specialized character in the overall context of location within a specific tissue. Spermatogenesis is a process constant of proliferation and meiosis, in which every daughter cell is compromised toward germ cell differentiation (spermatogonia, spermatocytes and spermatids) or to function in the renewal of its own population (spermatogonia).

It is widely accepted that the spermatogenic process is regulated by the gonadotropins follicle-stimulating hormone and luteinizing hormone which, in turn, are released by the gonadotropes-gonadotropin release hormone (GnRH). GnRHergic neurons located in the hypothalamus are regulated by other neurons, of which the nervous endings contact GnRHergic neurons (Figure 1). There is feedback among the sexual steroids produced by the testicles (progesterone, testosterone, and estradiol), the gonadotropes in the anterior hypophysis, and the hypothalamus.

Spermatogenesis occurs into the seminiferous tubules, out of which Leydig cells and blood vessels are located. In the seminiferous epithelium, the spermatogonium, located in the basal compartment, is the most primitive germ cell. Proliferation of spermatogonies occurs by mitosis. By the process of meiosis, the spermatocytes, located in adluminal compartment, give origin to the spermatids. Spermatids undergo a dramatic process of differentiation that converts them into the highly specialized sperm cells. Histologically, spermatogenesis progression is observed as a series of consecutives stages, each one characterized by a particular association of germ cells. A complete series of changes in cell associations (stages) arranged in the logical sequence of developmental progression is called the cycle of seminiferous epithelium. These associations develop and remain in one region of a seminiferous tubule. A segment of a tubule contains (in rodents) a single association; whereas, a complete series of segments constitutes a wave of seminiferous epithelium [1]. The number of stages and the type of associations is specie-specific. For example, there are twelve stages in mouse, fourteen in rat, and six in man. This classification divides a continuous process into discrete segments (Figure 2), then makes it possible to investigate the expression and role of individual factors along the spermatogenic process. Such an arrangement of the seminiferous epithelium means that inducing-differentiation factors are present in the seminiferous epithelium in a stage-specific manner. A distinct and well-defined population of germ cells interacts with Sertoli cells in a cyclic pattern. Sertoli cells secrete a large number of proteins and regulatory factors that are crucial for germ cell development [2], and apparently germ cells are needed to maintain that cycle of Sertoli cells [3, 4]. Spermatogonies/spermatocytes in the basal compartment of seminiferous epithelium are in contact with the basal lamina and Sertoli cells, whereas pachytene spermatocytes and spermatids are located in the adluminal compartment. Mature spermatozoa are located apically in Sertoli cells. Both basal and adluminal compartments are formed by tight junctions between adjacent Sertoli cells known as the blood-testis barrier (BTB) [5]. As germ cells move into the adluminal compartment, tight junctions between adjacent Sertoli cells from behind the germ cells, creating the BTB. The BTB segregates meiotic and postmeiotic cells into immunologically privileged adluminal compartment [5]. This cellular arrangement indicates that chemical messages stimulating development and differentiation of germ cells in adluminal compartment should be processed by Sertoli cells, and that germ cells in the basal compartment receive chemical messages distinct from those in the adluminal compartment.

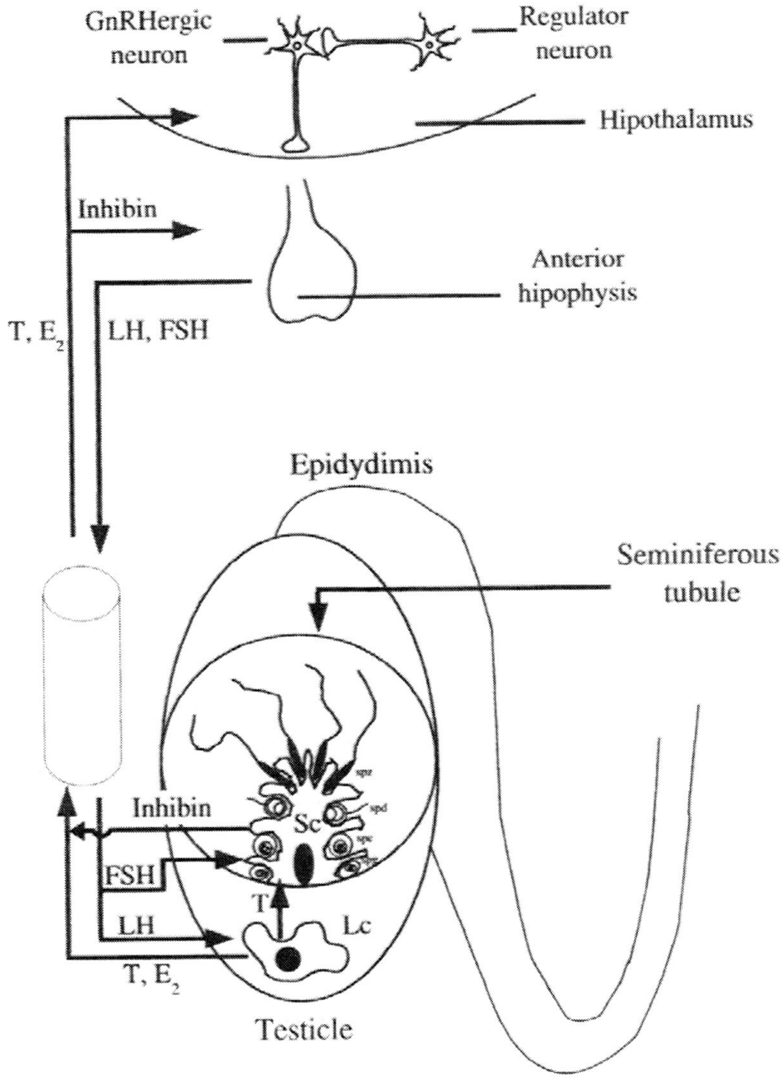

Figure 1. Schematic representation of the principal chemical messengers regulating spermatogenic function. T, testosterone; E2, estradiol; LH, luteinizing hormone; FSH, follicle- stimulating hormone; Sc, Sertoli cell; Lc, Leydig cell; spg, spermatogonium; spc, spermatocyte; spd, spermatid; spz, spermatozoon.

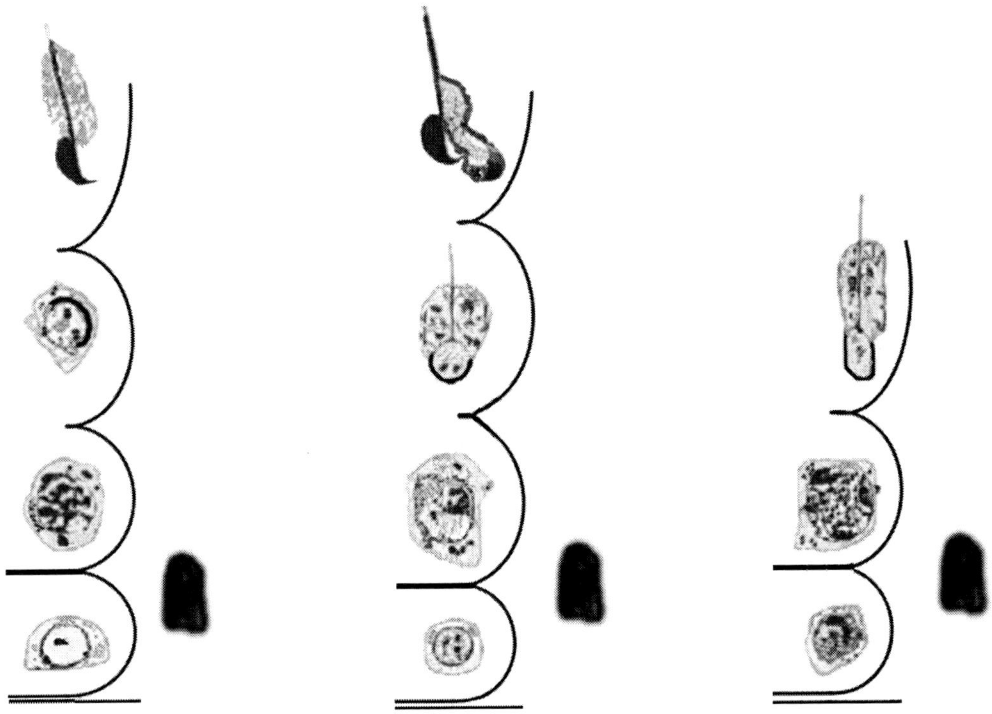

Figure 2. Germ cell associations in stages of mouse seminiferous epithelium. Germ cells with distinct morphology in stages VII-IX are depicted. All transformations (dynamic differentiation) occur in a segment of the seminiferous tubule. spg, spermatogonium; spc, spermatocyte; spdrd, round spermatid; spdel, elongating spermatid; spz, spermatozoid; Sc, Sertoli cell; Scn, Sertoli cell nucleus.

The Role of FSH in Spermatogenesis

It is well established that the FSH plays an important role in testicular development and spermatogenesis. In vivo FSH has been show as a germ cells survival factor [6, 7, 8]. In the adult rat and in humans, serum FSH levels remain relatively constant. However, the expression of FSH receptor (FSHR) on Sertoli cells varies more than three fold in a cyclical and stage-specific manner such that receptor levels are highest in stages XIII-II and minimal during stages VII-VIII [9, 10]. Because FSH receptor are found exclusively in the Sertoli cells, but not in germ cells themselves, it is likely that the FSH stimulation of Sertoli cells results in the induction of an intratubular factor essential for the survival of the male germ cells, as early suggested by Billig et al., [7].

FSH binding to its receptor is known to activate at least five signaling pathways in Sertoli cells: cAMP-PKA, MAP kinase, calcium, phophatidylinositol 3-kinase, and phospholipase A2 patways (reviewed in [11]). The testicular actions of FSH are mediated via a specific G protein-coupled cell surface receptor uniquely expressed in Sertoli cells [12]. Ligand-dependent activation of the FSHR initiates the production of intracellular cAMP [13] and Ca2 [14] second messengers. The levels of FSH-induced cAMP production in Sertoli cells closely follows the levels of FSH receptor with highest levels of cAMP observed in stages XIV-VI [15]. FSHR in perinatal animals induces a molecular signaling cascade that induces phosphatidylinositol 3-kinase/AKT pathway, it promotes aromatase expression and estradiol production, which stimulate the proliferation of Sertoli cells [16]. One target for the increase in cAMP and PKA is a class of transcription factors that bind to cAMP response elements (CREs). Specifically, the CRE binding protein (CREB) transcription factor is rapidly activated after being phosphorylated on serine 133 by PKA in response to FSH stimulation [17].

CREB may induce transcription factors required to activate others genes supportive of spermatogenesis [18], hormones that regulate spermatogenesis [19], and apoptotic factors [20, 21]. FSH and cAMP induce expression of the stem cell factor (SCF) in Sertoli cells, and there are three potential CREB-binding sites in the SCF promoter [21, 22]. It is knowed that in absence of SCF stimulation, spermatogonia and spermatocytes undergo apoptosis [23, 24].

The CREB transcripts in Sertoli cells fluctuates in a cyclical manner that depend on the specific cell association along the spermatogenic wave. In Sertoli cells of rats CREB mRNA is present in stages I-III of the seminiferous epithelium, highest in stages II-VI, and decreases to nearly undetectable levels during stages IX-XIV [25]. Sertoli cells do not appear to undergo apoptosis or necrosis when CREBm1 (mutant of CREB that cannot be phosphorylated on serine 133) is over expressed, implying that CREB is nor required for Sertoli cell survival [26]. In Sertoli cells, CREB is known to regulate directly or to be linked to the regulation of a number of genes required for differentiation of spermatozoa [18].

Because of the blood-testis barrier, the Sertoli cell must provide many factors required for the maintenance and development of germ cells [27]. Several genes that encode for proteins involved with microtubule and cytoskeleton rearrangement were identified as being regulated by FSH. These include actins, tubulins, lamin A, ankrin 3, and catenin alpha 2 [28]. The change in expression of few genes such as junctional adhesion molecule and scinderin whose products are involved in cell adhesion indicated a role for FSH in the adhesion of germ cells to Sertoli cells [28].

FSH has also been implicated in the expression of various isoforms of CREM (cAMP-responsive element modulator) that are expressed in spermatocytes and spermatids and are required for survival [29, 30]. However, as suggested by prior researchers [10], this regulation of germ cell CREM by FSH must be indirectly mediated trough as yet unidentified Sertoli cell factors. CREM is undetectable in prepubertal animals but highly abundant in adults [31]. CREM accumulates in haploid spermatids and is required for transcriptional activation of several post-meiotic genes [31, 32]. Most of these genes encode structural proteins required for differentiation of spermatozoa [18, 28]. On transgenic male rats -/- CREM germ cell development is arrested in spermiogenesis and the cell are eliminated by apoptosis [30, 33].

The CREB/CREM system can negatively autoregulate itself. Another CREM isoform, inducible cAMP early repressor (ICER), encodes a powerful repressor of cAMP-responsive genes [34]. In Sertoli cells, the only member significantly expressed is the ICER repressor, whereas, all the cAMP-dependent gene activation is carried out by CREB. In germ cells, however, the task of executing gene activation falls mainly on CREM. Seminiferous epithelium analysis of CREM-mutant male mice revealed post-meiotic arrest at the first step of spermiogenesis and a dramatic decline in post-meiotic gene expression. However, FSH and testosterone levels were not affected by the mutation [33].

FSH is generally considered a differentiation promoting agent for Sertoli cells [35]. This corresponds to ID proteins generally being considered as proliferation-promoting and differentiation-inhibiting factors. The ability of FSH to supress ID expression correlates with an increased differentiation and decreased proliferation of the cells [36]. A overexpression of ID and ID2 genes in a posmitotic, terminally differentiated cell type have the capacity to induce reentry into cell cycle [35].

The Role of Testosterone in Spermatogenesis

Testosterone, Androgen Receptor and Estrogen in the Seminiferous Epithelium

Hormonal regulation of the spermatogenic process occurs during three phases: initiation, maintenance and re-initiation [37]. Spermatogenesis in gonadotropin-deficient mice is qualitatively initiated by androgens [38]. Androgen is necessary for the completion of meiosis and differentiation of round spermatids into spermatozoa. If androgens are eliminated by hypophysectomy, there is a partial loss of round spermatids, with elongated spermatids observed [39], and if residual testosterone is eliminated by using a Leydig cell citotoxic such as dimethanesulphonate, or by a competitor of androgen such as flutamide, only a few round spermatids are observed and no elongated spermatids are present [40, 41]. It is thus clear that androgen plays a very important role in the development and differentiation of germ cells.

The role of androgen in spermatogenesis is mediated by androgen receptor (AR). Circulating androgens dissociate from carrier proteins, specifically sex hormone-binding globulin, prior to diffusing into target cells and binding to intracellular AR. The unliganded receptor is an inactive oligomer complexed to heat shock proteins (eg. Hsp90, Hsp70) and located in the cytoplasm. The oligomeric complex dissociates when bound to hormone, and the receptor undergoes a conformational change while being transporting to the nucleus, and while binding as a homodimer to DNA hormone-responsive elements [42]. AR is located in Leydig, peritubular myoid, and Sertoli cells, although localization in germ cells is controversial [43, 44, 45]. In this sense, some studies indicate that the presence of AR in germ cells is not necessary for normal germ cell development [46, 47] and fertility [46]. Paracrine communication between somatic and germ cells thus appears to be responsible for germ cell differentiation, although the mechanisms involved are poorly understood. AR protein expression in Sertoli cells varies as a function of the cycle of seminiferous epithelium, for example, in rat Sertoli cells, AR is first detected at late stage IV or early stage V, and high expression is maintained until spermiation in stage VIII and their expression disappears completely by stage IX[48, 49]; whereas in mice Sertoli cells AR expression is high in stages VI-VII an low in stage VIII-XII [50].

Sertoli, peritubular myoid, and Leydig cells have the ability to mediate the transcriptional effects of androgen, and receptor concentrations may be a limiting factor for responsiveness [51]. The cell-autonomous AR actions in Sertoli cells is an absolute requirement for androgen maintenance of complete spermatogenesis, and spermatocyte/spermatid development/survival depends critically on androgens. However, which factors are regulated by AR/androgen and how they stimulate spermatogenesis progression is poorly understand. Recently, the use of AR-knockout or ABP-overexpressing models and microarray technology have revealed which genes are AR-regulated and have shed light on the general role of AR/androgen interactions in the spermatogenesis process.

Lessons of Knockout Models and Other Models in AR Function

Studies using total or cell-specific AR-knockout male mouse lines have demonstrated a differential effect of AR in spermatogenesis. A Sertoli cell-selective knockout of AR increased germ cell apoptosis and grossly reduced expression of genes specific for late spermatocyte or spermatid development (AR exon 2 locus, Cre, Pem, A-myb, Pro-Acrosin binding protein, PT1, PT2, Protamin 1 and 2, anti-Mullerian hormone, ABP, cyclin A1 and sperm-1) [52, 53]. These findings indicate that AR expression and function in testicular cells other than germ cells, play a critical role in normal spermatogenesis. Differences in expression of cytoskeletal and extracellular matrix-related genes were found in Sertoli cell AR-knockout mice [54], and are related to the induction of a broad spectrum of functional defects, such as alteration in movements of developing germ cells, impaired functional integrity of the BTB, transport protein and paracrine factor production and/or secretion [55]. These defects impair nursery functions for developing cells and lead to the arrest of spermatogenesis before the second wave of meiosis. In total or Sertoli cell AR-knockout mouse lines, AR is essential for the completion of meiosis. In the total AR-knockout line, spermatogenesis does not progress beyond the pachytene spermatocyte stage (i.e. before meiosis II initiation, stage X), whereas Sertoli cell AR-knockout germ cells develop until the diplotene spermatocyte (approximately coincident with meiosis initiation, stage XI) [46, 53], and Leydig cell AR-knockouts reach the diplotene/meiosis II stage (round spermatid, stage XII). Interestingly, spermatogenesis is complete and the sperm produced are functional in germ cell AR-knockout mice [46]. Thus androgen/AR signaling in Sertoli cells plays the most important role in spermatogenesis [46]. Another hand, in vitro [56] and in vivo [46, 53, 57] non-functional AR leads to a diminished steroidogenic function and to spermatogenesis arrest, principally at the round spermatid stage.

Reduction of androgen levels in transgenic male mice overexpressing ABP increased the expression of a large number of genes, and only a small number were decreased [58], whereas in hypogonadal mice, testosterone treatment repressed rather than stimulated gene expression [59]. This phenomenon may represent a compensatory mechanism activated in testosterone-deprived Sertoli cells, or some of the activated genes may actually be negative regulators of Sertoli cell functions required for the support of spermatogenesis [58].

Chemical communication between androgen-producing Leydig and Sertoli cells is very important for the maintenance of spermatogenesis. Although androgen and AR have important roles in Sertoli cells, loss of functional AR in Leydig cells has a major influence on

Leydig cell steroidogenic function (i.e. testosterone production decreased) leading to spermatogenesis arrest, predominately at the round spermatid stage [46].

Androgens are converted irreversibly to estrogens by P450 aromatase (arom). Estrogen have two receptors (ERalpha and ERbeta) which are expressed differentially during male development [60]. In adult male testes, both ERalpha and ERbeta are expressed in spermatocytes, elongating spermatids, Sertoi cells and Leydig cells [61, 62]. whereas, arom and both estrogen receptor are present in sperm [63, 64, 65]. Hypogonadal (hpg) mouse have a congenital inability to synthetize GnRH, then do not show normal posnatal testicular development. This mouse has been used to study the mechanism of estrogens in spermatogenesis. In hpg mice estrogenic treatment induces qualitatively normal spermatogenesis via genomic estrogen receptor without role of AR [66, 67]. Interestingly, estrogenic treatment of hpg mouse induces a increase of circulating FSH. Espermatogenic effects of estrogen are induced principally by FSH than estrogen alone as demonstrated recently by [68]. However, as specified above, to estrogen act in spermatogenesis it is necessary almost low levels of androgens.

AR and Adherens Junctions in the Seminiferous Epithelium

Prior to puberty the Sertoli cells undergo active cell proliferation, and at the onset of puberty they become a terminally differentiated posmitotic cell population that support spermatogenesis. The molecular mechanisms involved in the posmitotic block of pubertal and adult Sertoli cells are unknown [35]. Sertoli cell fate is established in the embryonic gonad at the time of sex determination [69, 70] and is followed by a phase of rapid proliferation and differentiation. During puberty, occurs the final phase of Sertoli cell differentiation, which is marked by cessation of proliferation, and by irreversible changes in Sertoli cell morphology and physiology [71]. The changes associated with terminal differentiation of Sertoli cell at puberty include exit from the cell cycle and the formation of BTB [35]. This differentiated phenotype is needed for the proper microenvironment and cytoarchitectural support of the developing spermatogenic cells. Sertoli cell differentiation is accompanied by the expression of many gene products that are not present in immature cells [43, 72, 73, 74, 75, 76].

During spermatogenesis, basally located spermatogonia differentiate into the preletotene/leptotene stages of primary spermatocytes, and initiate meiosis. These primary spermatocytes must migrate from the basal compartment to the BTB in late stage VII to early stage IX of the cycle of seminiferous epithelium in mouse testis [77].

Loss of functional AR in Sertoli cells causes a broad spectrum of functional defects that lead to the arrest of spermatogenesis before the second wave of meiosis [53, 57, 78]. A cause of this phenomenon is the disruption of the BTB [55]. In Sertoli cell AR-knockout mice the expression of tight junction-related genes such as cystatin-TE [79], ocludin [55], claudin 3 [5] and claudin II [55, 79], is decreased, so it is clear that the absence of AR impairs functional tight junction formation and integrity.

In apical compartment of semiferous epithelium Sertoli cell interact with spermatids by a testis-adherens junction knowed as ectoplasmic specialization. Moreover, adherens junction participates also in BTB along tight junctions (Figure 3). In BTB adherens and tight junctions are restructuring to permit germ cells to move across to adluminal compartment and in apical compartment to permit full developed spermatozoa to be sloughed at spermiation [80]. The integrity of BTB cannot be compromised throughout spermatogenesis so that posmeiotic germ cell-specific antigens can be sequestered from the system circulation at all times [81].

It is well knowed that testosterone participates in BTB integrity and in spermiation failure. At date, using androgen-suppression model it has been observed that germ cell loss disruption of adherens junctions is limited to the Sertoli-germ cell interface without perturbing the BTB [81], and recently demonstrated that the transient opening of the BTB that facilitates germ cell movement is mediated via differential effects of testosterone and citokynes (such as TGFbetas) on the kinetics of endocytosis and recycling of integral membrane proteins (occludin, AM-A, and N-cadherin) at the BTB [82, 83, 84, 85].

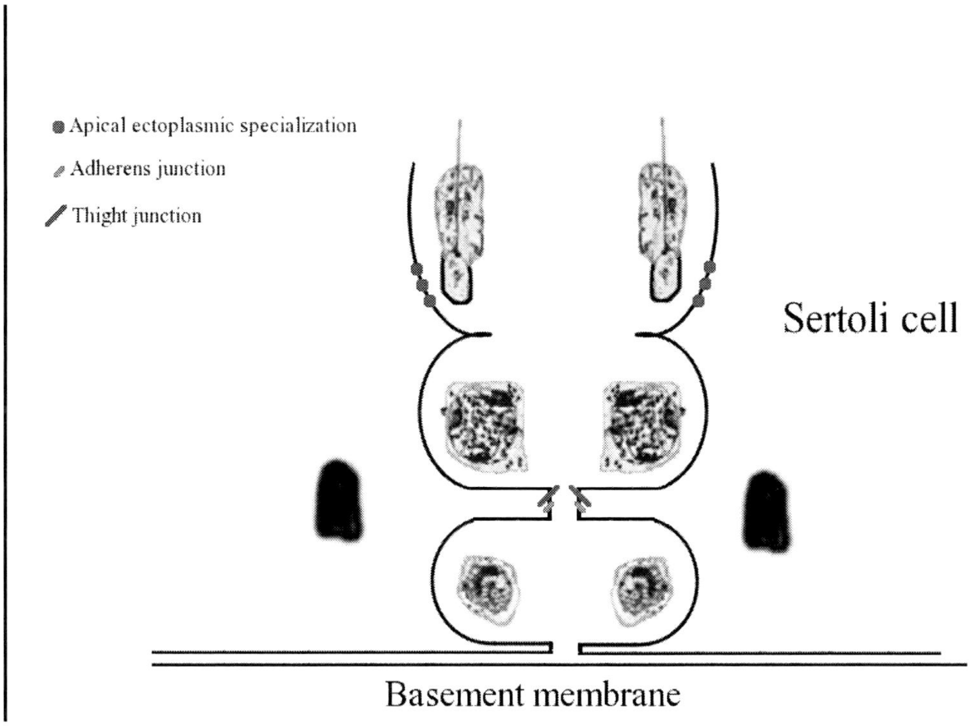

Figure 3. Schematic representation of adherens junction and tight junction in seminiferous epithelium. The ectoplasmic specialization in apical compartment is showed, is clear the relationship between Sertoli cell and spermatid elongating. Adheren junction and tight junction are part of the BTB that divide seminiferous ephitelium in basal and adluminal compartments.

Sertoli and Germ Cells as Regulators of the Cycle of the Seminiferous Epithelium

It is as yet not clear whether Sertoli or germ cells play the dominant role in regulating the seminiferous epithelium cycle. Timmons et al., [86] showed in WT mice that the somatic epithelial cycle can be maintained in the absence of germ cells for at least the first week of neonatal life, but Meng et al., [5] suggest that androgen could regulate the microenvironment within the seminiferous epithelium, creating conditions that are permissive, rather than instructive, for germ cell differentiation. Notably, rat germ cells transplanted into a mouse testis differentiate with rat cell kinetics [87]. The fact that embryonic stem cells can differentiate into germ cells in vitro in the absence of seminiferous epithelium supports the latter hypothesis [5].

An early research [88] suggested that there is Sertoli cell cycle, whereas and as Franca et al., [87] observed also germ cell cycles. However, the communication mechanisms that would permit synchronization of the cycles, and which are the molecular players involved in the dynamic cell differentiation (Sertoli and germ cells) are not known. However, a series of studies support parallel cycles. The absence of a functional AR in Sertoli cells prevents the progression of germ cell development [46, 53, 54] is indicative of a tight communication/synchronization of cycles between somatic and germ cells, and every germ-cell type expresses a group of genes in a stage-specific manner during spermatogenesis development [89, 90, 91]. Some of these genes could be expressed in all germ cells that are regulated during the cycle of seminiferous epithelium [89], which supports the idea that differential communication could synchronize Sertoli and germ cell cycles.

From all above information, androgen could trigger a transcriptional response in Sertoli cell, leading to instructive signals to the germ cells. Microarray studies on androgen function (AR-knockout [54], ABP-overexpression [58] or hypogonadal model [59]) show both up- and down-regulation of a great number of genes. However, at present only two genes are known to be expressed in Sertoli cells that have androgen-responsive elements that respond directly to androgens: the placental and embryo oncofetal gene Pem [92] and the protooncogene c-Myc [93]. Alternative mechanisms of androgen action, for instance, via conversion into estrogens [94] or via non-genomic pathways [95, 96, 97] thus must be considered to explain the development and differentiation of germ cells. Cheng et al. [96] and Fix et al., [97] demonstrated the activation of Src kinase and thus a MAPK cascade and CREB transcription factor by testosterone stimulus in Sertoli cells. Expression of three genes (LDH-A, CREB and Egr1) was observed in testosterone-stimulated Sertoli cells, none of which is regulated by androgen-responsive elements in their promoters, a finding that is consistent with the paradigm that androgen can activate Sertoli cell expression by means of MAP kinase pathway and CREB [97]. CREB and Egr1 are also regulated by a decrease in testosterone concentrations [58]. A scheme for testosterone signaling pathways in Sertoli cells has been proposed by Walker et al., [11].

Conclusions

The need for testosterone stimulation in meiotic/postmeiotic differentiation in germ cells is clear. However, the testosterone-induced factors involved in the communication/ synchronization between Sertoli and germ cells are largely unknown.

Gene expression data from FSH or testosterone-regulation demonstrate the complexity of the regulation of differentiation in seminiferous epithelium. To date, the need of FSH and testosterone in stage-specific development is relatively known, but spatial regulation along a tubule has not been explored. As mentioned above, a cell association develops and remains in one region of the seminiferous tubule, but it remains to be demonstrated how the chemical communication between adjacent Sertoli cells occurs, and particularly how a different association along a wave of seminiferous epithelium is established. Another layer of complexity is added to this problem by the occurrence of modulations in a tubule, i.e. the linking of consecutive segments of a seminiferous tubule with no descending order.

References

[1] Russell LD, Etllin RA, Sinha Hikim AP, Clegg ED. *Histological and histopathological evaluation of the testis.* Florida: Caché River Press; 1990.

[2] Griswold MD. The central role of Sertoli cells in spermatogenesis. *Semin Cell Dev Biol.* 1998 Aug;9(4):411–416.

[3] Jégou B, Pineau C. Current aspects of autocrine and paracrine regulation of spermatogenesis. *Adv Exp Med Biol.* 1995;377:67–86.

[4] Weinbauer GF, Wessels J. 'Paracrine' control of spermatogenesis. *Andrologia.* 1999 Sep;31(5):249–262.

[5] Meng J, Holdcraft RW, Shima JE, Griswold MD, Braun RE. Androgens regulate the permeability of the blood-testis barrier. *Proc Natl Acad Sci U S A.* 2005 Nov;102(46):16696–16700.

[6] Russell LD, Corbin TJ, Borg KE, De Franca LR, Grasso P, Bartke A. Recombinant human follicle-stimulating hormone is capable of exerting a bilogical effect in the adult hypophysectomized rat by reducing the numbers of degenerating germ cells. *Endocrinology.* 1993;133:2062–2070.

[7] Billig H, Furuta Y, Rivier C, Tapanaheim J, Parvinen M, Hsueh AJW. Apoptosis in testis germ cells: developmental changes in gonadotropin dependence and localization to selective tubule stages. *Endocrinology.* 1995;136:5–12.

[8] Ruwanpura SM, McLachlan RI, Stanton PG, Meachem SJ. Follicle-stimulating hormone affects spermatogonial survival by regulating the intrinsic apoptotic pathway in adult rats. *Biol Reprod.* 2008 Apr;78(4):705–713.

[9] Heckert LL, Griswold MD. Expression of follicle-stimulating hormone receptor mRNA in rat testes and Sertoli cells. *Mol Endocrinol.* 1991 May;5(5):670–677.

[10] Linder CC, Heckert LL, Roberts KP, Kim KH, Griswold MD. Expression of receptors during the cycle of the seminiferous epithelium. *Ann N Y Acad Sci.* 1991;637:313–321.

[11] Walker WH, Cheng J. FSH and testosterone signaling in Sertoli cells. *Reproduction.* 2005 Jul;130(1):15–28.

[12] Simoni M, Gromoll J, Nieschlag E. The follicle-stimulating hormone receptor: biochemistry, molecular biology, physiology, and pathophysiology. *Endocr Rev.* 1997 Dec;18(6):739–773.

[13] Means AR, Dedman JR, Tash JS, Tindall DJ, van Sickle M, Welsh MJ. Regulation of the testis sertoli cell by follicle stimulating hormone. *Annu Rev Physiol.* 1980;42:59–70.

[14] Gorczynska E, Handelsman DJ. The role of calcium in follicle-stimulating hormone signal transduction in Sertoli cells. *J Biol Chem.* 1991 Dec;266(35):23739–23744.

[15] Kangasniemi M, Kaipia A, Mali P, Toppari J, Huhtaniemi I, Parvinen M. Modulation of basal and FSH-dependent cyclic AMP production in rat seminiferous tubules staged by an improved transillumination technique. *Anat Rec.* 1990 May;227(1):62–76.

[16] McDonald CA, Millena AC, Reddy S, Finlay S, Vizcarra J, Khan SA, et al. Follicle-stimulating hormone-induced aromatase in immature rat Sertoli cells requires an active phosphatidylinositol 3-kinase pathway and is inhibited via the mitogen-activated protein kinase signaling pathway. *Mol Endocrinol.* 2006 Mar;20(3):608–618.

[17] Walker WH, Fucci L, Habener JF. Expression of the gene encoding transcription factor cyclic adenosine 3',5'-monophosphate (cAMP) response element-binding protein (CREB): regulation by follicle-stimulating hormone-induced cAMP signaling in primary rat Sertoli cells. *Endocrinology.* 1995 Aug;136(8):3534–3545.

[18] Sassone-Corsi P. Regulating the balance between differentiation and apoptosis: role of CREM in the male germ cells. *J Mol Med.* 1998;76(12):811–817.

[19] Najmabadi H, Rosenberg LA, Yuan QX, Bhatia N, Albiston AL, Burger H, et al. Transcriptional and posttranscriptional regulation of inhibin alpha-subunit gene expression in rat Sertoli cells by 8-bromo-3',5'-cyclic-adenosine monophosphate. *Mol Endocrinol.* 1993 Apr;7(4):469–476.

[20] Wilson BE, Mochon E, Boxer LM. Induction of bcl-2 expression by phosphorylated CREB proteins during B-cell activation and rescue from apoptosis. *Mol Cell Biol.* 1996 Oct;16(10):5546–5556.

[21] Taylor WE, Najmabadi H, Strathearn M, Jou NT, Liebling M, Rajavashisth T, et al. Human stem cell factor promoter deoxyribonucleic acid sequence and regulation by cyclic 3',5'-adenosine monophosphate in a Sertoli cell line. *Endocrinology.* 1996 Dec;137(12):5407–5414.

[22] Rossi P, Dolci S, Albanesi C, Grimaldi P, Ricca R, Geremia R. Follicle-stimulating hormone induction of steel factor (SLF) mRNA in mouse Sertoli cells and stimulation of DNA synthesis in spermatogonia by soluble SLF. *Dev Biol.* 1993 Jan;155(1):68–74.

[23] Packer AI, Besmer P, Bachvarova RF. Kit ligand mediates survival of type A spermatogonia and dividing spermatocytes in postnatal mouse testes. *Mol Reprod Dev.* 1995 Nov;42(3):303–310.

[24] Yan W, Suominen J, Toppari J. Stem cell factor protects germ cells from apoptosis in vitro. *J Cell Sci.* 2000 Jan;113 (Pt 1):161–168.

[25] Waeber G, Meyer TE, LeSieur M, Hermann HL, Gérard N, Habener JF. Developmental stage-specific expression of cyclic adenosine 3',5'-monophosphate response element-binding protein CREB during spermatogenesis involves alternative exon splicing. *Mol Endocrinol.* 1991 Oct;5(10):1418–1430.

[26] Scobey M, Bertera S, Somers J, Watkins S, Zeleznik A, Walker W. Delivery of a cyclic adenosine 3',5'-monophosphate response element-binding protein (creb) mutant to seminiferous tubules results in impaired spermatogenesis. *Endocrinology.* 2001 Feb;142(2):948–954.

[27] Jegou B, Sharpe RM. Paracrine mechanisms in testicular control. In: de Kretser D, editor. *Molecular biology of the male reproductive system.* Academic Press; 1993. p. 271–310.
[28] Sadate-Ngatchou PI, Pouchnik DJ, Griswold MD. Follicle-stimulating hormone induced changes in gene expression of murine testis. *Mol Endocrinol.* 2004 Nov;18(11):2805–2816.
[29] Foulkes NS, Schlotter F, Pévet P, Sassone-Corsi P. Pituitary hormone FSH directs the CREM functional switch during spermatogenesis. *Nature.* 1993 Mar;362(6417):264–267.
[30] Nantel F, Monaco L, Foulkes NS, Masquilier D, LeMeur M, Henriksén K, et al. Spermiogenesis deficiency and germ-cell apoptosis in CREM-mutant mice. *Nature.* 1996 Mar;380(6570):159–162.
[31] Foulkes NS, Mellstrom B, Benusiglio E, Sassone-Corsi P. Developmental switch of CREM function during spermatogenesis: from antagonist to activator. *Nature.* 1992;355:80–84.
[32] Sassone-Corsi P. CREM: a master-switch governing male germ cells differentiation and apoptosis. *Semin Cell Dev Biol.* 1998 Aug;9(4):475–482.
[33] Blendy JA, Kaestner KH, Weinbauer GF, Nieschlag E, Schütz G. Severe impairment of spermatogenesis in mice lacking the CREM gene. *Nature.* 1996 Mar;380(6570):162–165.
[34] Molina CA, Foulkes NS, Lalli E, Sassone-Corsi P. Inducibility and negative autoregulation of CREM: an alternative promoter directs the expression of ICER, an early response repressor. *Cell.* 1993 Dec;75(5):875–886.
[35] Chaudhary J, Sadler-Riggleman I, Ague JM, Skinner MK. The helix-loop-helix inhibitor of differentiation (ID) proteins induce post-mitotic terminally differentiated Sertoli cells to re-enter the cell cycle and proliferate. *Biol Reprod.* 2005 May;72(5):1205–1217.
[36] Chaudhary J, Johnson J, Kim G, Skinner MK. Hormonal regulation and differential actions of the helix-loop-helix transcriptional inhibitors of differentiation (Id1, Id2, Id3, and Id4) in Sertoli cells. *Endocrinology.* 2001 May;142(5):1727–1736.
[37] Weinbauer GF, Niechslag F. Hormonal control of spermatogenesis. In: de Kretser, editor. *Molecular biology of the male reproductive system.* Academic Press. San Diego; 1993. p. 101–142.
[38] Singh J, O'Neill C, Handelsman DJ. Induction of spermatogenesis by androgens in gonadotropin-deficient (hpg) mice. *Endocrinology.* 1995 Dec;136(12):5311–5321.
[39] Ghosh S, Sinha-Hikim AP, Russell LD. Further observations of stage-specific effects seen after short-term hypophysectomy in the rat. *Tissue Cell.* 1991;23(5):613–630.
[40] Kerr JB, Maddocks S, Sharpe RM. Testosterone and FSH have independent, synergistic and stage-dependent effects upon spermatogenesis in the rat testis. *Cell Tissue Res.* 1992;268(179-189).
[41] Franca LR, Parreira GG, Gates RJ, Russell LD. Hormonal regulation of spermatogenesis in the hypophysectomized rat: quantitation of germ-cell population and effect of elimination of residual testosterone after long-term hypophysectomy. *J Androl.* 1998;19(3):335–342.

[42] White R, Parker MG. Molecular mechanisms of steroid hormone action. Endocr *Relat Cancer*. 1998;5:1–14.
[43] Sar M, Lubahn DB, French FS, Wilson EM. Immunohistochemical localization of the androgen receptor in rat and human tissues. *Endocrinology*. 1990 Dec;127(6):3180–3186.
[44] Kimura N, Mizokami A, Oonuma T, Sasano H, Nagura H. Immunocytochemical localization of androgen receptor with polyclonal antibody in paraffin-embedded human tissues. *J Histochem Cytochem*. 1993 May;41(5):671–678.
[45] Bremner WJ, Millar MR, Sharpe RM, Saunders PT. Immunohistochemical localization of androgen receptors in the rat testis: evidence for stage-dependent expression and regulation by androgens. *Endocrinology*. 1994;135(3):1227–34.
[46] Tsai MY, Yeh SD, Wang RS, Yeh S, Zhang C, Lin HY, et al. Differential effects of spermatogenesis and fertility in mice lacking androgen receptor in individual testis cells. *Proc Natl Acad Sci U S A*. 2006 Dec;103(50):18975–18980.
[47] Johnston DS, Russell LD, Friel PJ, Griswold MD. Murine germ cells do not require functional androgen receptors to complete spermatogenesis following spermatogonial stem cell transplantation. *Endocrinology*. 2001;142(6):2405–8.
[48] Vornberger W, Prins G, Musto NA, Suarez-Quian CA. Androgen receptor distribution in rat testis: new implications for androgen regulation of spermatogenesis. *Endocrinology*. 1994 May;134(5):2307–2316.
[49] Zhu LJ, Hardy MP, Inigo IV, Huhtaniemi I, Bardin CW, Moo-Young AJ. Effects of androgen on androgen receptor expression in rat testicular and epididymal cells: a quantitative immunohistochemical study. *Biol Reprod*. 2000 Aug;63(2):368–376.
[50] Zhou Q, Nie R, Prins GS, Saunders PT, Katzenellenbogen BS, Hess RA. Localization of androgen and estrogen receptors in adult male mouse reproductive tract. *J Androl*. 2002;23(6):870–81.
[51] Ku CY, Loose-Mitchell DS, Sanborn BM. Both Sertoli and peritubular cells respond to androgens with increased expression of an androgen response element reporter. *Biol Reprod*. 1994 Aug;51(2):319–326.
[52] Gendt KD, Swinnen JV, Saunders PTK, Schoonjans L, Dewerchin M, Devos A, et al. A Sertoli cell-selective knockout of the androgen receptor causes spermatogenic arrest in meiosis. *Proc Natl Acad Sci U S A*. 2004 Feb;101(5):1327–1332.
[53] Chang C, Chen YT, Yeh SD, Xu Q, Wang RS, Guillou F, et al. Infertility with defective spermatogenesis and hypotestosteronemia in male mice lacking the androgen receptor in Sertoli cells. *Proc Natl Acad Sci U S A*. 2004 May;101(18):6876–6881.
[54] Denolet E, Gendt KD, Allemeersch J, Engelen K, Marchal K, Hummelen PV, et al. The effect of a sertoli cell-selective knockout of the androgen receptor on testicular gene expression in prepubertal mice. *Mol Endocrinol*. 2006 Feb;20(2):321–334.
[55] Wang RS, Yeh S, M CL, Lin HY, Zhang C, Ni J, et al. Androgen receptor in Sertoli cells is essential for germ cell nursery and junctional complex formation in mouse testis. *Endocrinology*. 2006;147:5624–5633.
[56] Hales DB, Sha LL, Payne AH. Testosterone inhibits cAMP-induced de Novo synthesis of Leydig cell cytochrome P-450(17 alpha) by an androgen receptor-mediated mechanism. *J Biol Chem*. 1987 Aug;262(23):11200–11206.

[57] De Gendt K, V SJ, Saunders PT, Schoonjans L, Dewerchin M, Devos A, et al. A Sertoli cell-selective knockout of the androgen receptor causes spermatogenesis arrest in meiosis. *Proc Natl Acad Sci USA.* 2004;101:1327–1332.

[58] Petrusz P, Jeyaraj DA, Grossman G. Microarray analysis of androgen-regulated gene expression in testis: the use of the androgen-binding protein (ABP)-transgenic mouse as a model. *Reprod Biol Endocrinol.* 2005;3:70.

[59] Sadate-Ngatchou PI, Pouchnik DJ, Griswold MD. Identification of testosterone-regulated genes in testes of hypogonadal mice using oligonucleotide microarray. *Mol Endocrinol.* 2004 Feb;18(2):422–433.

[60] Haeussler S, Wagner A, Welter H, Claus R. Changes of testicular aromatase expression during fetal development in male pigs (Sus scrofa). *Reproduction.* 2007 Jan;133(1):323–330.

[61] Pentikainen V, Erkkila K, Suomalainen L, Parvinen M, Dunkel L. Estradiol acts as a germ cell survival factor in the human testis in vitro. *J Clin Endocrinol Metab.* 2000;85(5):2057–67.

[62] Taylor AH, Al-Azzawi F. Immunolocalisation of oestrogen receptor beta in human tissues. *J Mol Endocrinol.* 2000 Feb;24(1):145–155.

[63] Aquila S, Sisci D, Gentile M, Middea E, Siciliano L, Andò S. Human ejaculated spermatozoa contain active P450 aromatase. *J Clin Endocrinol Metab.* 2002 Jul;87(7):3385–3390.

[64] Aquila S, Sisci D, Gentile M, Middea E, Catalano S, Carpino A, et al. Estrogen receptor (ER)alpha and ER beta are both expressed in human ejaculated spermatozoa: evidence of their direct interaction with phosphatidylinositol-3-OH kinase/Akt pathway. *J Clin Endocrinol Metab.* 2004 Mar;89(3):1443–1451.

[65] Rago V, Aquila S, Panza R, Carpino A. Cytochrome P450arom, androgen and estrogen receptors in pig sperm. *Reprod Biol Endocrinol.* 2007;5:23.

[66] Ebling FJ, Brooks AN, Cronin AS, Ford H, Kerr JB. Estrogenic induction of spermatogenesis in the hypogonadal mouse. *Endocrinology.* 2000 Aug;141(8):2861–2869.

[67] Ebling FJP, Nwagwu MO, Baines H, Myers M, Kerr JB. The hypogonadal (hpg) mouse as a model to investigate the estrogenic regulation of spermatogenesis. *Hum Fertil (Camb).* 2006 Sep;9(3):127–135.

[68] Baines H, Nwagwu MO, Hastie GR, Wiles RA, Mayhew TM, Ebling FJ. Effects of estradiol and FSH on maturation of the testis in the hypogonadal (hpg) mouse. *Reprod Biol Endocrinol.* 2008;6:4.

[69] Hacker A, Capel B, Goodfellow P, Lovell-Badge R. Expression of Sry, the mouse sex determining gene. *Development.* 1995 Jun;121(6):1603–1614.

[70] Lovell-Badge R, Hacker A. The molecular genetics of Sry and its role in mammalian sex determination. *Philos Trans R Soc Lond B Biol Sci.* 1995 Nov;350(1333):205–214.

[71] Jégou B. The Sertoli cell in vivo and in vitro. *Cell Biol Toxicol.* 1992;8(3):49–54.

[72] Ketola I, Anttonen M, Vaskivuo T, Tapanainen JS, Toppari J, Heikinheimo M. Developmental expression and spermatogenic stage specificity of transcription factors GATA-1 and GATA-4 and their cofactors FOG-1 and FOG-2 in the mouse testis. *Eur J Endocrinol.* 2002 Sep;147(3):397–406.

[73] Holsberger DR, Jirawatnotai S, Kiyokawa H, Cooke PS. Thyroid hormone regulates the cell cycle inhibitor p27Kip1 in postnatal murine Sertoli cells. *Endocrinology.* 2003 Sep;144(9):3732–3738.

[74] Law GL, Griswold MD. Activity and form of sulfated glycoprotein 2 (clusterin) from cultured Sertoli cells, testis, and epididymis of the rat. *Biol Reprod.* 1994 Mar;50(3):669–679.

[75] Schlatt S, de Kretser DM, Loveland KL. Discriminative analysis of rat Sertoli and peritubular cells and their proliferation in vitro: evidence for follicle-stimulating hormone-mediated contact inhibition of Sertoli cell mitosis. *Biol Reprod.* 1996 Aug;55(2):227–235.

[76] Norton JN, Skinner MK. Regulation of Sertoli cell differentiation by the testicular paracrine factor PModS: potential role of immediate-early genes. *Mol Endocrinol.* 1992 Dec;6(12):2018–2026.

[77] Russell LD. Movement of spermatocytes from the basal to the adluminal compartment of the rat testis. *Am J Anat.* 1977;148:313–328.

[78] Holdcraft RW, Braun RE. Androgen receptor function is required in Sertoli cells for the terminal differentiation of haploid spermatids. *Development.* 2004;131:459–467.

[79] Tan KAL, Gendt KD, Atanassova N, Walker M, Sharpe RM, Saunders PTK, et al. The role of androgens in Sertoli cell proliferation and functional maturation: studies in mice with total or Sertoli cell-selective ablation of the androgen receptor. *Endocrinology.* 2005 Jun;146(6):2674–2683.

[80] Wong CH, Xia W, Lee NPY, Mruk DD, Lee WM, Cheng CY. Regulation of ectoplasmic specialization dynamics in the seminiferous epithelium by focal adhesion-associated proteins in testosterone-suppressed rat testes. *Endocrinology.* 2005 Mar;146(3):1192–1204.

[81] Xia W, Wong CH, Lee NPY, Lee WM, Cheng CY. Disruption of Sertoli-germ cell adhesion function in the seminiferous epithelium of the rat testis can be limited to adherens junctions without affecting the blood-testis barrier integrity: an in vivo study using an androgen suppression model. *J Cell Physiol.* 2005 Oct;205(1):141–157.

[82] Zhang J, Wong CH, Xia W, Mruk DD, Lee NPY, Lee WM, et al. Regulation of Sertoli-germ cell adherens junction dynamics via changes in protein-protein interactions of the N-cadherin-beta-catenin protein complex which are possibly mediated by c-Src and myotubularin-related protein 2: an in vivo study using an androgen suppression model. *Endocrinology.* 2005 Mar;146(3):1268–1284.

[83] Xia W, Mruk DD, Lee WM, Cheng CY. Differential interactions between transforming growth factor-beta3/TbetaR1, TAB1, and CD2AP disrupt blood-testis barrier and Sertoli-germ cell adhesion. *J Biol Chem.* 2006 Jun;281(24):16799–16813.

[84] Yan HHN, Mruk DD, Lee WM, Cheng CY. Blood-testis barrier dynamics are regulated by testosterone and cytokines via their differential effects on the kinetics of protein endocytosis and recycling in Sertoli cells. *FASEB J.* 2008 Jan;.

[85] Yan HHN, Mruk DD, Cheng CY. Junction restructuring and spermatogenesis: the biology, regulation, and implication in male contraceptive development. *Curr Top Dev Biol.* 2008;80:57–92.

[86] Timmons PM, Rigby PWJ, Poirier F. The murine seminiferous epithelial cycle is prefigured in the Sertoli cells of the embryonic testis. *Development.* 2002 Feb;129(3):635–647.
[87] Franca LR, Ogawa T, Avarbock MR, Brinster RL, Russell LD. Germ cell genotype controls cell cycle during spermatogenesis in the rat. *Biol Reprod.* 1998 Dec;59(6):1371–1377.
[88] Elftman H. The Sertoli cell cycle in the mouse. *Anat Rec.* 1950;106:381–393.
[89] Anway MD, Li Y, Ravindranath N, Dym M, Griswold MD. Expression of testicular germ cell genes identified by differential display analysis. *J Androl.* 2003;24(2):173–184.
[90] Almstrup K, Nielsen JE, Hansen MA, Tanaka M, Skakkebaek NE, Leffers H. Analysis of cell-type-specific gene expression during mouse spermatogenesis. *Biol Reprod.* 2004 Jun;70(6):1751–1761.
[91] Clemente EJ, Furlong RA, Loveland KL, Affara NA. Gene expression study in the juvenile mouse testis: identification of stage-specific molecular pathways during spermatogenesis. *Mamm Genome.* 2006 Sep;17(9):956–975.
[92] Lindsey JS, Wilkinson MF. A testosterone- and LH-regulated homeobox gene expressed in mouse Sertoli cells and epididymis. *Dev Biol.* 1996;174:471–484.
[93] Lim K, Yoo JH, Kim kY, Kweon GR, Kwak ST, Hwang BD. Testosterone regulation of proto-oncogene c-myc expression in primary Sertoli cell cultures from prepubertal rats. *J Androl.* 1994;15:543–550.
[94] O'Donnell L, Robertson KM, Jones ME, Simpson ER. Estrogen and spermatogenesis. *Endocr Rev.* 2001 Jun;22(3):289–318.
[95] Silva FRMB, Leite LD, Wassermann GF. Rapid signal transduction in Sertoli cells. *Eur J Endocrinol.* 2002 Sep;147(3):425–433.
[96] Cheng J, Watkins SC, Walker WH. Testosterone activates mitogen-activated protein kinase via Src kinase and the epidermal growth factor receptor in sertoli cells. *Endocrinology.* 2007 May;148(5):2066–2074.
[97] Fix C, Jordan C, Cano P, Walker WH. Testosterone activates mitogen-activated protein kinase and the cAMP response element binding protein transcription factor in Sertoli cells. *Proc Natl Acad Sci U S A.* 2004 Jul;101(30):10919–10924.

In: Trends in Testosterone Research
Editor: Raymund E. Veritos
ISBN: 978-1-60456-127-2

Chapter V

Testosterone Depletion and Cognitive Impairment in Aging Men: A Possible Relationship Between Testosterone and Alzheimer's Disease?

Martine Simard [*] [1]***, Séverine Hervouet*** [2] ***and Hélène Forget*** [3]
[1] École de psychologie, Université Laval, and Centre de Recherche Université Laval-Robert-Giffard, Quebec City, Quebec, Canada
[2] École de psychologie, Université Laval, and Centre de recherche en cancérologie de l'Université Laval, Hôtel-Dieu de Québec (CHUQ), Quebec City, Quebec, Canada
[3] Département de psychoéducation et de psychologie, Université du Québec en Outaouais, Gatineau, Quebec, Canada, and École de psychologie, Université de Moncton, Moncton, New Brunswick, Canada

Abstract

Introduction: Animal research demonstrated a link between reductions in testosterone (T) levels, the development of the amyloid beta (Aβ) and tau (τ) proteins, and the presence of the APOEε4 allele. The Aβ and τ proteins are neuropathological characteristics whereas the APOEε4 allele is a risk factor for Alzheimer's disease (AD). On the other hand, several studies performed in men showed that a decline in T correlates with aging. Given that the risk to develop AD increases with age, some researchers proposed a relationship between the development of AD and reductions of T. Should this hypothesis be true, links should exist between aging, AD, cognitive deficits and depletion of T, and between T substitution treatment and cognition in elderly hypogonadal and AD men. The goal of this chapter was therefore to critically review the studies examining, in elderly hypogonadal and AD men, the T levels and cognitive functioning, and the effects of T substitution treatment on cognition.

[*] Address of correspondence: Dr. Martine Simard, École de psychologie, Pavillon Félix-Antoine Savard, Université Laval, Québec, Québec, G1K 7P4, Canada. E-mail : Martine.Simard@psy.ulaval.ca

Method: A search of MEDLINE and PsycInfo databases was conducted in order to identify articles published between 1994 and 2006. The key terms included "testosterone", "male hormone", "androgens", "gonadotropin", "cognition", "cognitive function", "Alzheimer's disease", "dementia", "aging", and "men". English-language, peer-reviewed articles were included. The populations of the reviewed studies were men aged of 50 years and greater. The studies assessing cognition and T levels had to use standardized measures, and were required to present diagnostic and/or control group comparisons. The treatment studies had to use at least placebo-control designs. Human single-cases were excluded.

Results: Analyses of the reviewed data showed that T levels were generally lower in the AD than healthy groups, and that elderly men with high T levels had better cognition than those with low T levels. Some studies however did not report any relationship between T levels and cognition. T substitution treatments generally yielded improvement in memory, executive and visuospatial functions in healthy elderly and AD men with and without hypogonadism.

Conclusion: Methodological limitations of the existing data include the lack of longitudinal studies, and small sample size in clinical trials for AD. However, there seems to be a relationship between pathological aging, cognitive impairment and reductions of T.

Keywords: Testosterone, androgens, Alzheimer's disease, cognition, aging.

Introduction

Alzheimer's disease (AD) is the most common cause of dementia in the elderly population. AD has affected 4.5 million individuals in the USA in 2000, and this prevalence will be three-fold in 2050 [1]. The prevalence estimates of the Canadian Study of Health and Aging have suggested that 5.1% of the Canadians aged 65 years and greater suffer from AD. If the prevalence estimates remain constant, 592,000 Canadians will present with AD by year 2021 [2]. The high prevalence of AD is thus an important international phenomenon.

Although the etiopathogenesis is still unknown, the neuropathological characteristics of AD, i.e. the senile plaques and neurofibrillary tangles, are relatively well described. Senile plaques are spheric and extracellular lesions presenting with amyloid deposits in their centers, which are associated with distorted neuronal processes called dystrophic neurites (Munoz et al. [3], for a review). The cerebral amyloid is principally made up of a protein called amyloid beta (Aβ) protein, a derived fragment of the transmembrane protein, amyloid beta protein precursor (A-βPP). In AD, this protein (Aβ) is produced in excess, accumulates in deposits, and thus constitutes the central part of the senile plaque. The neurofibrillary tangles (NFT) are intraneuronal lesions made up of abnormal neurofilaments. Biochemical analyses of these lesions have targeted the protein tau (τ) which is hyperphosphorylated (Touchon et al. [4], for a review). These neuropathological abnormalities precede and cause the neuronal deaths and losses observed in AD.

Many risk factors associated with AD have been identified over the past fifteen years, such as aging, being female, genetic factors related to chromosomes 21, 1, and 14, as well as the presence of the apolipoprotein gene (ApoE) coded on the chromosome 19 [3-6]. Aging itself is certainly the greatest risk factor. Recent research has identified two mechanisms related to aging that may potentially explain the development of the disease. On one hand, aging is associated with the production of free radicals which leads to an increase in βA deposits and aggregations, thus causing neurotoxicity. On the other hand, changes in the ribonucleic acid (RNA) messenger corresponding to the production of A-βPP are also involved in the development of AD (Munoz et al. [3], for a review).

Although AD is generally a random phenomenon, 5% to 10% of cases are autosomal dominant genetically transmitted[5]. Chromosome 21 codes A-βPP. When changes occur on this chromosome, there is an increase in βA. In addition, mutations on chromosomes 1 and 14 are often found in cases with familial AD. Interestingly, even if AD is a random phenomenon, a common genetic polymorphism affecting the apolipoprotein gene (ApoE) is strongly associated with a major risk of developing of AD, independently of age (Raber et al.[7], for a review). ApoE is a lipid protein coded by a gene on chromosome 19. The ApoE gene exists in 3 homologous allelic forms: ε2, ε3 and ε4. It was shown that an individual is five to fifteen times more likely to develop AD when the allele ε4 is present. On the contrary, the allele ε2 was shown to offer a modest protection against AD.[3,6]

Being female constitutes another risk factor for developing AD. This can be partly explained by the longer life expectancy generally found in women. ApoE4 interacts with female gender, further increasing the risk of AD and diminishing treatment efficacy in women. [8,9] In addition, hormonal changes, especially the decline in estrogen, are another plausible explanation for the development of AD. [10,11] Some research demonstrated that the estrogenic status in women modulates the metabolism of Aβ, the principal neurotoxic component of the cerebral amyloid associated with the disease. Low levels of estrogen would thus be associated with the increase of the beta-amyloid peptides, and high levels of estrogen would be associated with a reduction of the beta-amyloid peptides . [12,13]

More recently, several animal and laboratory research have demonstrated a link between reductions in testosterone (T) levels, the development of the amyloid beta (Aβ) and tau (τ) proteins, and the presence of the APOEε4 allele. [14-16] In addition, several clinical studies performed in men have shown that a decline in T correlates with aging. [17,18] Given that the risk to develop AD increases with age [1], some researchers have proposed that the depletion of T might be a supplementary risk factor for the development of AD. [19,20] Should this hypothesis be true, there should be some correlations between normal aging, depletion of T, T supplement treatment and cognition, as well as between AD, depletion of T, and improvement of cognitive functions following T supplement treatment.

Therefore, the principal goal of this chapter is to understand and also verify a possible relationship between the T levels, cognitive functioning and development of Alzheimer's disease in elderly men. In a first step to achieve this overarching goal, and to facilitate the comprehension of the reader regarding this matter, the hormonal mechanism and normal hormonal changes in elderly men will be briefly described. Then the selective literature review providing a biological and molecular rationale to our working hypothesis will be presented through brief sections describing the findings of some animal and human neuronal tissue culture studies establishing correlations between T levels, the development of the amyloid beta (Aβ) and tau (τ) proteins, and the presence of the APOEε4 allele. These sections will be followed by the results of the critical review on the clinical studies examining, in healthy elderly and AD men, the T levels and cognitive functioning (respectively sections 3.1 and 4.1), and the effects of T substitution treatment on cognition in healthy elderly men (section 3.2) and patients with AD (section 4.2). The following discussion will briefly summarize the data and address important clinical and research issues related to the topic.

Search Method

A comprehensive search of the computerized database MEDLINE, Current Content and PsycInfo has been conducted in order to identify articles published between January 1994 and May 2006, and investigating the relationship between T and cognition, T and AD, and T substitution treatment and AD. The following search key terms have been utilized: "testosterone", "male hormone", "androgens", "gonadotropin", "cognition", "cognitive function", "Alzheimer's disease", "dementia" and "men". Only English written articles published in peer-reviewed journals have been included. All the clinical studies included in the review had to be realized on an aging male population (aged 50-91 years). The studies presented in tables 1, 2 and 4 had to use standardized and well-validated neuropsychological tests. The clinical trials included in tables 2 and 4 were required to use at least a placebo-controlled study design in order to be reviewed. In the sections reviewing the results of animal and clinical studies, single-case studies were excluded.

Results of the Review

1. Male Hormonal Mechanism

1.1. Brief Review of the Physiology of the Hypothalamic-Pituitary-Gonadal Axis (HPG) in Men

In men, testes and adrenals secrete several male sex hormones called androgens. T is the most potent and abundant of the androgens and regulates a variety of bodily functions related especially to male reproductive function. Leydig cells, localized in the testes, produce T, while Sertoli cells promote spermatogenesis. The normal reproductive function is principally controlled by the action of two hormones of the anterior pituitary gland: the luteinizing hormone (LH) and the follicle-stimulating hormone (FSH). The LH and FSH are secreted in a pulsative manner under the influence of the gonadotropin-releasing hormone (GnRH) secreted by the hypothalamus. [21] A negative feedback loop of T towards the hypothalamus inhibits the hypothalamic secretion of GnRH, inhibiting the liberation of LH and FSH. Like most hormones, T is supplied to target tissues in the blood where much of it is bound transported to specific plasma proteins called *sex hormone binding globulin* (SHBG) and albumin.

T diffuses into the plasma in three fractions: 1) the free T (unbound to SHBG or to albumin); 2) the bioavailable fraction (composed of free fraction (FT) and fraction bound to albumin); and 3) total T (TT comprised of FT and bioavailable T (bT) [22,23]). The concentration of T in the plasma is generally very high in the morning, falling throughout the day, and reaching a minimum in the evening. [24,25]

T can be made biologically inactive by sex hormone binding globulin (SHBG), which does not permit it to bind to receptors. This antagonism is important because SHBG increases with aging, changes in hormone levels, and in various medical disorders. In fact, the FT and the albumin bound represent the fraction readily available for biological action. Consequently, only considering 'TT' levels may not reflect the T biologically active. [26]

1.2. Changing Androgen Levels in Elderly Men

Unlike menopausal women, men do not experience an abrupt interruption in reproductive functioning. However, it seems that average T levels decrease with age, especially after age 50. [17] In fact, the prevalence of bT deficiency in men aged 55 and over is as high as 50%.[27] Causal explanations for this age-related decline in T are complex and multifactorial. The most important change appears to be peripheral testicular deterioration, as evidenced by a reduction in the number of Leydig cells. The decrease in Leydig cells and secretion of T result in an increase in LH and FSH levels, causing the pulsative secretion of these substances (LH and FSH) to be irregular and of variable quantity. Changes occurring in the HPG axis are related to the asynchronic production of GnRH, and seem to influence the LH response. [18, 28, 29] Finally, a rise in SHBG concentration levels occurs with age, resulting in a reduction of FT and bT in the blood. [18]

To date, the exact parameters of the androgen deficiency (or hypogonadism) are still uncertain, although some authors provide a range of 'normality' for men (total T levels of 3-10 ng/ml or 10-35 nmol/L) and women (< 1ng/ml or < 3.5 nmol/L). [30] In elderly men, hypogonadism principally results in a dysfunction of the pituitary gland, and gonadotrophin deficiency. Thus, as men age, serum T levels tend to decline, and some older men develop a common syndrome called « andropause ».[21] While andropause does occur, it is still under diagnosed because its symptoms are similar to the normal effects of aging.

Several studies have shown that a decline in the bT fraction of plasmatic T correlates most strongly with aging and the physical and cognitive deficits that accompany it. [31, 32] As bT decreases with age, its effects on the body also decline. Clinical manifestations of hypogonadism in older men include a range of symptoms, such as diminished libido and sexual functioning, decreased muscle mass (sarcopenia) and bone density (osteoporosis), fatigue, irritability, and cognitive abnormalities. [18, 33, 34] Several studies have otherwise demonstrated the neuroprotective effect of T on the preservation of cognitive functions. [31, 35, 36]

2. Rationale for the Involvement of Testosterone in the Development of Cognitive Impairment and Alzheimer's Disease

2.1. Biological Rationale for the Involvement of Testosterone in Cognition

T is lipid soluble, thus it can enter cells throughout the body and nervous system regardless of whether there are androgen receptors (AR) in the cell. However, only in cells where it encounters a receptor does it form a complex that will influence protein synthesis in the nucleus of a neuron, and modify cell function. This modification can be in the form of specific changes in neurotransmitter production and release, synapse conformation that modifies efficacy, as well as many other possibilities. [26]

Animal studies have revealed that the mechanisms potentially underlying the association between androgen levels and cognition may be partly explained by the massive presence of androgen receptors (AR) in the telencephalon, and to a lesser extent, in the diencephalons. [37] Interestingly, the number of AR positive cells is greater in areas not considered to be primary components of the neural circuits involved in reproductive sexual behavior, and neuroendocrine regulation. [37] In nonhuman primates, AR have been found particularly numerous in the hippocampus, amygdala and prefrontal cortex, which are brain areas involved in learning and memory ([38, 39], for reviews). Moreover, androgens have been shown to have a functional impact upon neurons in the hippocampal formation, since they protect hippocampal pyramidal neurons from excitotoxicity both in vivo [40] and in vitro [41].

T has been shown to modulate neurotransmitters. For example, gonadectomy has selectively reduced acetylcholine levels in hippocampus and anterior cingulate cortex but not in other regions [42], and transiently decreased then increased dopamine innervation in cingulate cortex of rats [43]. T has also produced increased firing of serotonin neurons in male rats, although gonadectomy had no effect. [44]

In addition, in regions of the occipital cortex involved in visual discrimination tasks on which males outperform females [45], more AR immunoreactive neurons have been observed in male compared with female neonatal rats. [46] In contrast, no sex differences in AR-immunoreactive cell number have been observed in the anterior cingulate/frontal cortex, a region that has been proposed to undergo sexual differentiation in response to activation of estrogen receptors. [47, 48] These results suggest that the occipital and cingulate/frontal cortices may be differentially responsive to the effects of developmental exposure to androgens versus estrogens (DonCarlos et al. [37], for a review).

There is now evidence that androgens impact on the rate of development of specific cortical functions. In the studies of Goldman-Rakic (see Bachevalier and Hagger [49], for a review), it has been demonstrated that male infant monkeys outperformed females on an object discrimination reversal task that relies on the prefrontal cortex, and that androgens accelerate maturation of this brain region. Using a concurrent object discrimination task to measure learning of visual discrimination, a function attributed to the temporal cortex, Bachevalier and Hagger [49] showed that female infant monkeys outperformed males.

The above mentioned hormonal actions on brain structures are important in regards to the continuum of dementia, i.e. in mild cognitive impairment (MCI) and Alzheimer's disease. Neuropathological abnormalities [50] and atrophy of the hippocampal formation [51, 52] have been described in MCI and AD, and are consistent with verbal and spatial episodic memory deficits reported as the earliest symptoms of these two conditions [53-55] (Simard and van Reekum, [56], for a review).

The following sections will briefly present the research data on animal and human neuronal tissue cultures showing some correlations between T, βA, β-APP, tau (τ) protein, and the ε4 allele, all of which are factors in the development of AD.

2.2 Relationship between Testosterone and Alzheimer's Neuropathology

2.2.1. Animal and Neuronal Tissue Culture Research

Some evidence suggests that T may be implicated in the development of AD by exerting a neurotrophic action on the aging brain. [14, 16, 57, 58] Some laboratory studies have demonstrated that T influences some markers of AD. Upon examining neuronal cultures, Gouras et al. [57] reported that T treatment contributed to an increase in the secretion of non amyloidogenic β-APP fragment and a decrease in the secretion of Aβ. In addition, Papasozomenos and Shavanas [14] have determined that T prevented the hyperphosphorylation of τ, a component of AD.

Recently, researchers have indicated that the depletion of endogenous sexual steroid hormones in gonadectomized male rats resulted in increased brain levels of Aβ (the principal neurotoxic component of the cerebral amyloid found in AD), compared to male rats with intact gonads. These results suggested that T may also contribute to regulate the production of this protein. [16]

The observations of Pike [58] have supported the previous data by confirming that physiologic levels of T significantly protected cultured rat hippocampal neurons cells *in vitro* from cell death induced by the AD-related insult βA. This author explained that βA neurotoxicity has been significantly reduced by T via a rapid estrogen-independent mechanism which remained to be fully elucidated.

Another study has demonstrated that ApoEε4 male mice which had performed normally at baseline, presented major deficits in spatial learning and memory on the *water-maze test* following blockade of AR. The ApoEε3 male mice did not develop these difficulties. [15] Another study realized by the same team of researchers has also shown that castrated ApoEε4 male mice had impaired novel location recognition. [59]

2.2.2. Human Cell Culture and Pathological Research

Recently, a laboratory study has investigated whether androgens could prevent intracellular Aβ peptide (i$A\beta_{1\text{-}42}$) toxicity using primary cultures of human neurons. [60] The researchers have reported that physiological concentrations of androgens completely protected human neurons in primary cultures against microinjected i$A\beta_{1\text{-}42}$ toxicity. The mechanism underlying this relation might be that AR antagonists increase the level of heat shock protein 70 in the neurons. Heat shock protein 70 is a cell-protective agent considered as a molecular "chaperone" that can play a role in several neurodegeneration models. [61]

Rosario et al. [62] investigated T and estradiol levels in the postmortem brain tissues of elderly men with different neuropathological diagnoses. Three groups were compared: 1) neuropathologically normal (controls; n = 17); 2) AD (Braak stage 5-6; n = 19), and 3) mild neuropathological changes (Braak stage 2-3; n = 9). The authors have found that brain levels of T but not estradiol were significantly lower in AD compared with control subjects. They also have evidenced that brain levels of T were significantly reduced in men presenting with neuropathological characteristics consistent with an early stage of AD.

However, Twist et al. [63] have found that the T levels in the frontal cortex tissues were similar in AD patients (n = 5) and controls (n = 7). However the T levels were slightly, yet not significantly, lower in the temporal cortex of patients with AD compared to that of controls. The small sample size might be responsible for a lack of statistical power, and might perhaps explain the non significant results obtained by these authors.

Altogether, these studies suggest that gonadic hormones play a key role in the control of Aβ levels. It seems that an androgenic decline leads to an Aβ accumulation in some cerebral areas, and thus may represent a risk factor for the development of AD. In addition, T appears to offer some neuroprotection against neuronal injury, principally by reducing the secretion Aβ peptides and Aβ-induced neuronal toxicity.

2.2.3. Association between T Levels and ApoEε4

Hogervorst et al. [64] have investigated the link between T levels and the ApoEε4 allele in human subjects. In their study, two groups of males were compared i.e. a group with definite (autopsied) or probable AD ($n = 61$) and a control group ($n = 53$). Their results have revealed that T levels were lower in ApoEε4-positive controls than in those without ApoEε4. In addition, in men without ApoEε4, T levels were lower in subjects with AD compared to controls. The authors concluded that low T is a potentially modifiable risk factor, which may prove particularly relevant for ApoEε4 carriers at risk of developing AD.

Recently, the review of Raber [7] has suggested that androgens might be neuroprotective by antagonizing the detrimental effects of ApoEε4 on AR function. In fact, the author hypothesized that this consequence contributes to cognitive impairments such as deficits of spatial learning and memory, which are the principal cognitive functions impaired in early AD. This hypothesis has been confirmed by animal studies.[65] More research is however mandatory to elucidate the effects of ApoEε4 on AR function, and risks of AD.

2.2.4. Gonadotropin and AD

With age, men experience an increase in LH and FSH secretion. Surprisingly, the effects of increased circulating gonadotropin on the healthy aging brain have been scarcely explored. However, Bowen et al. [66] have attempted to elucidate the role of gonadotropin in the development and progression of AD. [66] In this study, serum concentrations of FSH, LH and T have been assayed in two groups of male subjects. The results revealed that the levels of circulating LH and FSH were significantly higher, and T was significantly lower in 40 patients with dementia, compared to 29 age-matched controls. The authors suggested that gonadotropins may contribute to the pathogenesis of AD.

Recently, Bowen et al. [67] have reported a significant increase in LH in the cytoplasm of pyramidal neurons and neurofibrillary tangles of AD brains ($n = 6$) compared to age-matched controls ($n = 7$). Unfortunately, given the small sample size, these results can hardly be generalized.

On the other hand, two studies did not find any difference between AD and control males in the average LH and FSH, using multivariate models controlling for age. [68, 69] According to Short et al. [69] the small sample size (AD, $n = 48$; healthy controls, $n=53$), and a type II error might have been responsible for their lack of significant results. However, the authors performed a paired analysis to clarify the differences among males, and have matched the AD patients within 3 years of age with a control group ($n = 38$). The rank sum tests were then statistically significant for LH ($p = 0.04$) but not for FSH.

The men studied by Hogervorst et al. [68] were younger than those studied by Bowen et al.. [66] This fact might have explained the discrepant results between the two studies, since gonadotropin levels increase with age. As presented earlier, LH concentrations increase when the T age-related decline occurs in men. The results of Hogervorst' study [68] thus have supported the "gonadotropin hypothesis" proposed by Gregory and Bowen [70] before these authors [68] controlled for the correlation between gonadotropin and age in the AD group. Following this control, there was no difference in gonadotropin concentrations between the AD and control groups. The "gonadotropin hypothesis" elaborated by Gregory and Bowen has primarily postulated that the detrimental effects attributed to estrogen could be attributed to an increase in LH.

A recent mechanistic link has been proposed by Casadesus et al. [71] to explain the evidence for the role of LH in the development of AD. Considering that an elevation of LH parallels the ectopic expression of cell cycle and oxidative markers that represent one of the initiating pathological changes preceding neuronal degeneration by decades, it is likely, given this temporal and spatial overlap with mitotic changes in AD, that elevations in LH are responsible for inappropriate cell cycle reentry in neurons. This hypothesis however does not preclude the involvement of other hormones of the HPG axis. Previous studies [70, 72] have shown that LH has mitogenic properties and could initiate the cell cycle abnormalities in neurons. LH receptors are present within the hippocampus, a brain region susceptible to modulate neurodegenerative changes. These observations possibly indicate an emerging role of LH in the development and progression of AD.

3. Clinical Studies on Testosterone Levels and Cognition in Healthy Elderly Men

3.1. Testosterone Parameters and Cognitive Function in Men

Table 1 presents the results of 11 studies that especially investigated the relationship between T parameters and cognitive functioning in healthy elderly men. Nine of these studies utilized a cross-sectional design and two of them a prospective longitudinal design. Five of these studies had a large sample including more than three hundred community-dwellings participants. Six studies had a small sample size (n from 24 to 79), and were thus at risk to lack statistical power.

Barret-Connor et al. [35] and Yaffe et al. [32] showed that the highest levels of bT were positively correlated with cognition, especially on tests of memory (BIMC, VRT), executive (TMT B), attention and working memory functions (MMSE- Spelling 'WORD' backwards; Digit Symbol). Aleman et al. [73] have found that TT was associated with good visuospatial construction praxis (Block Design), mental flexibility (Concept Shifting task) and working memory (Digit Symbol).

In a recent paper from the Massachusetts Male Aging population-based cohort study (n = 981) [74], least squares regression analyses were performed using working memory, speed/attention, and spatial ability tests as cognitive variables, and FT, TT, dehydroepiandrosterone (DHEA), dehydroepiandrosterone sulfate (DHEAS), androstanediol glucuronide (3 alpha-A-diol-gluc), LH, FSH, SHBG, prolactin, estrone, and cortisol as hormonal variables. In unadjusted models, the results showed that logged TT was positively associated with working memory (but was not associated with speed/attention or spatial relations). Logged 3 alpha-A-diol-gluc was positively associated with speed/attention tasks, and logged LH was negatively associated with speed/attention and spatial relation tasks. Logged FT, DHEA, and DHEAS were positively associated with increased functioning in all cognitive domains (working memory, speed/attention and spatial relations).

Hogervorst et al. [75] found a positive association between spatial recognition and total T. However, the other cognitive functions were not positively correlated with concentrations of sex steroids. These authors suggested that there may be a time window during which hormones show a positive relationship with certain cognitive functions in men (e.g. speed of information processing). In addition, several authors have identified an inverted U (quadratic) relationship between T and cognitive ability, suggesting an optimum T level for some cognitive functions. [76-78]

In the study of Burkhardt et al. [79] conducted in healthy elderly men., the APOEε4 carriers were significantly older (74.3 ± 5.3 years old) than the non carriers (69.5 ± 6.7), and there was a positive correlation between FT, APOEε4 and general cognitive functioning as measured with the CAMCOG-R. Executive and working memory functions were also positively correlated with FT and APOEε4. However, in APOEε4 non carriers, there were negative correlations between FT levels and performances on tests of executive, working memory and attention functions.

However, Perry et al. [80] concluded that bT was not an important determinant of cognitive function. The age range of the population (55-75 years) in the Perry study may explain the negative results. It is possible that by the age of 75, the bT concentrations do not drop sufficiently to produce significant alterations in cognition. In the study of Wolf and Kirschbaum [81], a negative correlation was reported between endogenous T levels and verbal fluency in older men, but this negative relationship became non significant when formal education and age were controlled for in the analyses. Finally, Carlson & Sherwin [82] did not find any association between T and any neuropsychological test in men.

All the studies presented in the previous paragraphs used a cross-sectional design, and three of them found no significant results. Interestingly, these three studies had a small sample size, thus it is possible that they lacked statistical power. However, even with significant positive results, cross-sectional designs cannot properly establish a causal relationship between depletions of the sex steroid hormones and cognitive deficits.

In order to overcome this limitation, Moffat et al. [83] used a longitudinal study design and demonstrated that FT may serve as a marker of cognitive performance, especially on tests of verbal and visual episodic memory, executive and spatial functions. These results thus clearly suggested a possible neuroprotective effect of T on brain and cognitive functions in elderly men.

Nevertheless, a recent longitudinal study [84] found no significant correlations between baseline sex hormones (T, estradiol, and estrone) concentrations and tests of executive functions, episodic and working memory, even when adjusting the SHBG concentrations. Because they found a significant positive relationship between T and cerebral volumes (frontal and parietal lobes), the authors concluded that the role for sex hormones in brain volume might predate potential associations between sex hormones and cognitive task performance.

In summary, despite some contradictory findings, it seems that bT is one of the markers of aging that correlates best with cognitive performance. One possible explanation is that bT crosses the hemato-encephalic barrier more easily than TT. Moreover, levels of TT in men decrease slowly with age, whereas bT levels decline abruptly.[85] For these reasons, it is possible to confer a protective role to bT that may improve some cognitive functions. Furthermore, some studies in the next section will show that T substitution have enhanced verbal, visuospatial, and memory functions in men who received it.

3.2. Testosterone Substitution Treatment and Cognitive Function in Healthy Elderly Men

In the past, research has better supported the role of estrogen than T in the preservation of cognitive functions. Estrogen hormone-replacement therapy (HRT) in women has been reported to have beneficial effects on cognitive abilities, particularly on verbal episodic memory, i.e. in short-delay free recall, long-delay recall and recognition. [86, 87] Moreover, HRT has been shown to reduce the incidence, and delay the onset of AD. [88, 89] The latter findings have nevertheless been refuted by three recent epidemiological studies that did not demonstrate the benefits of HRT (either using estrogen and progesterone or estrogen alone) in preventing dementia and cognitive decline in postmenopausal women. [90-92] Although considered controversial, these results may open the door to new debates.[93]

The questions regarding HRT may be equally applicable to men. In the previous section, several studies have demonstrated an association between serum levels of T and some cognitive functions (e.g., episodic and working memory, visuospatial ability) in elderly men without dementia, and the next sections will show that a depletion of androgen levels may be associated with dementia in aging males.

Meanwhile, in order to ascertain the impact of androgen levels on cognition in elderly men, researchers ideally have supplemented endogenous T levels by administering a T substitution treatment. Eight studies [94-101] assessing cognition following T treatment have been found in the literature (see table 2). Six clinical trials utilized a randomized double-blind placebo-controlled (R-DB-PC) design, and 2 studies, a double-blind placebo-controlled design. From 5 to 250 mg of T replacement therapy have been administered in 9 to 39 healthy elderly men during an average of 18.9 weeks (range: 1 to 48 weeks of treatment). In five studies [96-98, 100, 101], the participants had T levels in the lower normal limits according to the values of Pagana and Pagana [30], i.e. between 3-10 ng/ml or 10-35 nmol/L. Janowsky et al. [94] mentioned that their participants had T levels at baseline comparable with those reported for men in the same age range, whereas Janowsky et al. [95] reported that the FT levels of their participants at baseline was 50% lower than those of younger men. Finally, the elderly men included in the study of Sih et al. [99] were described as being hypogonadal.

Five out of 8 studies have shown that sex steroids can modulate some aspects of cognition. In these studies, T treatment increased spatial and/or verbal memory and/or visuospatial function (see the performance on Block Design). [94-98] On one hand, these results can be considered as strong evidence because the authors used a randomized double-blind placebo-controlled design (with the exception of the study of Janowsky et al. [95]).

On the other hand, all the studies had a small sample size, and thus possibly had reduced statistical power. However, multiple analyses were performed on several cognitive tests, and in these conditions, type I errors were more likely to occur. Furthermore, in the study of Kenny et al. [97], a large number of men discontinued their treatment before the end of the study. This situation might have explained that the cognitive results obtained by the T treatment group were not statistically different from the changes registered in the placebo group. In the clinical trial of Janowsky et al. [94], the hormone level measurement has not been performed at the same moment than the administration of cognitive tests. This was a strong limitation of their study.

Other authors [99-101] have found no association between T and cognitive function. Sih et al.[99] were unable to demonstrate any difference in verbal and nonverbal memory following T administration. The authors explained that the increase in estradiol levels, observed in the treatment group, could have contributed to mask the effects of T supplement on cognitive function. However, this study presented limitations. The investigators did not assess visuospatial functions whereas the biological rationale and previous literature reviews[102-103] strongly suggested a positive relationship between T and visuospatial functions such as spatial memory, visuoconstruction praxis and perceptual organization. In addition, the T treatment group had significant higher baselines scores than the placebo group on measures of cognitive function. Other limitations of this study included a small sample size altering the statistical power and a significant drop-out rate. Another study had a high percentage of drop-outs. In the study of Haren et al. [100], 25% of the enrolled men withdrew early before completing the protocol, which might have explained, at least partially, the negative results obtained by this group of researchers.

Surprisingly, in Wolf et al.'s [101] study, the placebo group showed a practice effect on the verbal fluency task, but the T group did not. These results suggested that T might have prevented the practice effect typically observed when the administration of the verbal fluency task is repeated at short time intervals. It is also possible that the short duration of treatment in this trial might have been responsible for the lack of beneficial effects on spatial cognition or memory.

Another study, (not presented in table 1), investigated the association between serum T concentrations and specific cognitive functions in newly diagnosed prostate cancer patients (n = 23) treated by androgen deprivation therapy (leading to castration T level [104]). Six months following the beginning of the treatment, visuomotor slowing, increased (slowed) reaction time on some attentional domains tasks, impairments on a vigilance test, delayed recall and speed of recognition for letters were observed. These deficits became statistically significant 12 months following the onset of the study. The findings of this study were interesting. On the contrary to previous treatment studies, the link between the levels of T and cognition was demonstrated by T deprivation. However, fatigue, a common side effect of cancer treatment, might have been responsible for these cognitive deficits.

4. Clinical Studies on Testosterone Levels and Cognition in Patients with AD

4.1. Studies Comparing Testosterone Levels in Patients with AD and Healthy Controls

Table 3 shows that seven cross-sectional studies have compared T levels between patients with mild to moderate AD and healthy elderly men. However, different conclusions have been drawn due to discrepancies in experimental designs, variability in techniques used to measure endocrinal parameters [105], presence of various covariates likely to influence androgen levels [109], and small sample size [106].

Three studies have reported lower T levels in men with AD compared to controls [66, 68, 107]. The results of another study [105] revealed lower FT and higher SHBG levels in patients with AD (n = 32) compared with healthy age-matched subjects (n = 32). These findings make sense since high SHBG levels reduce androgen and increase estrogen levels. However, the mechanism underlying the relation between higher than normal estradiol levels and AD is still unclear.

A recent study showed no difference on T, FAI and SHBG levels between control and AD groups. [108] However, when authors stratified analyses for age group (median split at 73 years of age), younger cases (n = 54) had lower FAI and SHBG than controls (n = 50) whereas older cases (n = 58) had lower levels of T than controls (n = 58). A paired analysis using logistic regression on patients with similar age was performed. The only factor that remained predictive of AD was a low baseline free androgen index (FAI). As the authors concluded, FAI could also explain the variance of many other risk factors for dementia and cognitive decline through its association, for example, with acute and chronic disease, vascular and thyroid problems, diabetes, as well as alcoholism. These concurrent factors have not been controlled for in this study.

Another study compared T, FT and FAI in AD cases and age-matched controls. [106] Surprisingly, the results have shown that AD cases had higher levels of T, FT and FAI than controls. These findings were clearly in contradiction with those of previous studies. In an attempt to explain this discrepancy, the authors suggested that the relative small sample size of the study prevented the results to reach statistical significance. In addition, the presence of uncontrolled confounding factors such as the body mass index, diet, and alcohol intake might have influenced the serum T levels.

Rasmuson et al. [109] conducted a study involving men and women. The results showed no significant difference between T and FT levels in the group of AD men only (n = 12) compared with the healthy control group (n = 10[109]). However, as pointed out by Hogervorst and Bandelow [110], the sample size in the study was too small, and required to be quadrupled for the results to reach statistical significance. Similarly, in the study of Okun et al. [111] no relationship between T levels and AD was found. They have measured plasma T levels in patients with AD (n = 50) and Parkinson's disease (PD, n = 68). The results showed that AD and PD cases compared to healthy controls had no greater decline in T. However, a larger sample size will be needed to confirm these results.

Table 1. Testosterone Parameters and Cognitive Functions in Healthy Elderly Men

Authors	Study design	N Characteristics Mean Age	Cognitive tests[a]	Androgen Parameters[b]	Results[c]
Barrett-Connor et al. [35]	CS Expl. analysis	547 P-based Cohort Community-dwelling men 70.2 ± 8.3 yrs	BIMC MMSE ('serial seven' + 'spelling "world" backward' analysed separately) VRT BSRT Semantic Fluency TMT B	TT bT	↑ levels of bT = ↑ scores on BIMC and BSRT ($p < 0.05$). Quadratic relations between TT and BIMC, and between TT and bT and "World" test, and between bT and VRT ($p < 0.05$).
Yaffe et al. [32]	CS	310 P-based listings 73.0 ± 7.1 yrs	MMSE TMT B Digit symbol	TT bT SHBG	Higher levels of bT = ↑ scores on all 3 cognitive tests ($p \leq 0.001$). ↑ levels of SHBG = ↓ scores on all tests ($p \leq 0.001$). No association between TT levels and cognitive scores (p = n.s).
Aleman et al. [73]	CS	25 Healthy older men 69.1 yrs (Range= 65-76)	WAIS BJLO Brus Reading test Block Design Digit Symbol Concept Shifting Task RAVLT	TT FT SHBG	Positive association between TT ($p < 0.01$) and SHBG ($p < 0.005$) on Block Design, Digit Symbol, and Concept Shifting Task.
Fonda et al. [74]	CS Analysis of Time 2 data	981 P-based Cohort- Men 62.6 ± 8.2 yrs	WAIS-R (BDS, DSS) Schaie-Thurstone AMAT	TT FT	Logged TT = ↑ on BDS and DSS (p unavailable) Logged FT = ↑ on each cognitive test (p unavailable)

Table 1. (Continued)

Authors	Study design	N Characteristics Mean Age	Cognitive tests[a]	Androgen Parameters[b]	Results[c]
Hogervorst et al. [75]	CS	145 Community-dwelling men + women 79 men 74.0 ± 6.1 yrs	CERAD 10 Word-List VPA test Graded Naming test CANTAB-Spatial Recognition PAL Pattern and Letter Comparison test	TT	Higher levels of TT = ↑ performance on Spatial Recognition test ($p < 0.01$)
Burkhardt et al. [79]	CS	45 Healthy elderly men APOEε4(+) and APOEε4 (-) subgroups 74.3 ± 5.8 yrs in ε4(+) 69.5 ± 6.7 yrs in ε4(-)	CAMCOG-R WMS-III (Paired Associates, Visual Reproduction, Letter Number Sequencing, Verbal Fluency tests) D-KEFS (Color-Word Interference Test)	FT SHBG	Significant interaction between FT and APOEε4 on CAMCOG-R ($p= 0.01$), and measures of executive functioning, working memory and attention (WMS-III + D-KEFS tests) ($p< 0.01$). Higher levels of FT associated with better general cognition in APOEε4(-) ($p=0.01$). Higher levels of FT associated with lower scores in tests of executive functioning, working memory and attention in APOEε4(+) ($p=0.02$).
Perry et al. [80]	CS	78 Community-dwelling men 65.6 ± 6.2 yrs	MMSE Exit Interview WCST TMT-B	bT	No significant correlation between bT and cognitive tests. Declining bT may be associated with impairment in executive function
Wolf and Kirschbaum [81]	CS	30 Community-dwelling men 69.0 ± 1.3 yrs	Verbal fluency City map task PAL Stroop Mental Rotation	TT	Low levels of TT associated with better verbal fluency but this negative association became a non significant trend when age and education were controlled for.

Table 1. (Continued)

Authors	Study design	N Characteristics Mean Age	Cognitive tests[a]	Androgen Parameters[b]	Results[c]
Carlson et Sherwin [82]	CS	24 Healthy older men 71.9 ± 5.9 yrs	WMS (PR, PA, VR, VPA, FM, DS, VMS) BSRT CR	TT	No correlation between TT and cognitive tests.
Moffat et al. [83]	LS Mean Follow-up= 9.7 yrs	407 Healthy elderly men Baseline age: 64.1 ± 9.4 yrs	BVRT MMSE Semantic Fluency Lexical Fluency TMT A and B CVLT (A, D, R) ROT Digit span	TT FT	Higher levels of FT = ↑ scores on BVRT ($p < 0.001$), on CVLT (A; $p < 0.001$, D; $p < 0.05$, R ; $p < 0.05$), on TMT A ($p < 0.05$) and TMT B ($p < 0.01$), and on ROT ($p < 0.001$). Higher levels of TT = ↓ on Digit Span backward ($p < 0.05$)
Lessov-Schlaggar et al. [84]	LS Range of follow-up: 10-16 yrs	348 Elderly men Twin pairs from P-based cohort	MMSE Digit Symbol TMT-A and B Stroop Lexical Fluency task CVLT BVRT	T SHBG Estradiol Estrone	No significant associations between baseline sex hormones (T, estradiol, and estrone) and follow-up cognitive performance, even when adjusting SHBG concentrations. However, significant positive relationship between T and cerebral volumes (frontal and parietal lobes).

P-based= Population-based; CS= Cross-sectional study; LS= Longitudinal study; yrs= years

[a] AMAT= Adult Mental Abilities Test; BJLO= Benton Judgement of Line Orientation test; BIMC = Blessed Information-Memory-Concentration test; BSRT= Buschke Selective Reminding Test; BVRT = Benton Visual Retention Test; CANTAB = Cambridge Neuropsychological Test Automated Battery; CERAD = Consortium to Establish a Registry for Alzheimer Disease; CR = Category Retrieval; CVLT = California Verbal Learning Test (A : words recalled, D : free recall delay, R : recognition accuracy); MMSE = Mini-Mental State Examination; MRT= Mental Rotation Task; PAL = Paired Associate Learning; RAVLT= Rey Auditory Verbal Learning Test; ROT = Card Rotation Test; TMT= Trail Making Test; VRT = Visual Reproduction Test; WAIS-R= Wechsler Adult Intelligence Scale-Revised (Backward Digit Span (BDS), Digit Symbol Substitution (DSS)); WCST= Wisconsin Card Sorting Test; WMS (PR, PA, VR, VPA, FM, DS, VMS) = Wechsler Memory Scale (Paragraph Recall, Paires-Associates, Visual Reproduction, Visual Paired Associates, Figural Memory, Digit Span, Visual Memory Span)

[b] TT= Total testosterone; BT= Biodisponible testosterone; FT = Free testosterone ; SHBG= Sex hormone binding globulin

[c] ↑ = increase; ↓ = decrease; n.s. = non significant.

Table 2. Cognitive Functioning of Healthy Elderly Men Receiving Testosterone (T) versus Placebo Treatment

Authors	Study Design [a]	No of participants T Tx/ Placebo/ Other	T Tx (mg) [b]	Duration of Tx (weeks)	Cognitive Tests [c]	Results [d]
Janowsky et al. [94]	R-DB-PC	27/ 29	15 (scrotal patch)	12	WAIS-R (Vocabulary, Block Design) CVLT WMS-R (Visual Reproduction) Groove Pegboard Test TMT	T group = ↑ spatial cognitive performance as assessed by the Block Design (p = ?)
Janowsky et al. [95]	DB-PC	10/ 9	150	4	SOPT	T group = ↑ working memory ($p = 0.02$) as assessed by the SOPT
Cherrier et al. [96]	R-DB-PC	13/ 12	100	6	Route test SALT OMDR PI Story Recall Block Design Stroop Verbal fluency	T group = ↑ spatial memory (Route Test), spatial ability (Block Design) and verbal memory (Story Recall) ($p < 0.05$ respectively)
Kenny et al. [97]	R-DB-PC	24/ 20	5 (scrotal patch)	48	Digit Symbol Digit Span TMT A-B	T group = ↑ performance on TMT B ($p < 0.01$)[¶]

Table 2. (Continued)

Authors	Study Design a	No of participants T Tx/ Placebo/ Other	T Tx (mg)b	Duration of Tx (weeks)	Cognitive Tests c	Resultsd
Cherrier et al. [98]	R-DB-PC	20/ 21/ 19*	100	6	Route Test Story Recall SOPT Stroop Verbal fluency	AT + T groups = ↑ spatial memory (Route Test : $p < 0.01$ respectively) T group = ↑ verbal memory (Story Recall : $p < 0.05$)
Sih et al. [99]	R-DB-PC	17/ 15	200	26	RAVLT RVDLT Semantic Fluency task	No difference between groups (p = n.s.) on the cognitive measures
Haren et al. [100]	R-DB-PC	39/ 37	80	48	TMT B Block Design MMSE	No difference between groups (p = n.s.) on the cognitive measures
Wolf et al. [101]	DB-PC	17/ 13	250	< 1	Route Test Story Recall Verbal Fluency Stroop Mental Rotation	Placebo group = ↑ verbal fluency ($p < 0.05$)

[a] R-DB-PC = randomized double-blind placebo control group design; DB-PC= double-blind placebo control group design

[b] T Tx = Testosterone treatment

[c] CVLT = California Verbal Learning Test; MMSE= Mini Mental State Examination; OMDR = Oculomotor Delayed Response; PI = Proactive Interference; RAVLT = Rey Auditory Verbal Learning Test; RVDLT = Rey Visual Design Learning Test; SALT = Spatial Array Learning Test; SOPT = Self-Ordered Pointing Test; TMT= Trail Making Test; WAIS-R = Wechsler Adult Intelligence Scale-Revised; WMS-R = Wechsler Memory Scale-Revised

[d] ↑ : higher or better; ? = missing information; n.s. = non significant;

* In this study, 3 groups were compared: 20 = T group (testosterone); 21 = placebo group; 19 = AT group (testosterone + anastrozole; block the conversion of T to estradiol)

¶ Trail-making B scores improved in the T group compared to baseline ($p < 0.01$) but no significant difference could be detected between scores from T and placebo groups ($p = 0.19$)

Table 3. Clinical Studies Examining Endocrine Parameters in Male Patients with Alzheimer's Disease and Healthy Elderly Men

Authors	Study Design	N AD/ HC	Severity of Dementia (AD)	Endocrine parameters[a]	Mean ± SD AD versus HC	Results
Bowen et al. [66]	CS-C	40/ 29	? AD in long-term care facilities	TT (nmol/ml)	256 ± 21 / 348 ± 26	Less T in AD patients ($p < 0.01$)
Hogervorst et al. [107]	CS-C	39/ 41	Minimal-to-Severe	TT (nmol/ml)	14.5 ± 5 / 18.0 ± 6	Less T in AD patients ($p < 0.005$) Lower TT more likely in AD men, independently of potential confounds
Hogervorst et al. [68]	CS-C	45/ 133	Mild-to-Moderate	TT (nmol/ml) SHBG (nmol/L)	13±6 /17 ± 8 43.9 ± 17.2 / 43.2 ± 18.3	Less T in AD patients ($p < 0.005$) Low TT and high SHBG levels= significant independent risk factors for AD
Paoletti et al. [105]	CS-C	32/ 32	Mild-to-Moderate	TT (ng/mL) FAI SHBG (nM/L)	4.17 ± 0.26 / 4.66 ± 0.23 5.27 ± 0.41 / 10.82 ± 1.10 87.03 ± 6.87 / 47.13 ± 4.29	Higher level of FT ($p < 0.01$) and SHBG ($p < 0.01$) in AD patients
Hogervorst et al. [108]	CS-C	50/ 46	Mild-to-Moderate	TT (nmol/L) FAI (nmol/L) SHBG (nmol/L)	15.46 ± 5.69 / 16.68 ± 7.64 0.33 ± 0.15 / 0.39 ± 0.18 44.18 ± 17.22 / 43.13 ± 21.89	No statistical difference between groups on the values Only FAI is a significant predictor for AD (O.R.=0.02, 95% CI= 0.01-0.47, $p < 0.05$

Table 3.(Continued)

Authors	Study Design	N AD/ HC	Severity of Dementia (AD)	Endocrine parametersa	Mean ± SD AD versus HC	Results
Pennanen et al. [106]	CS-C	14/ 16	Mild-to-Moderate	TT (nmol/L) FT (pmol/L) SHBG (nmol/L) FAI	16.2 ± 3.9 / 12.2± 4.8 199.4± 40.3 / 149.4 ± 36.2 58.2 ± 17.3 / 55.3 ± 21.8 29.7 ± 10 / 22.7 ± 4.4	Higher levels of TT ($p <$ 0.05), FT ($p < 0.001$) and FAI ($p < 0.05$) in AD patients
Rasmuson et al.[109]	CS-C	12 / 10	Mild-to-Moderate	TT (nmol/L) FT (?) SHBG (nmol/L)	17.8 ± 8.9 / 23.5 ± 4.7 0.7 ± 0.3 / 0.8 ± 0.2 27.4 ± 10.3 / 32.8 ± 12.8	No difference between T and FT levels in AD compared with HC
Okun et al.[111]	LS	50/ ?	?	TT (ng/mL)	60.1 / 35.0 (decline per every 10 years of age)	Greater decline in T levels in AD than community (p= 0.45)
Moffat et al.[113]	LS Mean follow-up= 19.1 yrs	574	N/A	TT (nmol/L) FTI SHBG	Approximate 26% reduction in the risk of AD for each 10-unit (nmol/nmol) increase in FTI	Diagnosis of AD associated inversely with FTI by itself and after adjustment for age, education, smoking status, body mass index, diabetes, any cancer diagnoses, and hormonal supplements

AD= Alzheimer's disease; HC= Healthy Controls; CS-C= Cross-sectional controlled; LS= Longitudinal Study; ?= Information not provided by the authors; N/A= Not applicable

[a] TT = Total Testosterone; SHBG = Sex Hormone Binding Globulin; FT = Free Testosterone; FTI= Free T Index.; FAI = Free Androgenization Index

Table 4. Cognition in Male Patients with Alzheimer's Disease or Mild Cognitive Impairment Receiving Testosterone versus Placebo Treatment

Authors	Study Design [a]	No of participants T Tx/ Placebo	T Tx [b]	Duration of Tx (weeks)	Cognitive Tests [c]	Results [d]
Tan and Pu [114]	R-PC (pilot)	T Tx= 5 AD / Placebo= 5 AD All patients= hypogonadal (TT< 7 nml/L)	200 mg every 2 wks	52	ADAS-Cog total CDT MMSE total	T Tx: ADAS-Cog ↑of 9.6 pts (6 mths post baseline; p= 0.02); MMSE ↑ (9 mths post baseline; p=0.02) CDT (n.s. ↑ at 9 mths post baseline) 1 T Tx drop-out (mth 9): aggressive + hypersexual behavior
Kenny et al. [115]	R-DB-PC (pilot)	T Tx= 6 MCI / Placebo= 5 MCI All patients= hypogonadal (bT < 128 ng/dl)	200 mg every 2 wks	12	CDT Digit Span MMSE TMT-B Verbal Fluency	No difference between groups (p = n.s.) No drop-out
Cherrier et al. [116]	R-DB-PC	T Tx=9 AD + 10 MCI Placebo=6 AD + 7 MCI (Mild-to-Moderate AD)	100 mg/wk	12	Route test WMS-R (SR) PI Stroop TMT-B Lexical Fluency task WAIS-R (Block Design)	T Tx = ↑ Route test [$F(2,24)= 3.29$, $p < 0.05$]; ↑ Block Design [$F(2,36)= 3.45$, $p < 0.05$]; compared to baseline + placebo T Tx= ↑ Verbal Memory compared with placebo (PI at wk 6; SR at wk 3) Drop-outs: 3 T TX, 1 Placebo

Table 4. (Continued)

Lu et al. [117]	R-DB-PC-PG	T Tx= 9 AD + 14 HC Placebo= 9 AD + 15 HC	75 mg/day of T-gel	24	MMSE total ADAS-Cog total CVLT long delay recall VMI BJLO WAIS-Block Design	AD-Placebo ↓ on VMI while AD-T Tx= baseline at end of study; HC-T Tx ↑ on VMI while HC-Placebo= baseline at end of study Drop-outs: 2 AD-T Tx , 4 HC-T Tx, 3 HC-Placebo

AD= Alzheimer's disease; MCI= Mild Cognitive Impairment; HC= Healthy Controls; wk= week; mth= month

[a] R-DB-PC = randomized double-blind placebo control group; R-DB-PC-PG= randomized double-blind placebo controlled, parallel groups

[b] T= Testosterone; Tx = Treatment; bT= bioavailable testosterone

[c] ADAS-Cog= Alzheimer's Disease Assessment Scale- Cognitive part; BJLO= Benton Judgement of Line Orientation test; CDT= Clock Drawing Test; CVLT = California Verbal Learning Test; MMSE= Mini Mental State Exam; PI = Proactive Interference; SR= Story Recall; TMT= Trail Making Test; VMI= Visual-Motor Integration; WAIS-R = Wechsler Adult Intelligence Scale-Revised; WMS-R = Wechsler Memory Scale-Revised

[d] ↑ : higher or better; ↓= deteriorated; ? = missing information; n.s. = non significant;

* In this study, 3 groups were compared: 20 = T group (testosterone); 21 = placebo group; 19 = AT group (testosterone + anastrozole; block the conversion of T to estradiol)

¶ Trail-making B scores improved in the T group compared to baseline ($p < 0.01$) but no significant difference could be detected between scores from T and placebo groups ($p = 0.19$)

Another study (not included in table 3) found that levels of total serum, FT, and SHBG were inversely correlated with levels of Aβ40 (i.e., amino-acid40) in 28 elderly men with memory loss (MCI) or dementia (n= 19 AD; n=3 with other dementia). The researchers concluded that the biochemical androgen status was associated with the level of expression of Aβ40 in the plasma, thus suggesting that a sub-clinical androgen deficiency enhanced the development of AD *in vivo*. [112]

Unfortunately, due to the cross-sectional nature of the aforementioned studies, it was impossible to determine whether a decrease in T was causative or consequential of AD. Moffat et al. [113] were the first authors to rigorously investigate the T /AD relationship using a prospective longitudinal design. In this study, 574 men aged from 32 to 87 years were followed every two years during an average of 19.1 years. Several samples of T and SHBG were collected throughout the course of this study. Diagnoses of AD were based on biennial physical, neurological, and neuropsychological evaluations. In this sample, 54 men were diagnosed with AD. The results revealed a significant association between long-term endogenous FT concentrations and subsequent AD diagnoses. Thus, these findings confirmed that free FT concentrations were a better predictor of AD than TT levels.

4.2. Cognitive Effects of Testosterone Substitution Treatment in Patients with Alzheimer's Disease or Mild Cognitive Impairment

Regarding the T substitution treatment in AD, only four studies have been found in the literature: one randomized placebo-controlled pilot study [114]; two randomized, double-blind, placebo-controlled trials [115-116], and one randomized, double-blind, placebo-controlled with parallel groups study [117] (see table 4). The four studies had a very small sample size (from 10 to 47 participants), and were thus at risk to lack statistical power. The participants presented either with Alzheimer's disease [114, 116, 117] or MCI [114, 116]. Only one study involved also healthy controls. [117] The treatment lasted from 12 to 52 weeks. In the first two studies that will be presented below, the participants were hypogonadal.

In order to verify whether T was involved in AD, Tan and Pu [114] selected 10 elderly hypogonadal males with AD from a sample of 36 men who recently received a diagnosis of AD, and then assessed their cognitive functions following the administration of T replacement therapy. Five of the hypogonadal patients were randomized to T treatment, and five, to placebo. The five patients with mild to moderate AD who received T replacements demonstrated an increase in T and bT levels, and registered an improvement in their cognitive functioning, particularly in their visuospatial skills. However, after nine months of treatment, a patient was withdrawn from the study because of aggressive and hypersexual behavior that could have been induced by the T substitution treatment.

Kenny and his collaborators [115] conducted a study on individuals presenting with mild-to-moderate cognitive impairment and did not find significant differences between the placebo (n = 5) and treatment groups (n = 6) on any cognitive score following the treatment. According to the authors, the sample was too small and the tests of cognitive performance assessing global cognitive functions (MMSE), construction praxis (CDT), verbal working memory (Digit Span), and executive functions (TMT-B and verbal fluency) might have lacked sensitivity to detect subtle cognitive changes in hypogonadal patients. This study had a number of limitations. First, the authors described their participants as presenting mild-to-moderate cognitive impairment, but given their cognitive scores at baseline, they were more likely to be demented. These patients might have presented another dementia than Alzheimer's disease, or a medical condition that may induce cognitive impairment, since the exclusion criteria were not stringent. Another strong limitation of this study was the fact that the total MMSE scores of patients in the T treatment group were significantly higher at baseline than those of patients in the placebo group.

In the study of Cherrier et al. [116], the T treatment and placebo groups both included patients with AD and MCI. All the participants had TT levels in lower normal limits. The results showed significant improvement in the T treatment group compared to baseline and the placebo group on tasks of visuospatial functions. Verbal memory, as measured with the proactive interference paradigm, was also improved in the T treatment compared with the placebo group. However, the drop-out rate in the T treatment group was 15.7% compared to 7.7% in the placebo group.

In the study of Lu et al. [117], the T treatment and placebo groups both involved patients with AD and healthy controls. The T levels of all participants were within normal limits. These authors did not find any real improvement following the T treatment. Instead, by the end of the trial, the performance of patients with AD in the placebo group declined on the visual-motor integration task whereas that of treated patients remained stable throughout the study. The drop-out rate was very high in the treated group (26%) compared with that of the placebo group (12.5%). This fact might raise the question of tolerability and safety of T treatment in individuals who do not present with hypogonadism.

Discussion

The goal of this chapter has been to improve our understanding, and to verify a possible relationship between low T levels, cognitive functioning and development of Alzheimer's disease in elderly men.

Clearly, there is a biological rationale for the involvement of T in cognition, especially in memory, executive and visuospatial functions (see section 2). There is also a strong biological rationale suggesting the implication of testosterone in the development of pathological and genetic abnormalities associated with AD. With age, decreased sex steroids may play an important role in deteriorations of the central and peripheral nervous system. The maintenance of serum levels could then preserve, to some extent, some cognitive functions in elderly men. Nonetheless, it is also possible that a reduction in T is a marker of "pathological aging" in general, and not necessarily a risk factor specific to AD. In order to clarify this issue, future research should examine the T levels in other populations suffering from various neurodegenerative dementias such as dementia with Lewy bodies, fronto-temporal lobar degeneration and Parkinson's disease with dementia.

A cross-sectional design might be useful to identify correlates and associated features of hormonal and cognitive impairment, and these findings may be quite informative. Therefore, despite some contradictory results, the evidence presented in this chapter suggests that T probably plays a role in some cognitive functions in elderly men, principally related to working and episodic memory, executive and spatial functions (see tables 1 and 2). These correlations between testosterone levels and cognition, and between the areas of improved cognition and T substitution therapy in healthy elderly men are congruent with the results of the studies presented in the section 2 on the biological rationale.

In addition, the findings of tables 3 and 4 have highlighted the possible involvement of T and sex hormones in general in the development and/or clinical symptomatology of AD. However, several methodological limitations will have to be overcome in the future. First, the nature of the cross-sectional design makes it impossible to infer a causal relationship between the low levels of T and the development of AD.

Moreover, most of the studies presented in Section 4.1 have only taken one T sample, and have postulated a relationship between T and AD. T serial levels are known to have large diurnal variability and may be influenced by several non controlled factors such as opioids, diet (body mass index), alcohol, physical activities, smoking, and the season, leading to interesting but yet premature conclusions in the reviewed studies. Thus prospective longitudinal studies are mandatory in order to clarify this question, and to replicate the results found in Moffat et al.[113] study.

The initiation of randomized-controlled clinical trials for the primary prevention of AD using T supplementation in men who present low androgens levels in middle age could be an interesting avenue for the future. In the present paper, several studies have explored the effects of T supplementation on cognitive function in healthy elderly men and patients with Alzheimer's disease or mild cognitive impairment. However, these treatments were often administered to patients who were not severely hypogonadal, and the duration of T treatment in healthy aging men was sometimes too short for the supplementation therapy to show significant effects on cognitive function. Even when some effects were registered, it was difficult to determine if they were maintained over a significant period of time, because the duration of the T substition was again too short.

On the other hand, hormone therapy replacement for men may increase, among other things, the risk of prostate cancer, atherosclerosis, hypertension, lipid alteration, sleep apnea, and strokes.[118] Although the benefit/ risk ratio of T replacement therapy in aging men is still unknown, the relatively high drop-out rates that have been found in the present chapter in studies involving non hypogonadal patients with AD and MCI [116,117] certainly indicate that clinicians and researchers should be cautious before prescribing T therapy in aging men. In future, it might be more appropriate to administer T replacement therapy in patients suffering from hypogonadism instead of providing T substitution to all cognitively impaired patients independently of their hormonal status. Carefully designed and monitored long-term clinical trials will contribute to evaluate the risks and benefits of T therapy.

Alzheimer's disease [119-121] as well as mild cognitive impairment [122-124] may present heterogeneous yet distinctive cognitive profiles. This suggests that the various cognitive presentations of AD may have different biological and/or hormonal causes. For example, several studies in this review have shown that sex hormones were associated with the preservation of episodic memory and learning in animals and humans. In another endocrinological realm, prolonged exposure to high cortisol levels has been found to harm working memory, decrease attention, and represent a risk factor for the development of neurodegenerative diseases. [125-127] An impairment or a decline in T could thus be the cause of one of these cognitive profiles, or could specifically be involved in other cognitive deficits associated with the parietal lobe, such as visuospatial ability. The sections on the biological rationale for the involvement of testosterone in cognition, as well as the results of the clinical studies herein presented certainly have provided a support to these possibilities.

One should also consider that several medical consequences may also be associated with androgen depletion in elderly men, for example, the development of diabetes [128] which is traditionally associated with a high risk of cerebral vascular lesion [129] , depression [130] and cognitive impairment [131,132] or hypothyroidism [133] which is also associated with some cognitive impairments [134] and affective symptoms. [135] Therefore, the cognitive impairments and dementia that follow androgen depletion could be due either to the reduction in androgen itself, or to its medical consequences. Further studies are needed in order to clarify this particular issue.

Conclusion

The results reviewed in this chapter have strongly suggested that a relationship between pathological aging, cognitive impairment and reductions of T exists. Methodological limitations of the existing data have included the lack of longitudinal studies, and small sample size. However, despite the limitations of the reviewed studies, the present chapter has highlighted the fact that future research should continue to investigate T levels and treatment in AD, and MCI populations. The role of T in the prevention and development of Alzheimer-type dementia is not yet completely elucidated.

Acknowledgments

This work was supported by a fellowship award (Séverine Hervouet) from the Canadian Institutes of Health Research. Dr. Simard is engaged in research supported by the Canadian Institutes of Health Research- Institute of Aging (grant # IAO-77374) and by a 2005 National Alliance for Research on Schizophrenia and Depression Young Investigator Award.

References

[1] Hebert, LE; Scherr, PA; Bienas, JL et al: Alzheimer disease in US population. Prevalence estimates using the 2000 census. *Arch. Neurol.* 2003, 60, 1119-1122.

[2] Anonymous. The Canadian Study of Health and Aging: risk factors for Alzheimer's disease in Canada. *Neurology.* 1994, 44, 2073-2080.

[3] Munoz, DG; Feldman, H. Causes of Alzheimer's disease. *Can. Med. Assoc. J.* 2000, 162, 65-72.

[4] Touchon, J; Portet, F. La maladie d'Alzheimer. Paris: Masson; 2002.

[5] Michel, B; Touchon, J; Becker, H et al: Neurodégénérescence et maladie d'Alzheimer, in Neurodégénérescence et vieillissement cérébral. Edited by Michel BF,Verdier JM. Marseille: Solal; 2004.
[6] Farrer, LA; Cupples, LA; Haines, JL et al: Effects of age, sex, and ethnicity on the association between apolipoprotein E genotype and Alzheimer disease. A meta-analysis. APOE and Alzheimer Disease Meta Analysis Consortium. *JAMA*. 1997, 278, 1349-1356.
[7] Raber, J. Androgens, apoE, and Alzheimer's disease. *Sci Aging Knowledge Environ.* 2004, 11, 1-11.
[8] Reed, T, Carmelli, D, Swan, GE et al. Lower cognitive performance in normal older adult male twins carrying the apolipoprotein Eε4 allele. *Arch. Neurol.* 1994, 51, 1189-1192.
[9] Farlow, MR. Alzheimer's disease: clinical implications of the apolipoprotein E genotype. *Neurology*. 1997, 48, S30-S34.
[10] Baldereschi, M; Di Carlo, A; Lepore, V et al. Estrogen-replacement therapy and Alzheimer's disease in the Italian Longitudinal Study on Aging. *Neurology*. 1998, 50, 996-1002.
[11] Matthews, K; Cauley, J; Yaffe, K; Zmuda, JM. Estrogen replacement therapy and cognitive decline in older community women. *J. Am. Geriatr. Soc.* 1999, 47, 518-523.
[12] Petanceska, SS; Nagy, V; Frail, D et al: Ovariectomy and 17beta-estradiol modulate the levels of Alzheimer's amyloid beta peptides in brain. *Neurology*. 2000, 54, 2212-2217.
[13] Tan, RS; Pu, SJ; Culberson, JW. Role of androgens in mild cognitive impairment and possible interventions during andropause. *Med. Hypotheses*. 2004, 62,14-18.
[14] Papasozomenos, S; Shanavas, A. Testosterone prevents the heat shock-induced overactivation of glycogen synthase kinase-3 beta but not of cyclin-dependent kinase 5 and c-Jun NH2-terminal kinase and concomitantly abolishes hyperphosphorylation of tau: implications for Alzheimer's disease. *Proc. Natl. Acad. Sci. U. S. A.* 2002, 99,1140-1145.
[15] Raber, J; Bongers, G; LeFevour, A et al. Androgens protect against apolipoprotein E4-induced cognitive deficits. *J. Neuroscience*. 2002, 22, 5204-5209.
[16] Ramsden, M; Nyborg, AC; Murphy, MP et al: Androgens modulate beta-amyloid levels in male rat brain. *J. Neurochem*. 2003, 87, 1052-1055.
[17] Alexandersen, P; Christiansen, C. The aging male: Testosterone deficiency and testosterone replacement. An up-date. *Atherosclerosis*. 2004, 173, 157-169.
[18] Lejeune, H; Dechaud, H; Pugeat, M. Contribution of bioavailable testosterone assay for the diagnosis of androgen deficiency in elderly men. *Ann. Endocrinol.* 2003, 64, 117-125.
[19] Zonderman, AB. Predicting Alzheimer's Disease in the Baltimore Longitudinal Study of Aging. *J. Geriatr. Psychiatry. Neurol.* 2005, 18, 192-195.
[20] Tan, RS; Pu, S-J. The andropause and memory loss: is there a link between androgen decline and dementia in the aging male? Asian Journal of Andrology 2001, 3, 169-174.
[21] Grant, NN; Anawalt, BD. Male hypogonadism in the primary care clinic. *Prim Care: Clinics in Office Practice* 2003, 30, 743-756.

[22] Seidman, SN; Roose, SP. The male hypothalamic-pituitary-gonadal axis: Pathogenic and therapeutic implications in psychiatry. *Psychiatr. Ann.* 2000, 30, 102-112.

[23] Seidman, SN. Testosterone deficiency and mood in aging men: Pathogenic and therapeutic interactions. *World J. Biol. Psychiatry.* 2003, 4, 14-20.

[24] Laycock, J; Wise, P. Essential Endocrinology. New York: Oxford University; 1996

[25] Weinbauer, GF; Gromoll, J; Simoni, M et al. Physiology of testicular function, in Andrology: Male Reproductive Health and Dysfunction. Edited by Nieschlag E Behre H. Berlin: Springer-Veriag; 1997.

[26] Janowski, JS. Thinking with your gonads: testosterone and cognition. *Trends in Cognitive Sciences.* 2006, 10, 77-82.

[27] Tenover, JL. Testosterone and the aging male. *J. Androl.* 1997, 18, 103-106.

[28] Morley, JE; Perry, HM 3rd. Androgen treatment of male hypogonadism in older males. *J. Steroid Biochem. Mol. Biol.* 2003, 85, 367-373

[29] Wespes, E; Schulman, CC. Male andropause: Myth, reality, and treatment. *Int. J. Impot. Res.* 2002, 14, S93-S98.

[30] Pagana KD, Pagana TJ. Diagnostic and Laboratory Test Reference 6th Edition. USA: Elsevier; 2002.

[31] Morley, JE; Kaiser, F; Raum, WJ et al. Potentially predictive and manipulable blood serum correlates of aging in the healthy human male: Progressive decreases in bioavailable testosterone, dehydroepiandrosterone sulfate, and the ratio of insulin-like growth factor 1 to growth hormone. *Proc. Natl. Acad. Sci. U. S. A.* 1997, 94, 7537-7542.

[32] Yaffe, K; Lui, L-Y; Zmuda, J et al. Sex hormones and cognitive function in older men. *J. Am. Geriatr. Soc.* 2002, 50, 707-712.

[33] Alexander, GM; Swerdloff, RS; Wang, C et al. Androgen-behavior correlations in hypogonadal men and eugonadal men. *Horm. Behav.* 1998, 33, 85-94.

[34] de Lignières B. L'andropause et sa prise en charge chez l'homme âgé. *Presse Med* 2002, 31, 1750-1759.

[35] Barrett-Connor, E; Goodman-Gruen, D; Patay, B. Endogenous sex hormones and cognitive function in older men. *J. Clin. Endocrinol. Metab.* 1999, 84, 3681-3685.

[36] Cherrier, MM; Plymate, S; Mohan, S et al. Relationship between testosterone supplementation and insulin-like growth factor-I levels and cognition in healthy older men. *Psychoneuroendocrinology.* 2004, 29, 65-82.

[37] Don Carlos, LL; Sarkey, S; Lorenz, B et al. Novel cellular phenotypes and subcellular sites for androgen action in the forebrain. *Neuroscience.* 2006, 138, 801-807.

[38] Janowsky, JS. The role of androgens in cognition and brain aging in men. *Neuroscience.* 2006, 138, 1015-1020.

[39] Yaffe, K. Testosterone and the brain: uncharted territory. *Lancet Neurol.* 2004, 3, 270.

[40] Ramsden, M.; Shin, TM; Pike, CJ. Androgens modulate neuronal vulnerability to kainate lesion. *Neuroscience.* 2003, 122, 573-578.

[41] Pouliot, WA; Handa, RJ; Beck, SG. Androgen modulates N-methyl-D-aspartate-mediated depolarization in CA1 hippocampal pyramidal cells. *Synapse.* 1996, 23, 10-19.

[42] Nakamura, N; Fujita, H.; Kawata, M. Effects of gonadectomy on immunoreactivity for choline acetyltransferase in the cortex, hippocampus, and basal forebrain of adult male rats. *Neuroscience*. 2002, 109, 473-485.

[43] Adler, A; Vescovo, P; Robinson, JK; Kritzer, MF. Gonadectomy in adult life increases tyrosine hydroxylase immunoreactivity in the prefrontal cortex and decreases open field activity in male rats. *Neuroscience*. 1999, 89, 939-954.

[44] Robichaud, M; Debonnel, G. Oestrogen and testosterone modulate the firing activity of dorsal raphe nucleus serotoninergic neurones in both male and female rats. *J. Neuroendocrinol*. 2005, 17, 179-185.

[45] Seymoure, P; Juraska, M. Vernier and grating acuity in adult hooded rats: the influence of sex. *Behav. Neurosci*. 1997, 111, 792-800.

[46] Nunez, JL; Huppenbauer, CB; McAbee, MD; Juraska, JM; Don Carlos, LL. Androgen receptor expression in the developing male and female rat visual and prefrontal cortex. *J. Neurobiol*. 2003, 56, 293-302.

[47] Shughrue, PJ; Stumpf, WE; MacLusky, NJ; Zielinski, JE; Hochberg, RB. Developmental changes in estrogen receptors in mouse cerebral cortex between birth and postweaning: studied by autoradiography with 11 beta-methoxy-16 alpha-[125I]iodoestradiol. *Endocrinology*. 1990, 126, 1112-1124.

[48] MacLusky, NJ; Walters, MJ; Clark, AS; Toran-Allerand, CD. Aromatase in the cerebral cortex, hippocampus, and mid-brain: ontogeny and developmental implications. *Mol. Cell Neurosci*. 1994, 5, 691-698.

[49] Bachevalier, J; Hagger, C. Sex differences in the development of learning abilities in primates. *Psychoneuroendocrinology*. 1991, 16, 177-188.

[50] Markesky, WR; Schmitt, FA; Kryscio, RJ; Davis, DG; Smith, CD; Wekstein, DR. Neuropathologic Substrate of Mild Cognitive Impairment. *Arch. Neurol*. 2006, 63, 38-46.

[51] Becker, JT; Davis, SW; Hayashi, KM et al. Three-dimensional Patterns of Hippocampal Atrophy in Mild Cognitive Impairment. *Arch. Neurol*. 2006, 63, 97-101.

[52] Gómez-Isla, T; Price, JL; McKeel, DW; Morric, JC; Growdon, JH; Hyman, BT. Profound Loss of Layer II Entorhinal Cortex Neurons Occurs in Very Mild Alzheimer's Disease. *J. Neurosci*. 1996, 16, 4491-4500.

[53] Morris, RG; Kopelman, M. The memory deficits in Alzheimer-type dementia: a review. *Q. J. Exp. Psychol*. 1986, 38A, 575-602.

[54] Linn, RT; Wolf, PA; Bachman, DL et al. The preclinical phase of probable Alzheimer's disease. *Arch. Neurol*. 1995, 52, 485-490.

[55] Tierney, MC; Yao, C; Kiss, A; McDowell, I. Neuropsychological tests accurately predict incident Alzheimer disease after 5 and 10 years. *Neurology*. 2005, 64, 1853-1859.

[56] Simard, M; van Reekum, R. Memory Assessment in Studies of Cognition-Enhancing Drugs for Alzheimer' Disease. *Drugs & Aging*. 1999, 14, 197-230.

[57] Gouras, GK; Xu, H; Gross, RS et al. Testosterone reduces neuronal secretion of Alzheimer's beta-amyloid peptides. *Proc. Natl. Acad. Sci. U. S. A*. 2000, 97, 1202-1205.

[58] Pike, CJ. Testosterone attenuates beta-amyloid toxicity in cultured hippocampal neurons. *Brain Res.* 2001, 919, 160-165.

[59] Pfankuch, T; Rizk, A; Olsen, R; Poage, C; Raber, J. Role of circulating androgen levels in effects of apoE4 on cognitive function. *Brain Res.* 2005, 1053, 88-96.

[60] Zhang, Y; Champagne, N; Beitel, LK et al. Estrogen and androgen protection of human neurons against intracellular amyloid beta1-42 toxicity through heat shock protein 70. *J. Neurosci.* 2004, 24, 5315-5321.

[61] Sakahira, H; Breuer, P; Hayer-Hartl, MK et al. Molecular chaperones as modulators of polyglutamine protein aggregation and toxicity. *Proc. Natl. Acad. Sci. U. S. A.* 2002, 99, 16412-16418.

[62] Rosario, ER; Chang, L; Stanczyk, FZ et al. Age-related testosterone depletion and the development of Alzheimer disease. *JAMA.* 2004, 292, 1431-1432.

[63] Twist, SJ; Taylor, GA; Weddell, A et al. Brain oestradiol and testosterone levels in Alzheimer's disease. *Neurosci. Let.* 2000, 286, 1-4.

[64] Hogervorst, E; Lehmann, DJ; Warden, DR et al. Apolipoprotein E epsilon4 and testosterone interact in the risk of Alzheimer's disease in men. *Int. J. Geriatr. Psychiatry.* 2002, 17, 938-940.

[65] Couse, JF; Korach, KS. Exploring the role of sex steroids through studies of receptor deficient mice. *J. Mol. Med.* 1998, 76, 497-511.

[66] Bowen, RL; Isley, JP; Atkinson, RL. An association of elevated serum gonadotropin concentrations and Alzheimer disease? *J. Neuroendocrinol.* 2000, 12, 351-354.

[67] Bowen, RL; Smith, MA; Harris, PLR et al. Elevated luteinizing hormone expression colocalizes with neurons vulnerable to Alzheimer's disease pathology. *J. Neurosci. Res.* 2002, 70, 514-518.

[68] Hogervorst, E; Combrinck, M; Smith, AD. Testosterone and gonadotropin levels in men with dementia. *Neuroendocrinol. Let.* 2003, 24:203-208.

[69] Short, RA; Bowen, RL; O'Brien, PC et al: Elevated gonadotropin levels in patients with Alzheimer disease. *Mayo Clin. Proc.* 2001, 76, 906-909.

[70] Gregory, CW; Bowen, RL. Novel therapeutic strategies for Alzheimer's disease based on the forgotten reproductive hormones. *Cell Mol. Life Sci.* 2005, 62, 313-319.

[71] Casadesus, G; Atwood, CS; Zhu X et al. Evidence for the role of gonadotropin hormones in the development of Alzheimer disease. *Cell Mol. Life Sci.* 2005, 62, 293-298.

[72] Davies, BR; Finnigan, DS; Smith, SK et al. Administration of gonadotropins stimulates proliferation of normal mouse ovarian surface epithelium. *Gynecol. Endocrinol.* 1999, 13, 75-81.

[73] Aleman, A; de Vries, WR; Koppeschaar, HP et al. Relationship between circulating levels of sex hormones and insulin-like growth factor-1 and fluid intelligence in older men. *Exp. Aging Res.* 2001, 27, 283-291.

[74] Fonda, SJ; Bertrand, R; O'Donnell, A et al. Age, hormones, and cognitive functioning among middle-aged and elderly men: cross-sectional evidence from the Massachusetts male aging study. *J. Gerontol. A Biol. Sci. Med. Sci.* 2005, 60, 385-90.

[75] Hogervorst, E; De Jager, C; Budge, M et al. Serum levels of estradiol and testosterone and performance in different cognitive domains in healthy elderly men and women. *Psychoneuroendocrinology*. 2004, 29, 405-421.
[76] Gouchie, C; Kimura, D. The relationship between testosterone levels and cognitive ability patterns. *Psychoneuroendocrinology*. 1991, 16, 323-334.
[77] Kimura, D; Hampson, E. Cognitive pattern in men and women is influenced by fluctuations in sex hormones. *Cur. Dir. Psychol. Sc.* 1994, 3, 57-61.
[78] O'Connor, DB; Archer, J; Hair, WM et al. Activational effects of testosterone on cognitive function in men. *Neuropsychologia*. 2001, 39, 1385-1594.
[79] Burkhardt, MS; Foster, JK; Clarnette, RM et al. Testosterone and Apolipoprotein E ε4 Status on Cognition in Healthy Older Men. *J. Clin. Endocrinol. Metab.* 2006, 91, 1168-1172.
[80] Perry, PJ; Lund, BC; Arndt, S et al. Bioavailable testosterone as a correlate of cognition psychological status, quality of life, and sexual function in aging males: Implications for testosterone replacement therapy. *Ann. Clin. Psychiatry*. 2001, 13, 75-80.
[81] Wolf, OT; Kirschbaum, C. Endogenous estradiol and testosterone levels are associated with cognitive performance in older women and men. *Horm. Behav.* 2002, 41, 259-266.
[82] Carlson, LE; Sherwin, BB. Steroid hormones, memory and mood in a healthy elderly population. *Psychoneuroendocrinology*. 1998, 23, 583-603.
[83] Moffat, SD; Zonderman, AB; Metter, EJ et al: Longitudinal assessment of serum free testosterone concentration predicts memory performance and cognitive status in elderly men. *J. Clin. Endocrinol. Metab.* 2002, 87, 5001-5007.
[84] Lessov-Schlaggar, CN; Reed, T; Swan, GE et al. Association of sex steroid hormones with brain morphology and cognition in healthy elderly men. *Neurology*. 2005, 65, 1591-1596.
[85] Demers, LM. Andropause: an androgen deficiency state in the ageing male. *Expert Opin. Pharmacother.* 2003, 4, 183-90.
[86] Jacobs, DM; Tang, MX; Stern, Y et al: Cognitive function in nondemented older women who took estrogen after menopause. *Neurology*. 1998; 50:368-373.
[87] Maki, PM; Zonderman, AB; Resnick, SM. Enhanced verbal memory in nondemented elderly women receiving hormone-replacement therapy. *Am. J. Psychiatry*. 2001, 158, 227-233.
[88] Kawas, C; Resnick, SM; Morrison, A et al. A prospective study of estrogen replacement therapy and the risk of developing Alzheimer's disease: the Baltimore Longitudinal Study of Aging. *Neurology*. 1997, 48, 1517-1521.
[89] Tang, MX; Jacobs, D; Stern, Y et al. Effect of oestrogen during menopause on risk and age at onset of Alzheimer's disease. *Lancet*. 1996, 348, 429-432.
[90] Espeland, MA; Rapp, SR; Shumaker, SA et al. Conjugated equine estrogens and global cognitive function in postmenopausal women: Women's Health Initiative Memory Study. *JAMA*. 2004, 291, 2959-2968.
[91] Shumaker, SA; Legault, C; Rapp, SR et al. Estrogen plus progestin and the incidence of dementia and mild cognitive impairment in postmenopausal women: the Women's

Health Initiative Memory Study: a randomized controlled trial. *JAMA*. 2003, 289, 2651-2662.

[92] Shumaker, SA; Legault, C; Kuller, L et al. Conjugated equine estrogens and incidence of probable dementia and mild cognitive impairment in postmenopausal women: Women's Health Initiative Memory Study. *JAMA*. 2004, 291, 2947-2958.

[93] Schneider, LS. Estrogen and dementia: insights from the Women's Health Initiative Memory Study. *JAMA*. 2004, 291, 3005-3007.

[94] Janowsky, JS; Oviatt, SK; Orwoll, ES. Testosterone influences spatial cognition in older men. *Behav. Neurosci.* 1994, 108, 325-332.

[95] Janowsky, JS; Chavez, B; Orwoll, ES. Sex steroids modify working memory. *J. Cogn. Neurosci.* 2000, 12, 407-412.

[96] Cherrier, MM; Asthana, S; Psymate, S et al. Testosterone supplementation improves spatial and verbal memory in healthy older men. *Neurology*. 2001, 57, 80-88.

[97] Kenny, AM; Bellantonio, S; Gruman, CA et al: Effects of transdermal testosterone on cognitive function and health perception in older men with low bioavalable testosterone levels. *J. Gerontol. A. Biol. Sci. Med. Sci.* 2002, 57A, 321-325.

[98] Cherrier, MM; Matsumoto, AM; Amory, JK et al. The role of aromatization in testosterone supplementation: effects on cognition in older men. *Neurology*. 2005, 64, 290-296.

[99] Sih, R; Morley, JE; Kaiser, FE et al. Testosterone replacement in older hypogonadal men: A 12-month randomized controlled trial. *J. Clin. Endocrinol. Metab.* 1997, 82, 1661-1667.

[100] Haren, MT; Wittert, GA; Chapman, IM et al: Effect of oral testosterone undecanoate on visuospatial cognition, mood and quality of life in elderly men with low-normal gonadal status. *Maturitas*. 2005, 50, 124-133.

[101] Wolf, OT; Preut, R; Hellhammer, DH et al: Testosterone and cognition in elderly men: a single testosterone injection blocks the practice effect in verbal fluency, but has no effect on spatial or verbal memory. *Biol. Psychiatry*. 2000, 47, 650-654.

[102] Christiansen, K; Knussman, R. Sex hormones and cognitive functioning in men. *Neuropsychobiology*. 1987, 18, 27-36.

[103] Sherwin, BB. Steroid hormones and cognitive functioning in aging men: A mini-review. *J. Mol. Neurosci.* 2003, 20, 385-393.

[104] Salminen, E; Portin, R; Korpela, J et al. Androgen deprivation and cognition in prostate cancer. *Brit. J. Cancer*. 2003, 89, 971-976.

[105] Paoletti, AM; Congia, S; Lello, S et al. Low androgenization index in elderly women and elderly men with Alzheimer's disease. *Neurology*. 2004, 62, 301-303.

[106] Pennanen, C; Laakso, MP; Kivipelto, M et al. Serum testosterone levels in males with Alzheimer's disease. *J. Neuroendocrinol.* 2004, 16, 95-98.

[107] Hogervorst, E; Williams, JH; Budge, M et al: Serum total testosterone is lower in men with Alzheimer's disease. *Neuroendocrinol. Let.* 2001, 22, 163-168.

[108] Hogervorst, E; Bandelow, S; Combrinck, M et al. Low free testosterone is an independent risk factor for Alzheimer's disease. *Exp. Gerontol.* 2004, 39, 1633-1639.

[109] Rasmuson, S; Näsman, B; Carlström, K et al. Increased levels of adrenocortical and gonadal hormones in mild to moderate Alzheimer's disease. *Dement. Geriatr. Cogn. Disord.* 2002, 13, 74-79.
[110] Hogervorst, E; Bandelow, S. The controversy over levels of sex steroids in cases with Alzheimer's disease. *J. Neuroendocrinol.* 2004, 16, 93-94.
[111] Okun, MS; DeLong, MR; Hanfelt, J et al. Plasma testosterone levels in Alzheimer and Parkinson diseases. *Neurology.* 2004, 62, 411-413.
[112] Gillett, MJ; Martins, RN; Clarnette, RM et al: Relationship between testosterone, sex hormone binding globulin and plasma amyloid beta peptide 40 in older men with subjective memory loss or dementia. *J. Alzheimer's Dis.* 2003, 5, 267-269.
[113] Moffat, SD; Zonderman, AB; Metter, EJ et al. Free testosterone and risk for Alzheimer disease in older men. *Neurology.* 2004, 62, 188-193.
[114] Tan, RS; Pu SJ. A pilot study on the effects of testosterone in hypogonadal aging male patients with Alzheimer's disease. *Aging Male.* 2003, 6, 13-17.
[115] Kenny, AM; Fabregas, G; Song, C et al: Effects of testosterone on behavior, depression, and cognitive function in older men with mild cognitive loss. *J. Gerontol. A Biol. Sci. Med. Sci.* 2004; 59:75-78.
[116] Cherrier, MM; Matsumoto, AM; Amory, S et al. Testosterone improves spatial memory in men with Alzheimer's disease and mild cognitive impairment. *Neurology.* 2005, 64, 2063-2068.
[117] Lu, PH; Masterman, DA; Mulnard, R. et al.Effects of Testosterone on Cognition and Mood in Male Patients With Mild Alzheimer's Disease and Healthy Eledrly Men. *Arch. Neurol.* 2006, 63, 177-185.
[118] Hijazi, RA; Cunningham, GR. Andropause: Is Androgen Replacement Therapy Indicated for the Aging Male? *Annu. Rev. Med.* 2005, 56, 117-137.
[119] Martin, A; Brouwers, P; Lalonde, F et al: Towards a behavioral typology of Alzheimer's patients. *J. Clin. Exp. Neuropsychol.* 1986; 8, 594-610.
[120] Boller, F; Forette, F; Khatchaturian, Z; Poncet, M; Christen, Y. Heterogeneity of Alzheimer's disease. BerlinSpringer-Verlag; 1992.
[121] Fisher, NJ; Rourke, BP; Bieliauskas, L et al: Neuropsychological subgroups of patients with Alzheimer's disease. *J Clin Exp Neuropsychol* 1996, 18, 349-370.
[122] Jacobson, MW; Delis, DC; Salmon, DP et al: Do neuropsychological tests detect preclinical Alzheimer's disease: individual-test versus cognitive-discrepancy score analyses. *Neuropsychology.* 2002, 16, 132-139.
[123] Petersen, RC; Doody, R; Kurz, A et al. Current concepts in mild cognitive impairment. *Arch. Neurol.* 2001, 58, 1985-1992.
[124] Petersen R. C. Mild cognitive impairment as a diagnostic entity. *J. Inter. Med.* 2004, 256, 183-194.
[125] Lupien, SJ; de Leon, M; de Santi, S et al: Cortisol levels during human aging predict hippocampal atrophy and memory deficits. *Nat. Neurosci.* 1998, 1, 69-73.
[126] Lupien, SJ; Nair, NP; Briere, S et al. Increased cortisol levels and impaired cognition in human aging: implication for depression and dementia in later life. *Rev. Neurosci.* 1999, 10, 117-139.

[127] McEwen, BS; de Leon, MJ; Lupien, SJ et al. Corticosteroids, the Aging Brain and Cognition. *Trends Endocrinol. Metab.* 1999, 10, 92-96.

[128] Laaksonen, DE; Niskanen, L; Punnonen, K et al. Testosterone and sex hormone-binding globulin predict the metabolic syndrome and diabetes in middle-aged men. *Diab. Care.* 2004, 27, 1036-1041

[129] Capes, SE; Hunt, D; Malmberg, K et al. Stress hyperglycemia and prognosis of stroke in nondiabetic and diabetic patients. A systematic overview. *Stroke.* 2001, 32, 2426-2432.

[130] Lyness, JM; Niculescu, A; Reynolds, CF 3rd; Caine, ED. The relationship of medical comorbidity and depression in older, primary care patients. *Psychosomatics.* 2006, 47, 435-439.

[131] Lopez, OL; Jagust, WJ; Dulberg, C et al. Risk factors for mild cognitive impairment in the Cardiovascular Health Cognition Study : Part 2. *Arch. Neurol.* 2003, 60, 1394-1399.

[132] MacKnight, C; Rockwood, K; Awalt, E; McDowell, I. Diabetes mellitus and risk of dementia, Alzheimer's disease and vascular cognitive impairment in the Canadian study of health and aging. *Dement. Geriatri. Cogn. Disord.* 2002, 14, 77-83.

[133] Velasquez, EM; Bellabarba, Arata G. Effects of thyroid status on pituitary gonadotropin and testicular reserve in men. *Arch. Androl.* 1997, 38, 85-92.

[134] Baldini, I; Vita, A; Mauri, M et al: Psychopathological and cognitive features in subclinical hypothyroidism. *Prog. Neuropsychopharmacol. Biol. Psychiatry.* 1997, 21, 925-935.

[135] Hendrick, V; Altshuler, L; Whybrow, P. Psychoneuroendocrinology of mood disorders. The hypothalamic-pituitary-thyroid axis. *Psychiatr. Clin. North Am.* 1998, 21, 277-292.

In: Trends in Testosterone Research
Editor: Raymund E. Veritos

ISBN: 978-1-60456-127-2

Chapter VI

A Soy-Free Diet Can Lower Testosterone Levels in Male Hamsters: Implications for Aggression Research

Timothy O. Moore[1]* and Mary Karom[2]
[1] Department of Psychology, Clark Atlanta University, Atlanta, GA, USA
[2] Departments of Biology and Psychology, Georgia State University, Atlanta, GA, USA

Abstract

Standard animal lab chow is soy-based, and diets rich in soy protein contain estrogen-like compounds called phytoestrogens. The purpose of this study was to explore the hormonal effects of a soy versus a soy-free diet on testosterone levels in male hamsters. In Experiment #1, thirteen adult male hamsters (110-125 g) were individually-housed, and then divided into a soy and a soy-free group. All hamsters had continuous access to food and water, and they were sacrificed after seven weeks. Blood was collected to measure testosterone levels and the testes were removed to analyze the morphology. There was a significant difference in testosterone levels between the Soy (9.11±1.26 ng/ml) and the Soy-Free group (3.89±0.27 ng/ml)[$t(11)=3.74$; $p<0.005$]. There was no difference in testes weight, but the dimensions were different between the Soy (251.2±6.9 mm2) and the Soy-Free group (229.5±6.8 mm2)[$t(13)=2.2$; $p<0.05$]. In Experiment #2, twenty adult male hamsters (110-125 g) were individually-housed and then divided into four groups: 1) Castrate+Soy; 2) Castrate+Soy-Free; 3) Sham Castrate+Soy; and 4) Sham Castrate+Soy-Free. Animals were sacrificed seven weeks after surgery and the diet manipulation. There were no detectable levels of testosterone in castrated males. However, the Sham+Soy (12.21±2.95 ng/ml) had significantly higher levels of testosterone compared to Sham+Soy-Free (3.92±0.8 ng/ml)[$t(9)=2.95$; $p=0.01$]. In sum, we have demonstrated that a soy-free diet lowered endogenous levels of

* Correspondence should be addressed to Timothy O. Moore, Ph. D., Department of Psychology, Clark Atlanta University, 223 James P. Brawley Drive, Atlanta, GA 30314. Tel: 404-880-6939; Fax: 770-879-0275; Email: tmoore@cau.edu.

testosterone, and we recommend that investigators evaluate the impact of phytoestrogens when investigating behavioral experiments that involve neurosteroids.

Introduction

Interpreting the results of experiments that are designed to investigate hormones and social behavior can be a challenge (Albers, Huhman and Meisel, 2002). Although researchers may make every attempt to design properly controlled experiments, there may be unseen factors that can affect social behavior. Hamsters are an excellent animal model to study interactions between conspecifics in a social setting. Although studies with hamsters can be controlled, diet is one particular extraneous variable that can affect experimental results. In the present study, the implication of diet and hormonal status will be addressed without the context of social behavior. The focal point of this investigation will be on soy products that contain estrogen-like compounds.

Estrogen-like compounds called phytoestrogens are found in soy-based animal diets. Soy products are used as the major protein source in all natural-ingredient, commercially available, rodent diets. The different types of phytoestrogens are isoflavones, coumestans and lignans. In soy-based animal diets, genistein and daidzein are specific isoflavones that can exert estrogen-like effects on behavior.

A recent literature review of hamster aggression and diet revealed less than four experiments that have been reported. The effects of leptin on the estrous cycle (Schneider, Goldman, Tang, Bean, Ji and Friedman, 1998) and the effects of bacteria against neoplasia (Lemonde, 1973) were conducted. However, our study investigating the neurobehavioral effects of phytoestrogens in male hamsters (Moore, Karom and O'Farrell, 2004) was the most recent publication to study the connection between diet and agonistic behavior in male hamsters.

We have consistently demonstrated that testosterone levels are lowered in hamsters fed a soy-free diet. This is a significant finding because testosterone is known to play a critical role in male aggression. If diet can manipulate endogenous levels of testosterone, it is pertinent that diet should be taken into consideration when conducting behavioral experiments.

Testosterone can be converted into estradiol by the enzyme aromatase. In addition, testosterone can be synthesized into 5-DHT by 5-alpha reductase. Therefore, the effects of testosterone may be exerted by either testosterone, 5-DHT or estradiol. Furthermore, the receptors for both testosterone and estrogen may influence agonistic behavior. There is abundant evidence from rodent experiments that testosterone can enhance aggressive behavior. The positive relationship has been primarily observed in mice and rats. In hamsters, this direct relationship has been inclusive (Moore, 2001).

For example, Syrian hamsters are spontaneously aggressive animals that have been used by numerous investigators to study the neural and hormonal control of aggression. Over the last three decades, studies examining the effects of gonadal hormones on intermale aggression in hamsters have produced conflicting results (for review see Albers et al., 2002). Some studies report that castration and/or administration of gonadal hormones to castrates can significantly influence the expression of at least some measure of aggression (Drickamer,

Vandenbergh and Colby, 1973; Grelk, Papason, Cole and Rowe, 1974, Payne, 1973; Payne, 1974; Payne and Swanson, 1971; Payne, 1972; Potegal, Blau, Black and Glusman, 1980; Vandenbergh, 1971), whereas other studies found no reduction in aggression following castration (Evans and Brain, 1974; Tiefer, 1970; Whitsett, 1975). The differences in the results of these studies may be due to the many different, and sometimes complicated, methodologies that have been used to study the effects of gonadal hormones on aggression in male hamsters.

In retrospect, seldom was there any mention that diet could be a contributing factor in hormone and aggression experiments. In most rodent experiments, the standard animal lab chow is soy-based. Diets rich in soy protein contain called phytoestrogens, and these compounds may indirectly alter physiology and behavior. Before we further investigate the behavioral effects of phytoestrogens, it is important that we understand the general physiological effects of phytoestrogens. In this study, we will explore the hormonal effects of a soy versus a soy-free diet on testosterone levels in male hamsters. The purpose of this investigation will be to explore if diet alone, and not in conjunction with agonistic behavior, can affect the hormonal status of male hamsters.

Method

Animals

Adult male hamsters (110-125 g) were purchased from Charles River Laboratory and housed in a light-dark cycle consisting of 14-h light and 10-h dark (lights off at 1000). Food and water were continuously available throughout all experiments. Upon arrival to our laboratory, experimental animals were isolated.

Diet Manipulation

Hamsters were divided into two groups: 1) the standard soy-based 5001 animal diet (Soy); and 2) the 5K96 casein-based diet (Soy-Free). The soy diet contained 460 ppm total isoflavones and the soy-free diet contained less than 1 ppm total isoflavones. The diets were purchased from LabDiet (Purina Mills). The casein-based diet is a natural ingredient diet, formulated to be used in experimental protocols where dietary estrogenic activity is a concern. It consistently analyzes less than 1.0 ppm total isoflavones (aglycone equivalents of genistein, daidzein and glycitein). The Purina Mills 5001 diet contains an equivalent of 810 μg/g total phytoestrogens (Brown and Setchell, 2001).

Experiment #1

Thirteen male hamsters were isolated and then divided into two groups: Soy and Soy-Free. Animals were sacrificed seven weeks after the diet manipulation.

Experiment #2

Twenty male hamsters were isolated and then divided into four groups: 1) Castrate+Soy; 2) Castrate+Soy-Free; 3) Sham Castrate+Soy; and 4) Sham Castrate+Soy-Free. Animals were sacrificed seven weeks after surgery and the diet manipulation.

Surgery

Hamsters were anesthetized in an enclosed Plexiglas chamber filled with isoflurane. Hamsters were shaved and the surgical area was cleaned with isopropropyl alcohol and betadine solution. A face mask was placed over the nasal region and isoflurane gas was continuously delivered for the entire surgical procedure. Hamsters were bilaterally castrated through a midline abdominal incision. After locating and retracting each testicle through the incision, the cremaster muscle was separated from the tail of the epididymis in order to maximally exteriorize the testicle and associated tissues. The ductus deferens, testicular vessels and associated fat were then twisted, ligated and crushed with hemostats distal to the ligature. The testicles were then removed and the stump was allowed to slip back into the abdomen. Neither the testicle nor the surrounding tissue was removed in sham castrates. The abdominal muscle was sutured in a simple continuous pattern and skin incisions were closed with wound clips. The suture material used for both the abdominal closure and the ligations was 4-0 polyglactin 90. Hamsters recovered from anesthesia in a heated room.

Radioimmunoassay

Using methods described elswhere (Albers and Prishkolnik, 1992), testosterone (T) levels were measured by radioimmunoassay (RIA) in blood samples obtained from the inferior vena cava after lethal injection of sodium pentobarbital. Briefly, 5 μl of serum from each sample was dissolved in 196 μl of 0.1 M phosphate-buffered saline (PBS) and extracted in 2 ml of ether. After extraction, each sample was assayed in duplicate, 50 μl antibody (ICN Biomedical, Costa Mesa, CA), and 50 μl of ^{125}I-labeled T (1800cpm), and was allowed to incubate overnight at room temperature. The reported cross-reactivities were as follows: T, 100%; DHT, 3.4%; androstenedione, 0.6%; androsterone, <0.01%, 17β-estradiol, <0.01%; estrone, <0.01%; progesterone, <0.01%. A dextran-coated charcoal incubation (20 min) removed unbound tracers. After centrifugation for 15 min at 4 degrees celcius, the supernatant was decanted and counted by an LKB1272 gamma counter. The intra-assay variability was approximately 10%.

Statistical Analyses

A Student's t-Test for independent samples was used to determine the difference between treatment groups. Data with more than two groups were analyzed by between-groups, one factor analysis of variance (ANOVA). When a significant effect was encountered, a Tukey HSD post hoc test was employed.

Results

Experiment #1

All hamsters were sacrificed seven weeks after the diet manipulation, and blood serum and testes were collected. Figure 1 illustrates a significant difference in testosterone levels between the Soy (9.11±1.26 ng/ml) and the Soy-Free group (3.89±0.27 ng/ml)[$t(11)=3.74; p<0.005$]. Although the production of testosterone was affected, an analysis of the testes provided intriguing results. There were no differences in testes weights, but the dimensions of the testes were different between the Soy (251.2±6.9 mm^2) versus the Soy-Free group (229.5±6.8 mm^2) [$t(13)=2.2$; $p<0.05$]. Figure 2 represents the testes dimensions.

Table 1. Comparison of body and testes weight when animals were sacrificed seven weeks post-diet manipulation

	SOY	SOY FREE
Body Weight	132.6±2.7	134.3±4.9
Testes Weight	3.3±0.01	3.4±0.0

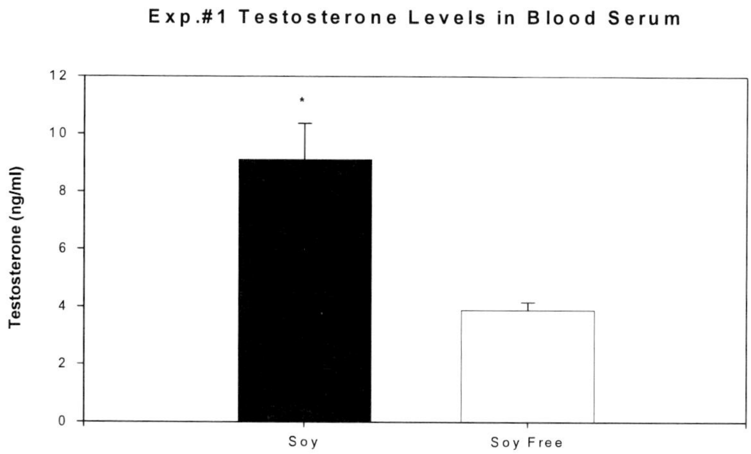

Figure 1. Following the administration of a soy (n=7) or a soy-free (n=6) diet for seven weeks, hamsters were sacrificed and testosterone was measured. An asterisk denotes a significant difference (p<0.005). Testosterone was higher in the Soy versus the Soy-Free group.

As stated, there was no difference in testes weight between groups and there was also no difference in the overall body weight at the time of sacrifice (see table 1). All hamsters had continuous access to food and water. Therefore, the diet was mainly controlled by the normal consumption of food by each animal. The amount of food consumed was not measured, but there was no difference in body weight between groups. Whether the diet was soy- or casein-based, there was equal growth between groups. However, endogenous hormones such as testosterone appeared to be sensitive to the diet manipulation.

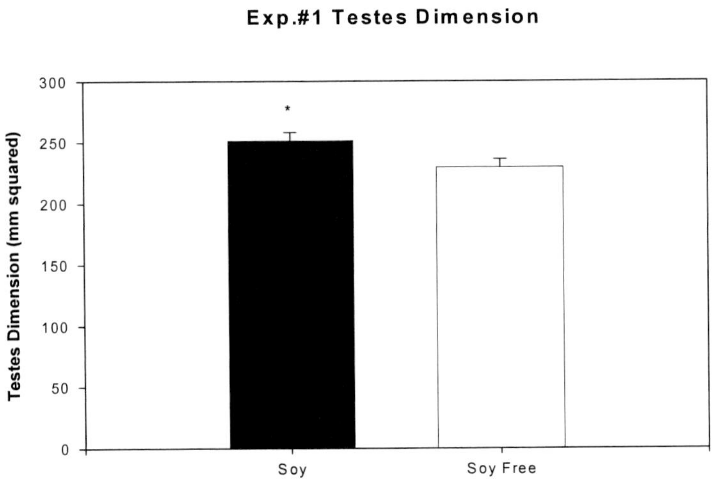

Figure 2. Following the administration of a soy (n=7) or a soy-free (n=6) diet for seven weeks, hamsters were sacrificed and the testes were removed and measured to analyze the size, weight and dimensions. An asterisk denotes a significant difference ($p<0.05$). The dimensions were slightly higher in the Soy group.

Experiment #2

An analysis was conducted between four different groups: Castrate+Soy; Castrate+Soy Free; Sham Castrate+Soy; and Sham Castrate+Soy-Free. Not surprisingly, there were no detectable levels of testosterone in castrated hamsters. According to our results, there was no evidence of any circulating testosterone in the blood serum of castrated hamsters. In contrast, the Sham Castrate+Soy group (12.21±2.95 ng/ml) had significantly higher levels of testosterone compared to the Sham Castrate+Soy-Free group (3.92±0.8 ng/ml) [$t(9)=2.95$; $p=0.01$]. The data are illustrated in figure 3

Since one half of the animals were castrated, we did not analyze the testes in Experiment #2. The weight was analyzed in figure 4 and we did observe the expectant increase in size over the seven week period for castrated hamsters. Although there were comparable weights between all four groups before and after the diet manipulation, we did observe a percent change within groups. For example, the Castrate+Soy group increased from 117g to 147g ($p<0.009$) and the Castrate+Soy-Free group increased from 123g to 153g ($p<0.09$). The Sham Castrate+Soy group increased from 120g to 132g ($p<0.002$), but the Sham Castrate+Soy-Free group did not have a significant increase from 125g to 153g ($p=0.13$) due to a high standard error of the mean.

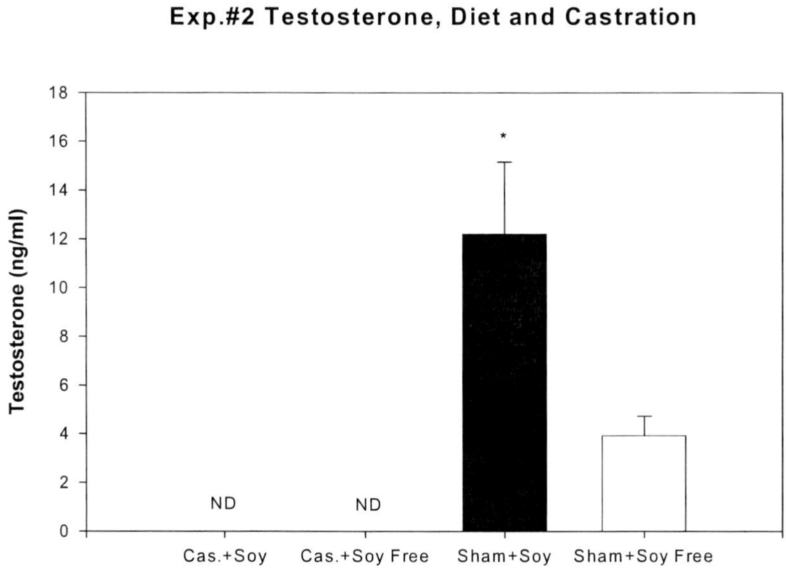

Figure 3. Twenty male hamsters were evenly divided into four groups. Hamsters were sacrificed seven weeks later and testosterone levels were measured. An asterisk denotes a significant difference ($p=0.01$) between the Sham+Soy and the Sham+Soy Free group. There were no detectable levels in castrates.

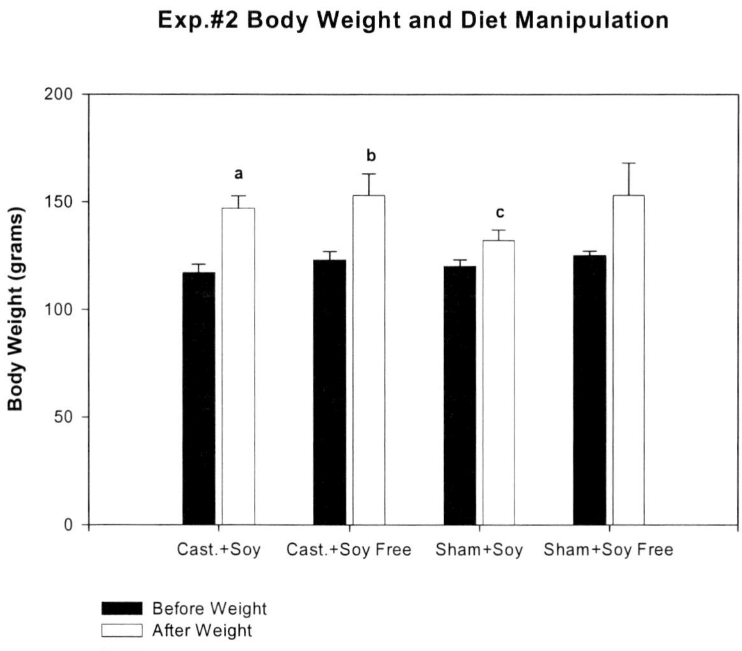

Figure 4. Body weight was measured before and after the diet and surgical manipulation. There was a significant change in weight for three out of the four groups. The letters (a, b and c) denote significance.

Conclusion

Our findings demonstrate that testosterone levels in male hamsters can be influenced by a standard, soy-based lab chow. The soy-free diet we used was casein-based, and we have consistently demonstrated that a soy-free diet can lower testosterone levels in the blood serum when compared to a diet containing soy. We did not measure consumption of the diet for each hamster, however, there was no difference between the weight of hamsters fed the different diets. The different levels of testosterone are more than likely due to the content of the food and not the amount of food consumed.

In hamsters, the only other published reports describing the influence of diet on physiology and social behavior have been with female Syrian hamsters fed leptin to study the effects on estrous cyclicity, social behaviors and ovulation rate (Schneider et al., 1998). Moreover, a very old study on the effects of bacteria against neoplasia in mice and hamsters was conducted (Lemonde, 1973). Our recent publication (Moore et al., 2004) has driven our research into uncharted territory. We can reliably suggest that diet should be taken into consideration when studying hormones and social behavior. In the analysis of behavior, the behavior may be indirectly altered by the diet and not the manipulated independent variable (e.g., lighting, opponent, phase, experience, surgical manipulation, etc.).

We have previously demonstrated (Moore et al. 2004) that the Soy-Free group had higher levels of vasopressin V1A receptor binding compared to the Soy group in the lateral septum. In contrast, the soy group had higher receptor binding in the lateral septum when compared to the soy-free group. We observed hormonal changes as a result of the diet manipulation and other research (Davis, 2002) investigating neuroanatomy suggests that soy products or phytoestrogens may be potent selective estrogen receptor modulators (SERMs). The summarized data are not conclusive, but there is speculation that phytoestrogens may exert both estrogenic and anti- estrogenic effects on estrogen receptors α and β. We did not measure any receptors in this study, but we can speculate that soy is affecting more than just blood serum concentrations of testosterone.

Interestingly, there was no difference in the weight of the testes between groups, but the dimensions were slightly different. In other words, the morphology of the testes may have changed from the diet manipulation, but the size was not affected. The change in morphology may have a connection to diet and cancer formation. For example, there has been an interest in potentially anticarcinogenic actions of isoflavones. Laboratory rats fed soy-enriched diets have less breast tumor development following stimulation with the directly- and indirectly-acting tumour-inducers (Messina, 1994).

Some investigators have directly exposed animals to specific phytoestrogens such as genistein and coumestrol. In a recent study, Wisniewski, Cernetich, Gearhart and Klein (2005) determined if exposure to genistein, during early periods of sex differentiation alters reproductive development and behavior in male mice. Aggressive behaviors were decreased, whereas defensive behaviors were increased in males that received the low dose genistein diet. According to Wisniewski et al.(2005), exposure to genistein during critical periods of sex differentiation results in concurrent and persistent demasculinization in male mice. In another study, the effects of coumestrol on estrogen receptor α knockout mice (ErαKO) was investigated (Jacob, Temple, Patisaul, Young and Rissman, 2001). The results demonstrated that coumestrol has antiestrogenic actions in the brain and pituitary and that ERα mediates these effects.

Other central nervous system mechanisms have also been studied. Androgen metabolizing enzymes, for example, are known to regulate neuroendocrine functions and reproductive behaviors, while calcium-binding proteins are associated with protecting against neurodegenerative diseases (Lephart, Thompson, Setchell, Adlercreutz and Weber, 2000). It was reported that consumption of phytoestrogens in rats via a soy diet for a relatively short interval can elevate plasma and brain phytoestrogen levels and decrease brain calcium-binding proteins without altering brain androgen metabolizing enzymes.

Lephart, Galindo and Bu (2001) were the first to show that life-long consumption of dietary phytoestrogens alters hypothalamic-pituitary-adrenal stress response in male rats. Phytoestrogen fed rats displayed significantly higher plasma ACTH and hippocampal glucocorticoid receptor levels when compared to phytoestrogen-free values. Similar to what we have presented in this study, the research by Lephart et al. (2002) provides critical evidence that soy-derived phytoestrogens have complex and beneficial effects on brain structure, function and behavior.

In sum, the neurobehavioral effects of dietary soy phytoestrogens cannot be overlooked in animal research. We must determine the importance of phytoestrogens given the recognized significance of estrogen in brain and neural disorders (Lephart et al., 2002). There is epidemiological, laboratory, and clinical evidence which indicates that phytoestrogens, like certain SERMs, have an antiproliferative effect on the breast, and positive effects on the lipoprotein profile and bone density (Brzezinski and Debi, 1999). If animal studies are to be the baseline for effects on humans, accurate assessment of the data will require researchers to consider the type of diet chosen for experimentation. In conclusion, there are potential benefits to human consumption of a soy-based diet. The research is not conclusive, but well controlled animal experiments will help to determine the beneficial as well as detrimental effects of phytoestrogens on human health.

Acknowledgments

In conjunction with the Center for Behavioral Neuroscience (NSF-STC #IBN-9876754), this work was supported by NIH Grant #NS37232.

References

Albers, H.E., and Prishkolnik, J. (1992). Sex differences in odor stimulated flank marking behavior in the Golden hamster (*Mesocricetus auratus*), *Hormones and Behavior*, 26, 229-239.

Albers, H.E., Huhman, K.L. and Meisel, R.L. (2002). *Hormonal basis of social conflict and communication. Hormones and Behavior*, 1, 393-433. Academic Press, New York.

Brown, N.M.and Setchell, K.D. (2001). Animal models impacted by phytoestrogens in commercial chow. *Laboratory Investigation*, 81, 735-747.

Brzezinski, A. and Debi, A. (1999). Phytoestrogens: the "natural" selective estrogen receptor modulators? *European Journal of Obstetrics and Gynecology and Reproductive Biology*, 85, 47-51.

Drickamer, L.C., Vandenbergh, J.G., and Colby, D.R. (1973). Predictors of dominance in the male golden hamster (*Mesocricetus auratus*). *Animal Behavior*, 21, 557-563.

Davis, S.R., (2002). Phytoestrogens in the context of SERMs. In *Contemporary Endocrinology: Selective Estrogen Receptor Modulators: Research and Clinical Applications* (Eds. Manni, A. and Verderame, M.F.) pp. 345-363, Humana Press, Totowa, NJ.

Evans, C.M. and Brain, P.F. (1974). Some studies on endocrine influences on aggressive behavior in the golden hamster (*Mesocricetus auratus* Waterhouse). *Progress in Brain Research*, 41, 473-480.

Grelk, D.F., Papson, B.A., Cole, J.E. and Rowe, F.A. (1974). The influence of caging conditions and hormone treatments on fighting in male and female hamsters. *Hormones and Behavior*, 5, 355-366.

Jacob, D.A., Temple, J.L., Patisaul, H.B., Young, L.J., and Rissman, E.F. (2001). Coumestrol antagonizes neuroendocrine actions of estrogen via the estrogen receptor α. *Experimental Biology and Medicine*, 226(4), 301-306.

Lemonde, P. (1973). Protective effects of BCG and other bacteria against neoplasia in mice and hamsters. *National Cancer Institute Monograph*, 39, 21-32.

Lephart, E.D., Thompson, J.M., Setchell, K.D.R., Adlercreutz, H. and Weber, K.S. (2000). Phytoestrogens decrease brain calcium-binding proteins but do not alter hypothalamic androgen metablozing enzymes in adult male rats. *Brain Research*, 859, 123-131.

Lephart, E.D., West, T.W., Weber, K.S., Rhees, R.W., Setchell, K.D.R., Adlercreutz, H. and Lund, T.D. (2002). Neurobehavioral effects of dietary soy phytoestrogens. *Neurotoxicology and Teratology*, 24, 5-16.

Lephart, E.D., Galindo, E. and Bu, L.H. (2003). Stress (hypothalamic-pituitary-adrenal axis) and pain response in male rats exposed lifelong to high vs. low phytoestrogen diets. *Neuroscience Letters*, 342, 65-68.

Messina, M. (1994). Soy intake and cancer risk: a review of the in vitro and in vivo data. *Nutrition and Cancer*, 21, 113-131.

Moore, T.O. (2001). Testosterone and male behavior: Empirical research with hamsters does not support the use of castration to deter human sexual aggression. *North American Journal of Psychology*, 3(3), 503-520.

Moore, T. O., Karom, M. and O'Farrell, L. (2004). The neurobehavioral effects of phytoestrogens in male Syrian hamsters. *Brain Research*, 1016, 102-110.

Payne, A.P. and Swanson, H.H. (1971). The effect of castration and ovarian implantation on aggressive behaviour of male hamsters. *Journal of Endocrinology*, 51, 217-218.

Payne, A.P. and Swanson, H.H. (1972). The effect of sex hormones on the agonistic behavior of the male golden hamster (*mesocricetus auratus* waterhouse). *Physiology and Behavior*, 8, 687-691.

Payne, A.P. (1973). A comparison of the aggressive behaviour of isolated intact and castrated male golden hamsters toward intruders introduced into the home cage. *Physiology and Behavior*, 10, 629-631.

Payne, A.P. (1974). A comparison of the effects of androstenedione, dihydrotestosterone and testosterone propionate on aggression in the castrated male golden hamster. *Physiology and Behavior*, 13, 21-26.

Potegal, M., Blau, A.D., Black, M. and Glusman, M. (1980). Effects of castration of male golden hamsters on their aggression toward a restrained target. *Behavioral Neural Biology*, 29(3), 315-330.

Schneider, J.E., Goldman, M.D., Tang, S., Bean, B., Ji, H. and Friedman, M.I. (1998). Leptin indirectly affects estrous cycles by increasing metabolic fuel oxidation. *Hormones and Behavior*, 33(3), 217-228.

Tiefer, L. (1970). Gonadal hormones and mating behavior in the adult golden hamster. *Hormones and Behavior*, 1, 189-202.

Vandenbergh, J.G. (1971). The effects of gonadal hormones on the aggressive behavior of adult golden hamsters (*Mesocricetus auratus*). *Animal Behavior*, 19, 589-594.

Whitsett, J.M. (1975). The development of aggressive and marking behavior in intact and castrated male hamsters. *Hormones and Behavior*, 6, 47-57.

Wisniewski, A.B., Cernetich, A., Gearhart and Klein, S.L. (2005). Perinatal exposure to genistein alters reproductive development and aggressive behavior in male mice, 84, 327-334.

In: Trends in Testosterone Research
Editor: Raymund E. Veritos
ISBN: 978-1-60456-127-2

Chapter VII

Behavioural Effects of Testosterone in Men: Directions for Future Research

Daryl B. O'Connor
Institute of Psychological Sciences, University of Leeds, Leeds, UK

As outlined in a later chapter in this collection, the association between testosterone, aggression and anger in humans has been the focus of substantial research attention over the last number of decades (e.g., Archer, 1991; Archer, Birring & Wu, 1998; Dabbs, Jurkovoic & Frady, 1991; Harris, 1999; O'Connor, Archer, Hair & Wu, 2002; O'Connor, Archer & Wu, 2004; Pagonis, Angelopoulos, Koukoulis & Hadjichristodoulou, 2006). Generally, these studies have either involved comparisons of testosterone levels and self-reported aggression between violent and non-violent groups or have been correlational in nature, investigating the degree of association between endogenous testosterone levels, aggression and hostile feelings in various samples of men (see Archer, 1991; Harris, 1999).

Moreover, these studies have shown conflicting results with much of the existing research being observational, retrospective and/or cross-sectional. As a consequence, it has proved difficult to render conclusions about causality. More recently there have been considerable developments with the publication of a number of carefully controlled, empirical investigations that have examined the effects of exogenous testosterone on anger and aggression outcomes in men (e.g., Anderson, Bancroft & Wu, 1992; Kouri, Lukas, Pope, 1995; O'Connor et al., 2002; 2004; Pope, Kouri & Hudson, 2000; Su et al., 1993; Tricker et al., 1996). In addition to including a wide range of self- and partner-reported behavioural outcome measures, these studies have experimentally manipulated testosterone levels into the supraphysiological range, using double-blind, placebo-controlled, cross-over designs. Despite these important methodological improvements there are a number of valuable directions that future research, into the effects of testosterone on behaviour, ought to pursue. These are discussed in turn.

Need for More Objective Assessments

Self- and partner-reported changes in behaviour are important and often represent the only methods available for assessing the effects of exogenous testosterone on aggression, anger and mood in naturalistic settings. Given that real-life incidents of human aggression are difficult to measure and record as they happen, researchers have to rely on indirect methods, which can broadly be divided into (1) laboratory procedures that simulate the sort of provoking situations that generate aggressive actions in the outside world and (2) reports of real-life aggression. In the latter case, the majority of studies have utilised psychometrically reliable and valid instruments such as the Aggression Questionnaire (Buss & Perry, 1992), the Profile of Mood States (McNair, Lorr, & Droppleman, 1992) or the Conflict Tactics Scale (Straus, 1979). To this list, a further less commonly used measure can be added, responses to hypothetical scenarios involving provocation – in other words, what people say they would do under situations which are likely to evoke anger (e.g., O'Connor et al., 2001; van Goozen et al., 1994). In the former case, researchers have incorporated laboratory-based measures of aggression such as the Point Subtraction Aggression Paradigm (PSAP; Cherek et al., 1996), which is a computerised provocation test that assesses aggressive responding.

However, it is important for future research to include more sensitive measures that may detect more subtle, but potentially clinically and pathologically significant changes in psychological outcomes. For example, administration of testosterone has been found to be associated with increases in the cognitive aspects of sexual functioning in men but not in interactional components such as sexual intercourse (e.g., Anderson, Bancroft & Wu, 1992; Alexander et al., 1997). Alexander et al (1997) found evidence of testosterone related changes in sexual arousal by measuring responses to a sexually explicit audiotape using a laboratory-based dichotic listening task. O'Connor, Archer, Hair and Wu (2001) also found exogenous testosterone to differentially influence cognitive functioning in men such that improvements in verbal ability were accompanied by reductions in spatial ability following testosterone treatment. Taken together, these findings indicate that behavioural effects of testosterone may be mediated via cognitive and attentional processes that are not tapped using traditional paper and pencil techniques.

More recently, Smith and Waterman (2003), using the dot probe and emotional Stroop tasks, found that violent offenders and aggressive individuals (as assessed by their self-reported anger scores) exhibited significant response biases to aggression words across both tests. These results indicated that processing biases may be associated with trait anger and aggression. In addition, pioneering research conducted by van Honk and colleagues (2001) has also shown that administration of a single dosage of testosterone (0.5 mg) has the capacity to induce an accelerative cardiac response (i.e., heart rate in beats per min) to angry faces in women. These authors suggest that specific changes in cardiac response may indicate aggression proneness and preparation for fight. To date, little or no research has examined whether supraphysiological increases in testosterone levels are associated with changes in aggression-related, attentional and cognitive processes or cardiac responses to anger-related stimuli.

Use of Daily Diary Designs

In addition to pursuing carefully designed studies in the laboratory, future research should also consider using innovative multi-level, daily diary methods in the real world. As outlined above, assessing real-life incidents of human aggression are difficult. However, using daily diaries allows researchers to identify more closely "real-time" occurrences or moments of change in study variables; reduce recall bias; decrease potential confounding by using participants as their own controls, and enable causality to be established in naturalistic settings (Affleck et al., 1999).

Previous research into the effects of testosterone on aggression outcomes has been overly reliant on cross-sectional methodologies that have used single indices (i.e., assessed aggressive behaviour 'generally' in a trait like manner) or 'snap-shot' measurements of aggressive behaviour (i.e., assessed self-reported aggression over the past four weeks). Such approaches have ignored the growing body of evidence showing that assessments of fluctuations in within-person daily events are important (cf., Nezlek, 2001; O'Connor, Jones, Conner, McMillan & Ferguson, 2008). In the area of testosterone and aggression, it remains a possibility that hormone-related changes in aggression, anger and mood are missed using conventional retrospective measures. This possibility is particularly relevant to studies that have examined the impact of therapeutic doses of testosterone (for male contraception or hormone replacement purposes) where changes may be relatively modest in size and/or infrequent, in contrast to studies of androgenic-anabolic steroid (AAS) abusers.

Using daily diary techniques, interval-contingent (i.e., assessments completed at the end of each day) or event-contingent methods (i.e., assessments completed in response to an event) can be employed, where the participants complete diaries each night at a fixed time period or during each day trigged by feelings or episodes of aggression/anger. This methodology facilitates the use of the powerful statistical technique known as multilevel random coefficient modeling (MRCM). This approach provides accurate analyses of multilevel data structures and would allow the modeling of day-to-day within-person effects *together* with the impact of between-person factors such as potential vulnerability variables such as age, violent history, AAS usage and trait impulsivity (cf., Nezlek, 2001; Snijders & Bosker, 1999). In standard MRCM nomenclature, future studies could be organized in a two level hierarchical structure with Level 1 being the within-person variation (e.g., daily patterns in aggressive behaviour, anger and mood) and Level 2 being the between-person variability (e.g., treatment condition, age, gender etc.).

Final Comments

Future research ought to carefully examine further the incidence of psychiatric symptoms in illicit AAS abusers. The converging evidence suggests that the existing findings may represent an underestimation of the true impact of AAS abuse in the general population. Many of the published studies have employed rigorous recruitment procedures and have screened out a large number of potentially 'high risk' participants. Therefore, the incidence rates in a population of AAS abusers may be substantially larger than those reported thus far in the scientific literature. In addition, given the relatively small sample sizes typically employed in AAS studies and the associated risk of type 2 errors (i.e., false negatives), it would be prudent for future studies to provide effect sizes for cases in which there are no significant differences between testosterone and placebo conditions. Effect sizes, unlike significance levels, are not influenced by sample size so it is possible to use them to assess the possibility that small- to medium-sized effects have not gone undetected by significance testing.

References

Affleck, G., Zautra, A., Tennen, H., & Armeli, S. (1999). Multilevel daily process designs for consulting and clinical psychology: A preface for the perplexed. *Journal of Consulting and Clinical Psychology*, 67, 746-754.

Alexander, G.M., Swerdloff, R.S., Wang, C., Davidson, T., McDonald, V., Steiner, B., & Hines, M. (1997). Androgen-behavior correlations in hypogonadal men and eugonadal men. I. Mood and response to auditory sexual stimuli. *Hormones & Behavior*, 31, 110-119.

Anderson, R.A., Bancroft, J., & Wu, F.C.W. (1992). The effects of exogenous testosterone on sexuality and mood of normal men. *Journal of Clinical Endocrinology & Metabolism*, 75, 1503-1507.

Archer, J. (1991). The influence of testosterone on human aggression. *British Journal of Psychology*, 82, 1-28.

Archer, J., Birring, S.S., & Wu, F.C.W. (1998). The association between testosterone and aggression among young men: Empirical findings and a meta-analysis. *Aggressive Behavior*, 24, 411-420.

Buss, A.H., & Perry, M. (1992). The aggression questionnaire. *Journal of Personality and Social Psychology,* 63, 452-459.

Cherek, D.R., Schnapp, W., Moeller, F.G., & Dougherty, D.M. (1996). Laboratory measures of aggressive responding in male parolees with violent and nonviolent histories. *Aggressive Behavior*, 22, 27-36.

Dabbs, J.M. Jr., Jurkovoic, G.L., & Frady, R.L. (1991). Salivary testosterone and cortisol levels among late adolescent male offenders. *Journal of Abnormal Child Psychology*, 19, 469-478.

Harris, J.A. (1999). Review and methodological considerations in research on testosterone and aggression. *Aggression & Violent Behavior*, 4, 273-291.

McNair, D.M., Lorr, M., & Droppleman, L.F. (1992). *EdITS manual for the Profile of Mood States*. Educational and Industrial Testing Service, San Diego: California.

Nezlek, J.B. (2001). Multilevel random coefficient analyses of event- and interval contingent data in social and personality psychology research. *Personality and Social Psychology Bulletin*, 27: 771-785.

O'Connor, D.B., Archer, J., & Wu, F.C.W. (2004). Effects of testosterone on mood, aggression and sexual behavior in young men: A double-blind, placebo-controlled, cross-over study. *Journal of Clinical Endocrinology & Metabolism*, 89, 2837-2845.

O'Connor, D.B., Archer, J., & Wu, F.C.W. (2001). Measuring aggression: self-reports, partner reports and responses to provoking scenarios. *Aggressive Behavior*, 27, 79-101.

O'Connor, D.B., Archer, J., Hair, W.M., & Wu, F.C.W. (2001). Activational effects of testosterone on cognitive function in men. *Neuropsychologia*, 39, 1385-1394.

O'Connor, D.B., Archer, J., Hair, W.H., & Wu, F.C.W. (2002). Exogenous testosterone, aggression, and mood in eugonadal and hypogonadal men. *Physiology & Behavior*, 75, 557-566.

O'Connor, D.B., Jones, F., Conner, M., McMillan, B., & Ferguson, E. (2008). Effects of Daily Hassles and Eating Style on Eating Behavior. *Health Psychology*, in press.

Pagonis, T.A., Angelopoulos, N.V., Koukoulis, G.N., & Hadjichristodoulou, C.S. (2006). Psychiatric side effects induced by supraphysiological doses of combinations of anabolic steroids correlate to the severity of abuse. *European Psychiatry*, 21, 551-562.

Smith, P., & Waterman, M. (2003). Processing bias for aggression words in forensic and nonforensic samples. *Cognitive & Emotion*, 17, 681-701.

Snijders, T., & Bosker, R. (1999). *Multilevel analysis*. London: Sage.

Straus, M.A., Hamby, S.L., Boney-McCoy, S., & Sugarman, D.B. (1996). The revised Conflict Tactics Scales (CTS2): Development and preliminary psychometric data. *Journal of Family Issues*, 17, 283-316.

van Goozen, S.H.M., Frijda, N.H., Kindt, M., & van de Poll, N.E. (1994). Anger proneness in women: development and validation of the anger situation questionnaire. *Aggressive Behavior*, 20, 79-100.

van Honk, J., Tuiten, A., Hermans, E., Putman, P., Koppeschaar, H., Thijssen, J., Verbaten, R., & van Doornen, L. (2001). A single administration of testosterone induces cardiac accelerative responses to angry faces in healthy young women.*Behavioral Neuroscience*, 115, 238-242.

In: Trends in Testosterone Research
Editor: Raymund E. Veritos

ISBN: 978-1-60456-127-2

Chapter VIII

The Neuroendocrinology of Testosterone – Sociosexual Behavior Relations

George T. Taylor*, Joshua Dearborn and Susan Fortenbury
Behavioral Neuroscience, Univ. of Missouri, St. Louis, MO 63121 USA.

Abstract

Steroids produced in the periphery have long been of interest to reproductive biologists. The emergence of neuroendocrinology as a dominant subfield of behavioral studies appeared to demote steroids to a lesser status than the exciting neuropeptides that clearly interacted with many regions of the brain. Seminal findings in recent years, however, have propelled the study of steroids back onto center stage. In this chapter we identify the seminal findings and describe why they are revolutionary. These new findings have demonstrated steroids have the capacity to modify the structure and function of brain regions both related to and unrelated to reproduction. The consequences on behavior are likely to be profound. This chapter focuses on one steroid, testosterone, because it occupies a strategic position in the metabolic cascade of the sex steroids. It is a position that can influence the actions of androgens and estrogens, as well as the adrenal precursors of testosterone and the recently identified neurosteroids, on the brain and behavior. We believe future research will reveal testosterone to have behavioral effects extending well beyond those related to reproduction. Still, the massive literature on testosterone – sociosexual behavior provides a solid background on which to begin that work.

* Correspondence concerning this article should be addressed to George T. Taylor, Ph.D. Professor of Psychology & Director of Behavioral Neuroscience, University of Missouri - St. Louis, One University Blvd. St. Louis, MO 63121 U.S.A. Tel: (314) 516-5475; Fax: (314) 516-5392; E-mail: geot@UMSL.edu.

Section I. Introduction

Reproductive function, most notably sexual behavior, has been the meat and potatoes of behavioral endocrinology for over a century. Androgens, and especially testosterone (TS), have been front and center for much of the century.

The first experimental manipulation of the endocrine system often cited in textbooks is of a demonstration of castrated roosters being implanted with testes. The treatment restored the color and size of their combs, as well as fully restored crowing, fighting and sexual behaviors. Later, an aging researcher reported rejuvenation of sexual prowess with an implant of an aqueous solution from crushed testes of experimental animals injected into his own abdominal cavity (Wilson 2000). Few can watch today's television commercials on topical TS without smiling and thinking how little times have changed.

These early studies point to four important features that defined much of the research in endocrinology for the next decades. First, there was a clear focus on practical therapeutic application to humans. Understanding the basic biology of sex hormones was only of secondary interest. Second, the studies demonstrated a fundamental research paradigm of endocrinology – ablation and hormone replacement as the experimental manipulation with functional restoration as the outcome measure. Third, the studies focused on the relation of a hormone to function and dysfunction of systems related to reproduction. A special focus was on sociosexual behaviors, defined as behaviors related to successful reproduction. Finally, the hormones on which most attention was placed were the sex steroids. It was TS and males in the early days, but today there has been at least equal focus on estrogens and progesterone in females.

Later still came the recognition that a non-sex steroid, corticosteroid, was intimately involved in the response to stressors. The bind that tied corticosteroids to sex steroids were the findings that stress could suppress reproductive physiology and function. Without doubt, steroids were firmly entrenched into the field of behavioral endocrinology (Beach 1981).

Behavioral neuroendocrinology emerged as the dominant subfield with a handful of seminal findings in recent decades These results have made it clear that steroids do more than simply maintain peripheral structures and reflexively activate subcortical brain regions to initiate regulatory behaviors. The seminal findings suggest sex steroids do more, much more.

One of the more satisfying outcomes is to give contemporary legitimacy to a behavioral biologist with interest in the steroids. The new findings also allowed researchers to move beyond the simple correlational studies of circulating TS and behavior. We now can understand better puzzling findings from the earliest days in behavioral endocrinology. More important, the seminal findings have thrust the brain into a central position in the study of steroids.

Our goal in this chapter will be to address the current status of TS and behavior in relation to the recent findings. We will use reproductive behaviors as the exemplary literature because that is surely the most complete. There are already excellent reviews of endocrine - sociosexual behavior relations (Archer 1994, Baum 2002, Meisel and Sachs 1994, Meston, 2000). Rather than presenting another similar review, we have organized topics to emphasize the changes in thinking induced by the seminal findings as they have impacted the study of TS. We characterize these findings as "revolutionary" for several reasons. 1) The findings were more or less unexpected. 2) They introduced a level of complexity for the study of steroid - behavior interactions that few would have envisioned in the early days of endocrinology. 3) They provided a searchlight to guide our study of the fundamental mechanisms in the brain responsible for the steroid – behavior correlations.

It is our hope that the reader who persists to the end of this chapter will better appreciate the neuroendocrine complexities researchers have encountered in the study of a seemingly simple hormone – behavior interaction. Emphasis will be primarily on male animal models and men, although the emerging role of TS on female behaviors will be discussed where appropriate. Finally, the chapter may also prove helpful to students and researchers in behavioral neuroendocrinology because similar complexities likely apply to other hormone – behavior relations.

I.1. Sexual Behaviors can be Separated into Motivation and Performance Behaviors

A first step in digesting the large literature on sexual behavior is to distinguish its two separate components, motivation and performance. Sexual motivation refers to measures of the male's interest to engage in sexual activity, sometimes referred to as sexual arousal or libido. Sexual performance is the effectiveness of the male to initiate and complete a copulatory bout. The two components of sexual behavior involve distinct, quantifiable behaviors.

Successful reproduction requires the male to be sufficiently motivated to find a receptive female. Clever methods have been adopted to quantify intensity of sexual motivation in laboratory animals. One example is a small treadmill on which a male mouse must continue to run to stay nearby the stationary female (Craigen and Bronson 1982). More commonly, the measure of motivation is latency to initiate a mount of the female (Meisel and Sachs 1994) or time spent near an inaccessible estrous female (Taylor, *et al* 1991). Sexual motivation in females can be assessed also by time spent near a reproductive male or by recording solicitations, a species-specific set of behaviors used in the pre-copulatory phase (Taylor, *et al* 1989).

Copulation can be more easily observed than motivation in animal models. There are a number of distinct behaviors that can be independently measured, most notably latencies and frequencies of mounting, intromissions and ejaculations (Taylor and Weiss 1987). The single behavioral marker of receptivity in the female is lordosis, the bent-back positioning by the female, exposing her genitals and allowing the male to penetrate her.

In humans, the most common measures of both sexual interest and activity are self-reports, either from recall or a diary. There are a number of sophisticated recording instruments available to researchers, but they are intrusive and have limited use. Self-reports remain most convenient and most popular.

I.2. Distinct Brain Pathways have Evolved for Sexual Motivation and Performance in Males

The two components of sexual behavior also involve different underlying neural systems. An exemplary experiment (Everitt 1990) demonstrated the different neural systems underlying sexual motivation and performance. Male rats pressed a bar to deliver a receptive female rat into his chamber. After training, the medial preoptic area (MPOA) of the hypothalamus was lesioned in one group of males. The animals continued to bar press for the female but no longer would attempt to mount and copulate with her. Both amygdalae were lesioned in a second group. These males no longer bar pressed to produce the receptive female. If she was placed inside the chamber, however, the male readily copulated. The suggestion is clear that an intact MPOA is necessary for normal copulatory performance whereas the amygdala is intimately involved in sexual motivation.

That experiment, and many others before and afterwards (Pfaus 1996), have demonstrated that the CNS ultimately holds the key to understanding sexual function in both males and females. The structures in the brain most often cited as being directly related to the control of male sexual behavior are the olfactory tubercles, corticomedial nuclei of the amygdaloid complex, bed nucleus of the stria terminalis (BNST), and the hypothalamus, especially the medial preoptic area (Baum 2002, Cooke, *et al* 1999b, Dominguez and Hull 2005).

Circulating levels of TS and the other sex hormones readily cross the blood brain barrier and, joined by a host of neurotransmitters and neuropeptides involved in reproduction, exert profound influence on the activity of these structures (Hull, *et al* 1999, McEwen, *et al* 1995). The evidence is overwhelming that TS is critical for the organization and activation of sexual motivation and performance of males. We present in the next section five findings (highlighted in bold and listed as II.1, II.2 and so forth) that changed, indeed revolutionized, the study of steroid physiology and behavior.

Section II. Findings that Revolutionized the Study of Neuroendocrinology of Testosterone – Behavior Relations

II.1. Fetal Testosterone Organizes Male Brain Circuitry

The influence of TS on the brain begins early. Beginning in the prenatal phase and continuing as the brain and periphery develop in the neonate, TS or its absence determines sexual differentiation. Early exposure to TS permanently masculinizes the male for an array of behavioral and physiological functions. The fetal and postnatal periods of testicular activity have profound effects on male sexual differentiation, whereas in the female early sexual development occurs without influence of ovarian function. In the absence of circulating TS, the mammalian brain and urogenital systems are feminized and de-masculinized.

Other data confirm male perinatal physiology being more reactive than that of females to sex hormones. Testosterone is being released in the male fetus long before the hypothalamic – pituitary - gonadal (HPG) axis has matured. Still, the HPG axis is fully functional in the male rat during the last days of gestation (Huhtaniemi 2000). In the first hours after birth, only the male experiences a burst of TS that increases circulating titers to near adult levels for a short period of time (Timiras and Cons 1982). This dramatic increase may or may not have consequences for later adult sociosexual behaviors (McGivern, *et al* 1998). By contrast, the fetal ovary is in a quiescent state, and its endocrine activity begins in earnest only with the first signs of puberty.

Sex steroidal influences lay relatively dormant in the postnatal animal until puberty. Then the same sex hormones, along with surges of gonadotropins and neuropeptides, activate the circuits organized during fetal development. This two phase influence of TS on behavior is the now classic organizational – activational model (Arnold and Gorski 1984, Phoenix, *et al* 1959). Fetal organization of sexually dimorphic brain morphology and circuitry can be observed in behaviors prior to puberty. Examples are the sexually dimorphic play and cognitive behaviors of prepubertal animals (Hodes and Shors 2005, Taylor 1980a). Clearer differences emerge with the activation of the circuitry by pubertal hormones. The results are gender-typical adult sociosexual behaviors, as well as influences on an array of non-reproductive behaviors.

The organizational – activational concept remains a powerful guide and is treated today as dogma by most neuroendocrinologists (Hall, *et al* 2004). However, there are several refinements of the original organizational – activational model that are based largely on the rodent brain (Ball and Balthazart 2006). For example, a key step suggested by rodent studies is that metabolism of TS to estradiol is necessary to induce a masculine organization of the brain. There is little evidence, however, to indicate that step is necessary in primates. Testosterone is likely directly responsible for the masculinization of the primate brain (Breedlove and Hampson 2002, Cooke, *et al* 1999a). Nonetheless, these findings point out the importance of the metabolic cascade for the synthesis of steroids for understanding the influence of TS on sociosexual behaviors.

II.2. Estradiol is a Metabolite of Testosterone

The metabolic cascade of steroidal hormones is remarkably complex and details remain unclear (Ball and Balthazart 2006, Occhiato, *et al* 2004). One basic feature is that the two primary metabolites of TS are estradiol (E2) and dihydrotestosterone (DHT). Thus, TS may directly activate steroid-sensitive tissues or be metabolized to either E2 or DHT which in turn activates the tissue. Whether TS or its metabolites activate the target cell is dependent upon the presence or absence of specific enzymes. Aromatase is responsible for converting TS to E2 and 5alpha-reductase converts TS to DHT (Payne and Hales 2004).

In tissue containing aromatase, and that includes many brain regions, the result is that TS is a prohormone in adult males. The direct effect on function is after TS is metabolized to E2 and E2 binds the estrogen receptor (Adkins-Regan 1981, Cooke, *et al* 1998). Evidence comes from the many reports with experimental animals showing E2 alone could restore sexual behaviors of castrated adult males (Baum 2002). For example, castrated male rats were injected either with TS, E2 or DHT. Only DHT failed completely to restore the animals' sexual behaviors (Johnston and Davidson 1972).

More recent work has confirmed that it is the conversion of TS to estrogen that is the critical step (Ball and Balthazart 2006). Blocking aromatase activity or injecting an anti-estrogen into the MPOA blocked the activation of male-typical sexual behavior by TS. Administering an estrogen directly to the MPOA in castrated animals activated male-typical sexual behavior.

Not to be outdone, DHT had its own surprise. It turns out to be a more potent androgen than TS. Upon conversion of TS to DHT in many peripheral sites, DHT binds the androgen receptor with higher affinity (Martini, *et al* 1990).

DHT also can magnify the effects of TS, as exemplified with its role in maturation of the penis at puberty. During adulthood, DHT also has primary responsibility for maintaining normal function of many of the secondary sex characteristics, as well as pathological conditions. Benign prostatic hyperplasia, prostate cancer, acne, androgenic alopecia in men, and hirsutism in women are all related to DHT production (Occhiato, *et al* 2004).

Originally, it seemed that DHT and E2 had divided the androgenic labor (Bonsall, *et al* 1992, Martini, *et al* 1990). The idea was of DHT being the active metabolite in peripheral tissues and E2 being the metabolite in the brain. Thus, E2 was the steroid most responsible for behavior in males. Supporting data came from administering DHT to a castrated rat. When given peripherally, DHT was less effective than TS in activating sexual behavior in castrated male rats (Butera and Czaja 1989). Integrity of the penis was maintained, but DHT did little to restore sexual behavior. Administering E2 did the opposite for a castrated male. Penile morphology was disturbed, but sexual motivation was intact (Sachs, *et al* 1984).

Such parsimony is rare in endocrinology, and it was not to last long. In rodents, it appears TS influences sexual behaviors of the males after it is converted to E2 while, in the brains of primates, it is TS interacting directly with the AR that underlies male sexual behaviors (Michael, *et al* 1987). We now know also that DHT is found in abundance in the brain (Bonsall, *et al* 1985), along with concentrations of the 5alpha-reductase enzyme converting TS to DHT (Cooke, *et al* 2003). Clearly, DHT influences brain structure and function. The functional dichotomy for DHT and E2 was officially put to rest with findings that E2 plays a critical role in male peripheral structures and functions (Akingbemi 2005, Sharpe 1998).

II.2.1. There are two Metabolic Pathways for Synthesizing Testosterone

TS is the major androgenic steroid in circulation, with the Leydig cells of the testes as the principal source of the hormone in males. The adrenal glands supplement TS synthesis by secreting the hormone precursors androstenedione (ANDRO), dehydroepiandrosterone (DHEA) and its sulfate (DHEAS). Adrenal steroids are converted to TS in peripheral tissues, often in the skin or fat (Payne and Hales 2004).

The role of the adrenal precursors of TS, especially DHEA, in normal physiology is of considerable recent interest (Beck and Handa 2004). Development of a mature adrenal gland, known as adrenarche, typically begins in children between 6 and 8 years of age, i.e., well before the onset of puberty. One functional outcome is the appearance of pubic hair.

Interestingly, the dramatic increase in levels of the adrenal precursors of TS occurs without corresponding increases in the other adrenal steroids, corticosteroids and mineralocorticoids. Peak levels of DHEA are found in adult humans during the 20s and 30s and decline progressively thereafter.

Steroidogenesis of androgens, ovarian steroids and adrenal corticosteroids involves many of the same precursors. Two pathways are used for the synthesis of TS. The typical, preferred pathway is cholesterol –> pregnenolone –> progesterone –> 17alpha-hydroxyprogesterone –> ANDRO –> TS (Lieberman and Prasad 1990). A secondary route however is from pregnenolone –> DHEA –> ANDRO –> TS.

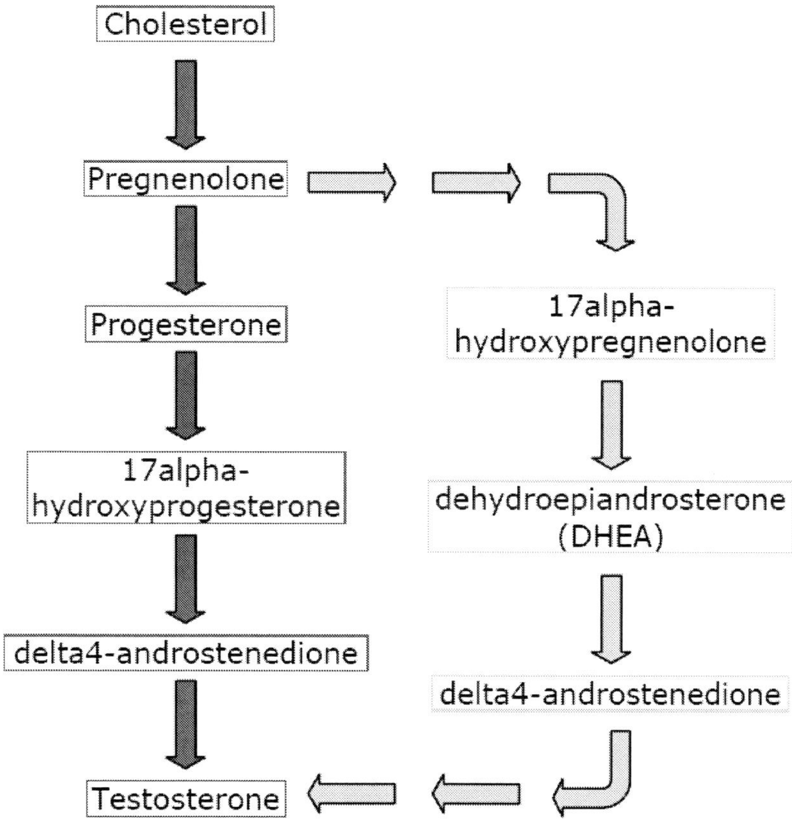

Figure 1. Metabolic cascade for the synthesis of testosterone and its potent metabolites, estradiol and dihydrotestosterone. The primary pathway is represented by the blue arrows.

II.2.2. Supplements of the Adrenal Precursor Androstenedione do not Increase Testosterone

A fundamental question about steroid metabolism is under what conditions is the secondary pathway used in place of the preferred pathway? We do not know. We do know, however, that there are surprising outcomes from manipulating precursor levels that may involve switching between the two pathways. For example, ANDRO supplements would seem to predict increased levels of TS by providing more precursor for increased production of TS. The enzyme responsible for converting ANDRO to TS, 17beta-hydroxysteroid dehydrogenase, is found in most body tissues. Androstenedione is also produced by some plants and has been marketed as a product for increasing blood TS concentrations, that is, as a natural alternative to anabolic steroid use. At least that was surely the thinking of baseball player Mark McGwire and other professional athletes who were self-administering ANDRO.

However, the interconversion of ANDRO and TS and metabolism to other bioactive steroids is complex. The results are often surprising. For example, supplements of a TS precursor may not have the expected effects on TS or its functions (Arlt, *et al* 1999, King, *et al* 1999). Oral ANDRO supplements revealed none of the expected increases in serum TS nor did it promote muscle strength (Birchard 1999). We also were surprised by our findings when castrated male rats were administered ANDRO. In TS restored castrates, concomitant ANDRO treatments suppressed androgen-sensitive behaviors (Taylor, *et al* 1994).

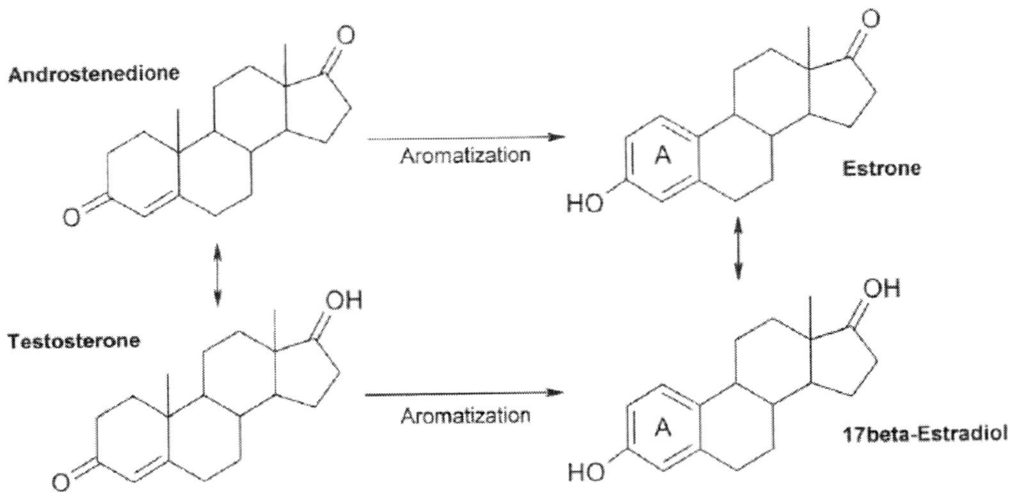

Figure 2. Metabolic cascade for the two possible pathways for the metabolism of androstenedione (ANDRO).

The key may be that in addition to serving as a precursor to TS, ANDRO is closely connected to estrogens (King, *et al* 1999). Androstenedione can be converted directly to an estrogen, specifically estrone, thereby completely bypassing testosterone (Labrie, *et al* 1998, Welt, *et al* 2006). Alternatively, because TS is also aromatized to E2, it also is possible that increased production of TS following ANDRO administration may result in increased aromatization, which would further attenuate any increase in the blood TS concentration (King, *et al* 1999). Sure enough, a study of young men with normal TS values confirmed the increased estrogen levels. The only steroids to increase with oral ANDRO supplements were serum E2 and estrone (King, *et al* 1999).

II.2.3. Female Sexuality May be More Sensitive to the Adrenal Precursor DHEA

Androstenedione, however, has not received the research attention lavished on the other major TS precursor synthesized by the adrenal glands. DHEA appears to be a more potent precursor and perhaps serves both reproductive and non-reproductive functions.

DHEA and its sulphate DHEAS are easily detected in circulation of humans, although only with some difficulty in rodent models. DHEAS serves as reservoir for DHEA and the conversion is via cellular sulfatase. DHEA can then serve as a precursor for a number of other steroids, including ANDRO, TS, and E2 (Chen, *et al* 2005).

One set of findings that has focused attention on DHEA and DHEAS is that both show a progressive decline in adults with age that corresponds to physical aging. Circulating levels of DHEA and DHEAS are dramatically reduced in aged primates, including humans.

There has been considerable discussion recently over whether to consider DHEA a hormone. At this time, DHEA is more appropriately referred to as a steroid, a prohormone or an androgen precursor (Dhatariya 2005, Labrie, *et al* 2005). It is not an androgen nor is it a hormone. DHEA does not bind to either the estrogen or androgen receptor and, therefore, it has no direct androgenic activity. Unlike other major steroids, a receptor for DHEA or one of its metabolites has not been definitively isolated in the reproductive system or in the brains of animal models (Johannsson, *et al* 2002). Consequently, the problem of proponents of DHEA therapies is to identify a cellular mechanism of action for DHEA (Widstrom and Dillon 2004). One possibility is that DHEA exerts functional effects by neuromodulation and improvement in endothelial cell function (Piroli, *et al* 2002). Another is DHEA may act as a neurosteroid by binding a cell membrane-bound receptor in the brain. Unfortunately however, this potential receptor is yet to be isolated (Widstrom and Dillon 2004).

Still, the best evidence is that DHEA plays an important role in the periphery by its role as a precursor for the peripheral synthesis of TS, DHT, and E2. Levels of DHEA predict androgen and estrogen concentrations in peripheral tissues, although they have little effect on circulating levels of the sex hormones (Chen, *et al* 2005). Other possible influences on the periphery include enhancement of the immune system, antagonism of corticosteroids, and involvement in cellular pathology and even obesity. Williams (Williams 2000) has reviewed the literature on each of these possible functions as well as critiquing the mechanisms suggested for DHEA influences on the periphery.

More relevant here is to consider the role of DHEA in sociosexual behaviors. Interestingly, there has been more enthusiasm for a DHEA – sexuality relation in females than in males. This may reflect the notable paucity of findings supporting a clear role for DHEA in males. For example, a study of sexual behaviour in young healthy eugonadal men also assayed adrenal and testicular sex steroids. Serum DHT concentration was the only independent hormonal predictor of their sexuality (Mantzoros, *et al* 1995).

In an experiment with animals, we treated castrated rats daily for 4 wks with adrenal steroids in the presence or absence of restorative doses of TS (Taylor, *et al* 1994). DHEA, DHEAS, and ANDRO were administered as cyclodextrin complexes to mimic the pharmacodynamics of the endogenous products. DHEA supplements alone were unable to maintain integrity of sociosexual responses and androgen target tissues after castration

(Beyer, *et al* 1973). More remarkable was that DHEA suppressed the normal restorative functions of TS therapy to the castrated animals.

The story is quite different in females, especially in postmenopausal women. That low levels of circulating DHEA have been demonstrated in women with diminished libido and other symptoms of sexual dysfunction has suggested the use of DHEA as a supplement to increase androgenic activity (Saltzman and Guay 2006). Acute DHEA exposure, however, induced no changes on subjective (self-report) or physiological (vaginal photoplethysmograph) sexual responses to erotic stimuli in premenopausal women (Meston and Heiman 2002). Chronic DHEA treatment was more successful in women with androgen deficiency due to hypopituitarism. Oral DHEA raised the serum levels of DHEAS to normal age-related reference ranges, but only slightly increased TS titers. Despite subnormal TS levels, the DHEA treated women increased their initiation of sexual activity (Johannsson, *et al* 2002).

II.2.4. Testosterone is Important for Sexual Motivation in Women

Testosterone appears to have been adopted by the female endocrine system for some aspects of successful reproduction. Aggression is possibly one behavioral example (Dabbs and Hargrave 1997), but sexual motivation is more likely. Although not without controversy, TS seems to play an important role in sexual interest exhibited by the female (Federman 2004).

Most of the supporting data comes from studies of women because it proves more difficult to assess initiation of a sexual encounter in animal models. One reason is that non-human females are solicitous of sex only when in estrus, which makes separating the effects of TS from other sex hormones difficult. Moreover, there are surprisingly few studies of animal models in which previously untreated adult females are treated with TS and behavior is measured. An exception is an experiment by Van de Poll and colleagues (VandePoll, *et al* 1988). Female rats treated for 14 days with exogenous TS spent more time near a male than untreated control females. Interestingly, urinary marking by the females increased immediately upon injection of TS.

The steroid metabolic cascade revealing that E2 is a metabolite of TS suggested two conclusions. Testosterone, the prototypical masculine hormone, is a requisite precursor for the estrogens found in females (Goldstein, *et al* 2004). And, that one may find detectable amounts of unmetabolized TS in circulation of females.

Subsequent assays of serum confirmed the existence of TS in females. Indeed, levels of TS were surprisingly high, higher even than circulating estrogens. Although at levels that are approximately 10% of the titers found in males, women typically have more absolute amounts of TS in circulation than E2 (Miller, *et al* 2001, Miller 2002). This is partly because E2 is synthesized at low rates. Androgens are quantitatively the predominant sex steroid in women, circulating in the micromolar and nanomolar concentration range, compared with picomolar levels of estrogens (Sarkola, *et al* 1999, Young, *et al* 2000).

In the male, the majority of TS production occurs in the testes. In the female, 25% of TS is produced in the adrenals, 25% in the ovaries, and 50% in the peripheral tissues from precursors released from the adrenals and ovaries (Bachmann 2002).

Serum levels of TS follow a pattern of increases and decreases across the menstrual cycle that somewhat mimic the rise and fall of estrogens (Dougherty, *et al* 1997, Miller, *et al* 2001). Peak levels are found at mid-cycle and remain detectable throughout the cycle.

The next question is whether TS activates brain processes underlying reproduction and non-reproduction function in females. The answer suggested is yes for both functions. For example, data from a recent study of ovariectomized rats were that hippocampal neurons responded to TS in a similar manner to the influence of E2 on dendritic morphology in the hippocampus, a brain region critical for learning and memory (Leranth, *et al* 2004a).

Other findings suggested an impact of circulating TS on female sexual behavior. A correlational study of premenopausal women with or without complaints of sexual dysfunction revealed lower adrenal precursors and TS of the latter group (Guay, *et al* 2004). Indeed, the predominant symptom of women with androgen deficiency is loss of sexual desire (Davis 1999). Low TS levels may accompany a variety of conditions in women of reproductive age, including hypothalamic amenorrhea, hypopituitarism, premature ovarian failure, and premenstrual syndrome, as well as glucocorticosteroid or oral estrogen therapies (Kalantaridou and Calis 2006). Consequences of androgen insufficiency include various peripheral changes such as increased vasomotor flushing, loss of bone and muscle mass and replacement of muscle with adipose tissue, as well as a pattern of declining sexual functioning. Along with decreased sexual motivation, there is a reduction of sexual fantasy and enjoyment; , diminished sexual arousability, and decreased vaginal vasocongestion in response to erotic stimuli (Bachmann 2002).

The more common cause of androgen decreases is simply aging. Serum androgen levels exhibit a progressive stepwise decline from 20 to 49 years of age (Guay, *et al* 2004). Women in their forties have approximately half the level of circulating total TS as that of women in their twenties (Dennerstein, *et al* 2002).

The best evidence for a TS – sexual motivation relation is the value of TS therapy on the sexual vitality of postmenopausal women (Shifren 2004, Somboonporn, *et al* 2005). Although the evidence for TS as fundamental to low sexual interest in younger women has proved more inconclusive (Guay, *et al* 2004, Nyunt, *et al* 2005), there is greater support from androgen treatments of postmenopausal women (Davis 1999).

For example, Sherwin et al. (Sherwin, *et al* 1985) assessed sexual functioning in menopausal women administered TS over a 3 months period. It was clear that exogenous androgen enhanced the intensity of sexual desire and arousal and the frequency of sexual fantasies. However, the results were limited to sexual motivation rather than sexual activity. This may be a reflection only that sexual activity involves non-endocrine factors such as marital status, partner interest and past experiences.

Postmenopausal women volunteers were administered either oral estrogens with or without concomitant androgen for eight weeks in a double-blind study. Sexual function was assessed with a questionnaire. Results were that sexual desire, satisfaction and frequency increased significantly more in the group receiving androgen than in women receiving by estrogen only or estrogen-progestin therapy (Sarrel, *et al* 1998). Finally, in a single-blind study TS was administered by implants for 2 years to postmenopausal women. Results indicated significantly greater scores for sexual activity, satisfaction, pleasure, and orgasm compared with controls (Davis, *et al* 1995).

An unanswered question is whether TS directly increases arousability in women or if it must be first converted to E2 (Bancroft 2005). In the latter case, it would suggest that estrogen therapy would have the same effect on sexual motivation. The studies cited above suggest that not to be the case. Sexuality of postmenopausal women was greater with a combination of TS and estrogen compared to women receiving estrogen alone (Davis, *et al* 1995, Dobs, *et al* 2002). More recently (Davis, *et al* 2006) there was a report that an aromatase inhibitor in combination with TS therapy had no significant effect on sexual restoration in women. The suggestion is that it is TS acting on the androgen receptor and that is the key to sexual motivation in women.

II.3. Androgen Receptors are Found in Structures Both Related and Unrelated to Reproduction

Molecular biology has allowed identification of receptors for steroidal hormones and for localizing concentrations of the receptors in tissues throughout the body. Estrogen receptors (ER) and androgen receptors (AR) were found in the periphery and brains of both genders of common laboratory animals. Surprisingly the receptors appear in brain regions responsible for reproduction as well as in brain regions with little relation to reproduction (Nyborg, 1994).

It came as a further surprise to many of us to learn that there is no specific TS receptor. The receptor is the more generic androgen receptor (AR). As already noted, TS serves both as an active hormone and as a prohormone. Genetic evidence indicates that TS and DHT work via a common intracellular receptor (Wilson, *et al* 2002). Testosterone has good affinity for the AR, but, interestingly, DHT has a notably higher affinity for the androgen receptor. Either directly or after conversion to E2 or DHT, TS interacts with sex steroid receptors to produce both peripheral and central activation that underlies sociosexual behaviors in the male.

In the periphery, steroid receptors are found in a remarkable variety of tissues, from muscle and bone to cranial motor nuclei to the cornea and retina of the eye (Wickham, *et al* 2000). Some of the influences of TS on these structures appear to require aromatization, bone for example, and others not, muscle for example (Bronwyn, *et al* 2003). The greatest concentration of AR, however, is where one would expect to find it, in the reproductive tract. Estrogen receptors are often found co-localized with the AR, for example in the testes (Carreau, *et al* 2003). The result is that TS and its metabolites are integral in maintaining the structure and function of peripheral structures involved in normal male sexual function (Goldstein, *et al* 2004). More specifically, TS directly impacts sexual behaviors by its effects on peripheral neurons that trigger and complete copulatory reflexes (Keast 1999). The influence on genital organ sensitivity plays an important role in sexual arousal and orgasm.

II.3.1. Distribution of Androgen Receptors in the Brain

In the rodent brain, conversion of androgens into estrogens by aromatase is a key mechanism by which TS regulates many physiological and behavioral processes, including the activation of male sexual behavior, brain sexual differentiation and negative feedback effects of steroid hormones on gonadotropin secretion (Balthazart and Ball 1998). Therefore, cells that express steroid hormone receptors are integral to the action of gonadal hormones and represent essential components of the mechanism underlying masculinization of the brain.

Neurons with ARs in their nuclei are distributed widely in many regions of the brain including the preoptic area of the hypothalamus, septal area-bed nucleus, amygdala, and brain stem (Bonsall, *et al* 1985). ARs are also concentrated in areas of the brain that are not primarily involved in reproduction, such as the basal forebrain, hippocampus, caudate putamen, midbrain raphe and brainstem locus coeruleus (McEwen 2001).

The brain regions most closely related to male-specific sexual behaviors are located in various limbic structures and in the olfactory system. Most critical are the hypothalamus and amygdala. Testosterone and its metabolites interact with steroid receptors in hypothalamic limbic structures, where they elicit conscious perception and pleasurable reactions by influencing the release of specific neurotransmitters.

Although traditionally believed to be only in subcortical regions, ARs are also found in cortical and subcortical brain regions unrelated to reproduction, notably the hippocampus. AR immunoreactivity and binding are very similar in rat hippocampus as in the sexual behavior-dependent hypothalamus. ARs are concentrated in the CA1 region, an area that plays a major role in learning and memory (Xiao and Jordan 2002). That ARs are present also on axons and dendrites in cerebral cortex highlights the likelihood that androgens play an important and novel extra-nuclear role in neuronal function (DonCarlos, 2003}. This lays the groundwork for other surprises that have changed the way neuroendocrinologists think about sex steroids and behavior.

II.3.2. Gender Differences in Steroid Receptors Predict Sexual Behavior Differences but not Dimorphic Non-reproductive Behaviors

When neuroendocrinologists talk about "brain sex" or a brain being organized as masculine or feminine, it could mean many things. It could mean males and females having more neurons in certain brain areas, leaving those areas larger. It could mean having the same number of neurons but the neurons are connected differently leaving neurotransmitter pathways wired differently. It could also refer to the different numbers of steroid receptors in masculine and feminine brains with those receptors being distributed differently. Or it could refer to a brain region that metabolizes the same hormones differently. The net result of all these possibilities is that the same hormone, whether it be TS or estrogen or another hormone, delivered to the brain of an adult can lead to sexually dimorphic behaviors (Resko and Roselli 1997, Simerly 2002).

Still, much of the interest has centered on size differences and on receptor differences, likely because they are the easiest to quantify. Only a couple of size differences exist, most famously is the clearly larger size of the higher vocal center (or HVC) in male songbirds (Nottebohm and Arnold 1976). There are reports of subtle size differences in brain regions between men and women. The amygdala and hypothalamus appear to be larger in men. Both regions are also the same regions that contain high concentrations of steroid receptors (Hamann 2005).

It is notable that the both androgen and estrogen receptors are detected in the same brain regions in males and female animal models. ARs are found in neuroanatomical areas of both genders in the medial hypothalamic area, ventromedial and dorsomedial nucleus, preoptic area, arcuate nucleus, amygdala and regions of the hippocampus, arcuate-median eminence and BNST, with the greatest AR density reported in the preoptic and hypothalamic areas, septum and amygdala of these animals.

Receptor numbers differ in the expected direction in some brain regions. The two subtypes of estrogen receptor (ER), designated as ER-alpha and ER-beta, are distributed differently in male and female brains (Shughrue, *et al* 2000). Although ER-beta is found in the hippocampus of male and female rats, females have higher concentrations (Zhang, *et al* 2002).

Using 4 strains of male and female mice Lu (Lu, *et al* 1998) found sexually dimorphic receptor concentrations in various brain regions. Males had a higher absolute number of AR than females. Concentrations of AR were higher in males in brain regions associated with male-typical sexual behaviors, e.g., BNST and MPOA. AR decreased significantly with castration. Indeed, most differences in AR numbers between the sexes are detected in hypothalamic nuclei and other structures related to reproduction (Chen and Tu 1992, Lu, *et al* 1998).

In many non-reproductive structures, however, there are surprisingly few or no sex differences in distribution and concentrations of ERs and ARs (Michael, *et al* 1995, Scott, *et al* 2000). Moreover, where there may be sex differences, there is no clear functional logic for the existence of different receptor numbers. An example is the AR findings from autopsies of a small number of men and women between 20 years and 39 years (Fernandez-Guasti, *et al* 2000). Again, ARs were found in high numbers in both male and female hypothalamus. However, men had higher AR concentrations in the suprachiasmatic nucleus of the hypothalamus, a region generally agreed to be related to diurnal activity rather than sexual behavior.

The presence of large numbers of ER and AR in both sexes would seem to pose interpretation problems for relating dimorphic functions to the steroid receptor. High concentrations of ERs in males can be explained, however, by the metabolism of TS into E2 in brain tissues to interact with ERs. Notably, amounts of aromatase are higher in many brain regions of male animal models than of females (Lu, *et al* 1998, Roselli and Resko 1997). The presence of high concentrations of ARs in the brains of females is more puzzling (Xiao and Jordan 2002).

II.4. Steroids act through Genomic AND Non-genomic Mechanisms

Steroid hormones are unique endocrine products in the way they interact with nuclear DNA. This capacity allows for many of the distinctive features of steroids to induce the long-lasting changes that are observed, for example, the surge of TS with the oncoming breeding season in feral animals or the onset of puberty in humans.

In the past decade another mechanism for influences on brain and behavior has been identified. In addition to the well-established nuclear action of steroid receptors, membrane-associated receptors for gonadal steroid hormones have been discovered. This finding has revolutionized the way we think of steroids, recognizing rapid actions of steroids that could not be attributed to transcriptional regulation. Considerable evidence has now accumulated to support the existence of these nonnuclear receptors. Our ideas have now been broadened to recognize gonadal steroid receptor action via extranuclear sites.

II.4.1. The Classic Mechanism for Steroidal Influence is Genomic and Slow

It has been known for some time that TS and the other steroids have direct influence on DNA transcription in the nucleus of target cells. The result is that the genomic effects are slow because it requires time for the multiple steps to initiate DNA activation and subsequent protein synthesis to initiate functional changes. Genomic changes, consequently, are long-lasting.

Steroidal hormones belong to a ligand-activated nuclear receptor family. Members of this family have been defined by their ability to bind to specific DNA sequences in promoter regions of hormone responsive genes.

Unbound TS in circulation enters a cell and binds the androgen receptor (AR) to form a steroid ligand. Prior to confronting TS, the AR is loosely bound to a protein in the cellular cytoplasm or nucleus. Surprisingly, the exact location of the steroid-hormone receptor is not known. What is known is that TS diffuses into the cell and binds the receptor and the TS – AR complex then diffuses into the cell nucleus. The TS - AR complexes bind to specific sequences of DNA called steroid-response elements, as well as to nuclear-receptor coactivators or repressors (Gruber, *et al* 2002). Upon binding to these hormone response elements in the DNA, the receptors are capable of exerting powerful modulatory effects on transcription of specific genes.

The outcomes are prominent changes in neural morphology and function. Testosterone surges are linked to an increase in neuron somal size, neuritic growth, plasticity and synaptogenesis in both motoneurons of the spinal nucleus of the bulbocavernosus muscle in the reproductive system of males and several populations of pelvic autonomic neurons (Bialek, *et al* 2004). The genomic influences of TS are now known to extend beyond the reproductive system. Changes in lateralized function of the hemispheres and hippocampal activation are but two examples.

Castration of adult rats is reported to induce a decrease of dendritic spines in the CA1 region of the hippocampus (Leranth, *et al* 2004b). Castration also reduced numbers of acetylcholine neurons in some cortical areas, and 4 weeks of exogenous TS restored the cholinergic pathways in the adult rats. These data suggest that the presence or absence of TS profoundly influenced the cholinergic population in cortical and subcortical areas of the adult rat brain (Nakamura, *et al* 2002). These and other data have led to the speculation that TS is a neuroprotective agent (Frye and McCormick 2000).

One final word on androgen receptors and it has a familiar ring. There is more complexity than researchers had hoped. The concept of a single hormone activating a single receptor is being replaced by a more complex model (Vanderschueren and Bouillon 2000). The picture emerging is of the original hormonal signal undergoing transformation in the target tissue from processes such intracellular enzyme activities, receptor concentration and function, and post-receptor cross-talk. The result is modulation of the original signal and fine-tuning of the biological response.

II.4.2. A second Mechanism for Steroidal Influence is Non-genomic and Fast

Steroids are usually identified as genomic regulators. Recently a body of evidence has accumulated demonstrating specific membrane effects more akin to neurotransmitter activities. That is, steroids can help coordinate neural firings by interacting with both membrane and intracellular receptors. The resulting rapid modulation of cellular activity is measured in seconds or minutes and suggests a non-genomic role for certain steroids. Rapid steroid synthesis and metabolism have been found to exist in the CNS, and downstream effects can be seen in both the central and peripheral nervous systems.

The mechanism for rapid, non-genomic action is suggested by the findings that ARs are present on axons and dendrites within the mammalian central nervous system. AR expression in axons was identified in the rat brain at the light microscopic level and details confirmed at the ultrastructural level. AR-immunoreactive axons were observed primarily in the cerebral cortex and were rare in regions where nuclear AR expression is abundant. This suggests that there are separate functional systems for the genomic and non-genomic influence of the sex steroids. The observation that ARs are present in axons and dendrites highlights the possibility that TS plays an important and novel extra-nuclear role in neuronal function (DonCarlos, *et al* 2003).

Current levels of circulating steroids can induce changes in neural morphology that would appear to be too fast to be genomic. The best example comes from estrogen and female rats. The rapid rise and fall of estrogen during the 4-day estrous cycle of f rats is accompanied by equally rapid increases and decreases in numbers of dendrites in certain hippocampal regions (Woolley 1998). Significantly, those are the same regions responsible for certain types of memory.

The implications that steroids have fast, membrane-mediated influences on the brain function are nothing short of revolutionary. That steroids can have acute, momentary actions opens a new avenue of thinking about the brain. The pharmaceutical industry has been among the first to recognize the potential of non-genomic steroidal actions. A prominent example is that sex steroids may contribution to brain plasticity.

II.4.3. Steroids Play a Role in Brain Plasticity

Neuroscientists use the word "plasticity" to refer to brain tissues that maintain the capacity for structural changes in mature animals. That TS and the other sex steroids could contribute to brain plasticity is a remarkable development for several reasons.

To set the scene, recall the original organizational - activational model. The suggestion is that organizational effects are structural and irreversible, whereas activational effects were functional and reversible. The thought was that once fetal development and its sensitive periods to TS had passed, the organized morphology of the brain would not change with changes in circulating adult hormones.

The activational component, on the other hand, was considered labile and modifiable, say by castration or hormone supplements. The hormonal influences that activated a function after puberty, sexual motivation for instance, were completed without changing integrity of the long-ago established structures. As long as those masculinized brain tissues have sufficient current levels of TS from the adult testes, we would see normal male sexual functioning. Remove the testes and TS and we would observe sexual behaviors beginning a downhill slide. Brain anatomy does not change with castration, but the behavior activated by TS does.

In general, the structural – functional distinction between organization – activation roles of the model have been largely upheld today. But, the line between function and structure has been blurred in the brain. Current research on the effects of gonadal steroids on the brain and spinal cord indicates that these agents can have profound trophic effects on many aspects of neuronal functioning. As example, TS induced structural remodeling of the neuromuscular junctions of the peripheral nervous system in the male rat reproductive tract (Gordon, *et al* 1990). Cranial nerves also show morphological sensitivity to androgens. Some of these effects may be genomic and some non-genomic. Regardless of the mechanism of action, the consequences are notable on cell survival, growth and metabolism, elaboration of processes, synaptogenesis, and neurotransmission (Jones, *et al* 1999).

Still, the best evidence that some structures in the brain maintain plasticity to hormones is the capacity of hormones to change the physical structure of the adult hippocampus. Specifically, features of hippocampal anatomy can be molded by current levels of ovarian hormone in cycling female rats. The initial findings were of neural morphology rapidly changing with fluctuations of endogenous sex hormones in adult female rats (Woolley, *et al* 1993). More recently, ovariectomized rats administered TS induced similar increases in dendritic spines (Leranth, *et al* 2004a). Male brains may or may not undergo similar changes. These data highlight both the plasticity of the adult brain and the importance of hormone fluctuations on the brain during the activational phase (Breedlove and Jordan 2001).

There are good reasons, however, to believe that the male brain will show less plasticity than female brains, and that TS will be less likely to be as important of a player as ovarian hormones. A key difference between male and female brains is that only the females undergo dramatic endocrine fluctuations over days. It is probably accurate to suggest that even neuroendocrinologists have not fully appreciated the dramatic differences between a fluctuating endogenous hormonal stimulus experienced by females and a more or less constant one experienced by males (Taylor and Pitha 1988).

II.5. The Brain Synthesizes its own Steroids

We have known for decades that steroid hormones influence the brain. That is to say, a sex hormone released by the far-away gonads is pumped in the blood to the brain where it binds a steroid receptor. But, it has been recognized only in the past decade or so that the brain appears to be producing its own steroids. This has led, among other things, to a confusion of terms.

Terminology in the steroid hormone literature has not shown ideal consistency. The result is confusion about the definitions of steroids in the periphery and the CNS (Stoffel-Wagner 2001). We have already introduced one example, DHEA, which is referred to erroneously as an androgen or as a hormone.

"Biologically active steroids" are steroids that have the ability to bind to a steroid receptor in the periphery or the CNS. Examples are TS, E2, progesterone and corticosteroid.

"Neuroactive steroids" are those substances that bind to a steroid receptor in the CNS. All the aforementioned steroids also meet the criterion for neuroactive steroids.

But the brain synthesizes its own steroids for local use in the brain. These became known as "neuroactive steroids" (Baulieu 1998), i.e., steroids used by the brain for both reproductive and non-reproductive functions. The most important feature is that neurosteroids are synthesized directly in the brain. The neuroactive steroids are not the familiar steroids, and include DHEA and progesterone metabolites such as allopregnanolone. Likely neurosteroids use non-genomic mechanisms to quickly modify brain activity and behavior (Rupprecht and Holsboer 1999). The terminology details may seem like splitting of hairs, but it is an important distinction because there are revolutionary implications in the concept of a neurosteroid.

One implication is that, rather than relying entirely on the peripheral endocrine organs for its hormones, the brain has evolved the capacity to synthesize its own steroids (Corpechot, *et al* 1981, Mellon 1994). This can be demonstrated by removing the peripheral organs, adrenals and gonads, and the amounts of neurosteroid in the brain do not change (Baulieu 1997). Economically, neurosteroids are synthesized mostly from the same precursors and enzymes as used for peripheral synthesis.

Another implication is perhaps more profound and has the potential to open a new chapter for steroidal influence on brain and behavior (Engel and Grant 2001). The mammalian brain has adapted both peptides and steroids used in reproduction for other neural functions. The ancient hormones synthesized in the periphery now have a new role. Rather than evolving completely new substances for complex behaviors such as memory or mood, steroids have been hijacked by the brain for other uses (Belelli and Lamber 2005, Birzniece, *et al* 2006).

Section III. Circulating Testosterone and Sociosexual Behaviors

III.1. Testosterone in Circulation shows wide between and within Individual Differences

A basic tenet of endocrinology is that endocrine products are released from glands to be carried by the bloodstream to target tissues some distance away. Sometimes this bloodstream is nearby and served by a specially evolved vascular source, a so-called portal system. The direct portal connection between hypothalamus and anterior pituitary is an important example. Much more commonly, the blood delivery system is general circulation, and that is almost always the source obtained for analyses of the steroids. There are myriads of methods to collect blood from experimental animals (Weiss, *et al* 2000), including the one familiar to human patients.

Once blood is drawn from men and assayed, the serum reveals only 2% found in the bloodstream is so-called unbound or free TS. That is, the portion of TS that is not bound to a protein, either albumin or sex hormone binding globulin (SHBG). The free fraction has traditionally been viewed as the source of biologically active TS that could enter cells and interact with a receptor. For example, aging men experience both reduced free TS and increased levels of SHBG (Swerdloff and Wang 2004). Much has been made of this observation. This includes a comparison of bound and free TS in patients with probable Alzheimer's disease with the conclusion that only free TS is significantly lower in male patients (Moffat, *et al* 2004).

Now it seems that albumin bound TS can be uptaken by cells and dissociated from the protein to interact with the receptor. Moreover, the bound form is a type of reservoir of TS that may actually facilitate the entry of hormone into the cell (Goldstein and Sites 2002). The result is that a considerable portion of the TS in circulation actually is in a readily bioactive form in males. The anxiety of researchers and clinicians over bound and free TS is probably unwarranted (Davidson, *et al* 1982). Serum TS levels and free TS are often highly correlated in healthy males (Stalenheim, *et al* 1998).

III.1.1. Within Individual Assays revealed that Testosterone is Released in Pulses throughout the Day and Night

In the mid-1970s an important discovery was made about the way that gonads release their hormones into circulation. Release is not by slow leakage but in a series of episodic bursts throughout the day (Bartke and Dalterio 1975, Sodersten, *et al* 1983). Soon, the findings were extended to other endocrine glands, including those outside the HPG axis (Linkowski, *et al* 1985, Penny 1985, Samuels, *et al* 1990). This pattern became known as pulsatile release. The term continues to be used to distinguish circadian pulses from the gradual increases in hormone known as surges that occur, for example, in males of seasonal breeding species or with the advent of puberty in boys.

Recognition of the ubiquity of pulsatile release of endocrine products forced researchers to better control sampling protocols. Most prominent was to measure hormone levels at the same time of the day. With that control in place, however, it was possible to make comparisons among and within males.

Little TS is stored in the testes and newly synthesized TS is quickly released into the bloodstream in 6-10 pulses of different amplitudes per day in men. The pattern is variable both between males and over days in the same male. Still, in men there is a fairly reliable TS pulse early in the morning, around daybreak. The pulse-generator responsible for the pattern of pulsatile release of TS is unknown, but we do know it is more than simply the HPG axis. Specifically, neurons projecting from various subcortical brain regions influence the amplitude and frequency of hypothalamic gonadotropin releasing hormone (GnRH) released from the hypothalamus into the pituitary (Abbud, *et al* 1999, Scott, *et al* 1997).

One result of this pulsatile feature is that hormone sensitive tissue responds best to aperiodic stimulation. Indeed, a continuous stream of hormone can produce a paradoxical suppression of target tissue activity (Southworth, *et al* 1991). That feature has made its way into hormone therapies as GnRH agonists are used to suppress the downstream release of luteinizing hormone and, thus, TS (Matthews, *et al* 1998, Rosler and Witztum 1998).

III.1.2. Differences in Endogenous Testosterone between Males do not Explain Differences in Sexual Behavior

Reports of within individual variability were quickly followed by findings of considerable variability between individual males. Testosterone values in healthy young males of many species, including humans, range over values that differ significantly. In men the lower limit for normative values is 300 ng/ dl but the values may range to 900 ng/ dl or more (Howell and Shalet 2001). Upon reflection, individual differences in TS were not surprising. Males within a social group differ, of course, along many physical and behavioral continua. Some of these differences are androgen dependent, including sexual behaviors. Yet, the surprise was that in normal adult males the wide individual variability in circulating TS levels did not seem to be linked in any meaningful way with individual differences in any aspects of sexual behavior (Meston and Frohlich 2000, Schiavi and White 1976).

Of course, a certain amount of TS is necessary for normal sexuality. Castrated animal models and men (Greenstein, *et al* 1995) typically experience dramatic decreases in all measures of interest and performance. In gonadally intact males, hypogonadism is also associated with low level of male sexual behavior (Gray, *et al* 1981, Sternbach 1998).

Yet repeatedly the findings from studies of intact laboratory animals and men are that individual differences in endogenous TS levels and measures of sexual behaviors are not significantly related (Damassa, *et al* 1977, Meston and Frohlich 2000). Phoenix and Chambers for instance have made an exhaustive study of the sexual behaviors of rhesus monkeys and laboratory rats. One dominant theme is their conclusion that circulating TS is not the key factor in individual differences in the sexual behaviors of intact young or old males (Chambers and Phoenix 1992). Even administering exogenous hormone to elevate TS titers of so-called sexually sluggish young male monkeys failed to improve their performance (Phoenix and Chambers 1986).

The same absence of a TS – sexual behavior relation appears to hold for non-traditional animal models. A study of male and female meerkats (Carlson, *et al* 2004) reported no rank-related differences in circulating levels of TS among males. Dominant, breeding males and females, however, did have significantly higher cortisol levels than the subordinates, non-breeding meerkats.

Similar conclusions have been reported for men (Brown, *et al* 1978, Schiavi and White 1976, Zitzmann and Nieschlag 2001). The former study employed collection of two samples taken a week apart from 101 young adult men. Serum TS concentrations in the two samples were highly correlated, indicating good reliability and consistency. However, there was no correlation with their self-reported frequencies of sexual behaviors. The conclusion was that differences among men in circulating TS concentration within the normal range do not account for differences in sexual interest or activity (Brown, *et al* 1978).

One finds data in the literature suggesting a positive correlation of TS and sexuality (Knussmann, *et al* 1986). However, the bulk of the data supports the original conclusions. There is little correlation between circulating levels of the hormone and performance measures.

There are many possible explanations for the absence of correlation between resting TS and sexual behavior. One possibility is differences in nocturnal hormone pulses that are not typically measured. After finding the usual absence of a correlation between TS levels and copulation in rhesus monkeys, the researchers measured nocturnal hormone titers (Michael, *et al* 1984). They found that the most sexually active males had less of a nadir of the circadian rhythm at night, thus maintaining a higher level of TS during sleep. The implication is that, considered over the entire day, the TS levels were higher in the more sexually active male.

Another possibility is that the relation is in the opposite direction, that is, sexual activity increases TS in males rather than TS increasing the behavior. Sure enough, sexually experienced male rats have larger testes and higher TS levels (Frankel 1984, Taylor, *et al* 1985) compared to virgin males. However, the increases of TS appear to be only observed with chronic sexual contact. Testosterone is not released with copulation. Measurement of various hormones in male rhesus monkeys following copulation revealed no acute increases in circulating TS (Phoenix, *et al* 1977). Only cortisol increased in the monkeys. Although it was with masturbation, the same result for TS was reported after orgasm in men. Only prolactin increased (Kruger, *et al* 2003).

Interestingly this same relation, or absence of a relation, may not hold for females. As noted in a previous section, it is likely that TS is responsible for libido in women. Although there are far fewer studies of women than men, resting levels of TS appear to be related to self-reports of sexual interest in women (Sherwin, *et al* 1985).

III.1.3. Rather than a Dose-response Model, a threshold Model may be more accurate for the Testosterone - Behavior Relations

These findings led to the conclusion that the relation of TS and sexual behavior, and likely all behaviors, were better described by a threshold hormone model than a dose-response model. Simply the idea is that, once a threshold is passed, increases in circulating TS will have no further effects on behavior (Buena, *et al* 1993, Ewing, *et al* 1979, Isidori, *et al* 2005).

One prediction from the threshold model is that TS restored castrates will show similar sexuality as before the surgery. That is, exogenous TS to a formerly sexually active castrated male will restore his sexual behavior, but only to his previous level. The data support that prediction (Phoenix and Chambers 1986).

Additional evidence for the threshold model is that when TS levels are manipulated to ensure high or low TS values within the normal male range, sexuality of the two groups are the same (Buena, *et al* 1993, Taylor, *et al* 1985). In the former study, two groups of healthy men were treated for 9 weeks with a GnRH agonist to slightly suppress or exogenous TS to slightly increase TS serum levels. Sexual function evaluated by daily dairies revealed no significant differences in overall scores or in subcategories of intensity of sexual feelings or sexual activity between the two groups. The authors' conclusion was that a minimal value of TS above threshold was sufficient to fully restore sexual behavior in men (Buena, *et al* 1993).

The threshold model remains a dominant concept today despite mounting evidence that some behaviors, including aspects of sexual behaviors, may show a dose-response relation to TS (Gray, *et al* 2005). The threshold vs. dose-response issue continues to define much of the research in this area, both basic research and applications to clinical populations. More recently the debate has included the effects of TS supplements to eugonadal men, defined as healthy males with normal endocrine functions (O'Connor, *et al* 2004). That controversy surrounds the consequences from use and abuse of anabolic steroids, as well as the value of supplement of TS to healthy men. Those issues will be addressed in the last sections of this chapter.

An important feature of the literature reviewed above is to emphasize that the typical paradigm is a study of baseline or steady-state hormone. Researchers refer to this as "current levels" or "prevailing levels" of hormone in serum. Better perhaps is "resting levels" because it focuses on the key concept that the values reported are the serum steroidal titers of a male in a normal, unstimulated condition. And the threshold model seems to most accurately describe current TS levels – sociosexual behavior relations in males.

III.2. Acute and Chronic Changes in TS Induce Behavioral Changes

The conclusion that resting TS levels of healthy males are seldom informative in explaining individual differences in behavior would seem to place a cloud on further research on TS – behavior relations. There is, however, another way to ask questions about the relation. Rather than resting levels, for instance, do changes in TS induce reliable changes in behavior? Given the proclivity of experimentalists and clinicians to manipulate, it is not surprising that the changing hormone literature is much larger, with more interesting outcomes, than the literature on resting hormone titers.

III.2.1. Momentary Changes in Testosterone can Change Sexual Function

As discussed at length above, a basic principle of steroid endocrinology is that the primary pathway for influencing behavior is genomic. The result is that, in most situations, TS and the other steroids are unlikely to show a momentary relation to behaviors. Rather hormones help set the conditions that a behavior will occur in the presence of a specific stimulus (Wade 2006). This is because most steroid effects require some period of time to influence the genome.

There have been clever attempts to identify the time period. One example in humans was with women exposed to a dose of TS while watching pornographic films. Sublingual intake of exogenous TS was followed by a sharp increase in plasma TS levels within 15 minutes. The circulating levels declined gradually over the next 90 minutes to reach baseline values. Only 3 to 4 hours after reaching peak levels was there a significantly increased genital responsiveness (Tuiten, *et al* 2000). These data suggest behavioral changes can occur within a few hours, although the time period is likely longer for other steroid – behavior relations.

The time delays of the classic genomic activity of steroids raised the puzzle of how it was possible for sudden changes in TS to have an immediate effect on physiology and behavior (Sachs 1997). Such momentary changes have been demonstrated in a variety of experimental paradigms.

Males of many species experience a rapid increase in TS levels to the appearance of a receptive female, her odors or even an environment in which the male had previously copulated (Fukada, *et al* 1988, Huang, *et al* 1989, Taylor 1980b). Those males may also exhibit an immediate increase in sociosexual behaviors (Taylor, *et al* 1984). These results also point out the important concept of hormone – behavior relations being a two-way street.

Environments and behavior can modify the endocrine milieu which, then, can influence the behavior sensitive to the hormone (Aluja and Torrubia 2004).

More recent studies have confirmed the influence of the environment, as well as providing additional neurophysiological evidence of a rapid activation of neural activity to receptive females. For example, using nuclear fos immunoreactivity as a marker of neuronal activation (Kelliher, *et al* 1999), male rats were exposed to the soiled bedding of the female. Those males showed significantly more neuronal fos immunoreactivity than clean-bedding control males in the nucleus accumbens, medial amygdala, BNST and MPOA. Even greater neuronal fos responses were detected in these brain regions in males allowed to mate.

Molecular changes in the brain with acute exposure to exogenous TS include an experiment in which androgen receptor concentrations were examined in castrated adult male rats and gonadally intact females (Xiao and Jordan 2002). Animals received an injection of either TS propionate or vehicle 2 hours prior to sacrifice. AR receptor numbers within the CA1 region of the hippocampus increased in both genders to the acute TS injection. Interestingly, the increases were greater in the left hippocampus than the right, but only in the males, suggesting a sex difference in laterality of AR in hippocampal structure and function.

Still, the most important conclusion for our discussion is that the rapid rise in AR numbers point to a non-genomic effect of steroids in the hippocampus. Additional evidence comes from findings that a single acutely stressful event quickly enhanced dendritic spine density in the male hippocampus but reduced density in the female hippocampus (Shors, *et al* 2001).

Rapid behavioral changes to acute changes in circulating steroids have been reported in other paradigms. These include increased aggression in male rats to acute increases in corticosteroids (Haller, *et al* 2000), and an immediate response by women to a recently formed metabolite of TS. This is in the form of attraction to the odors of androstenol from men that is found in the apocrine glands located in the axillae of the skin in the armpits and pubic region (Kohl, *et al* 2001).

A more titillating behavioral example is the so-called Coolidge effect (Dewsbury 1981). This refers to the reinstitution of copulation in sexually satiated males with the introduction of a new, unmated female. In this paradigm, a male is allowed to copulate to exhaustion, identified by the male refusing to attempt to initiate another copulation. However, removal of that female and replacement with a novel, receptive female is quickly followed by renewed, vigorous copulation. This procedure can be repeated several times with a new female and the same male, with the same result.

The implication is of a momentary rise in TS followed by an immediate behavioral change. The most likely explanation is for non-genomic activities of steroid hormones. We know now that steroids, including androgens, have the capacity for membrane-induced activation of neurotransmitter pathways underlying behavior (Frye 2001). Steroid receptors on the presynaptic and postsynaptic neurons can quickly influence neural activity and, thus, behavior.

Another mechanism for fast changes in sexual responsiveness of the male changes to momentary changes in TS is an indirect effects. We have demonstrated that female rats prefer a male with high TS levels. Intact females given a choice between inaccessible castrated males restored with different amounts of TS preferred to spend time near the higher TS male

(Taylor, *et al* 1982). It is possible that the adaptive value of a sudden pulse of TS in the male is that the female will be more responsive to the male, thus increasing his sexual prowess.

III.2.2. Chronic Changes in Testosterone are Likely to Change Sexual Function

Most of the research on changing levels of hormone, however, has looked at long term TS exposure. This is in recognition that typically steroid hormonal changes slowly modify sexual behavior.

Chronic hormonal changes can be either from natural changes or experimentally induced changes. Most often the changes are to increase circulating hormone. Puberty or increases during a breeding season represent natural elevation of TS. Exogenous administration to castrated animals or hypogonadal men represent the most studied groups for behavioral changes accompanying chronic increases in TS titers. Natural declines with aging are a notable instance of decreases in circulating TS.

An interesting study group are men convicted of felonies for sexually deviant behaviors. Often they are pedophiles. Studies of surgical castration in a large study of 104 sex offenders found highly significant decreases in sexual arousal or performance in 90% of the men. Further studies of recidivism indicated a significant decrease in sex offenders following castration (Stone, *et al* 2000).

Still, it is notable that castrated males do not immediately lose sexual capacity (Baum, *et al* 1986). In male rats, the decline in copulatory performance takes a time course that is the reverse of the normal sequence of mounting without intromission, multiple intromissions followed by ejaculation. With castration of the rat, the first copulatory response to be lost is ejaculation and the last to be lost is mounting (Davidson 1966). Actually the very first sexual response, sexual motivation, is the last to be lost, and may never disappear entirely in castrated males, most notably men. The same is observed with a pharmacological agent that blocked the conversion of TS to E2 in the brains of male rats. All aspects of sexual behavior were eventually disrupted, but again the ordering of behavioral disruption was the sequence of ejaculation to sexual motivation (Bonsall, *et al* 1992).

The point is that a sudden and dramatic decrease in TS requires time to impact most androgen – sensitive structures and, especially, behaviors. In the following sections, we will consider paradigms that underline the importance of significant changes in circulating TS and the impact on sexual behaviors.

III.2.3. Aging Represents a Natural Chronic Decrease in Testosterone and Sexual Function

In assessing the behavioral consequences of changes in circulating hormone levels and sexual behavior, a good place to start is with the aging male literature. Studies with non-human animals and humans have repeatedly confirmed the informal observations of many of us; aging is accompanied by a decrease in sexual behavior. Sexual performance declines earlier and more dramatically with aging than does sexual interest, but both performance and motivation show declines (Bancroft 2005, Taylor, *et al* 1996). There is also a progressive and systematic decrease in systemic TS in males (Lupo-DiPrisco and Dessi-Fulgheri 1980,

Seidman 2003). Endocrine aging is less dramatic than the menopause of women, but aging exacts a toll on males and androgen-sensitive functions.

In a study of gonadally intact 22-24 months old male rats in good general health, we used multiple measures of sociosexual behavior and reproductive physiology to demonstrate that even healthy aging is accompanied by endocrine declines (Taylor, *et al* 1996). The untreated old animals showed clear decrements on all 13 measures of hypothalamic – pituitary – testicular function. This included reduced TS titers and decreased sexual activity.

The same is reported for a retrospective and prospective evaluation of sexual function and behavior in 77 healthy married men aged 45 to 74 years. There were significant age-related decreases in sexual desire, sexual arousal and activity, and increases in erectile problems. Aging also was negatively correlated with TS (Schiavi, *et al* 1991).

III.2.4. Hormone Therapy to Aged Males Increases Sexual Behaviors

There may or may not (Haren, *et al* 2002, Mazur, *et al* 2002) be a clearly identifiable causal relation between the two events, but a logical step for treatment of low sex hormone levels and reduced sexuality accompanying aging is hormone supplementation (Hayes 2000). There is understandable reluctance for clinicians to recommend TS therapy for aging men, given the well-known androgen sensitivity of the vulnerable prostate gland (Hijazi and Cunningham 2005). Nonetheless, given the success in experimental animals, TS supplementation for aging men remains an attractive therapy (Swerdloff and Wang 2004).

Clearly, androgen sensitive reproductive structures in older male animal models maintain sensitivity to additional TS (Chambers, *et al* 1991, Chubb and Desjardins 1984). The bulk of the data confirm benefits of TS to older males (Davidson, *et al* 1982, Schiavi, *et al* 1997). Treated males do not experience complete recovery to the behaviors of young males, but treated old males show more sexual interest and, to a lesser extent, increased copulatory capabilities.

Benefits of androgen therapy are accrued best in aged animal models and humans that are free of the diseases of old age (Wespes and Schulman 2002) and in aging males suffering the lowest TS levels (Corona, *et al* 2004). Not surprisingly, supplementation during middle age may be most effective. Testosterone supplements to 13 months old male rats, an ontogenetic period that models middle age in men, successfully increased most aspects of sexual behavior (Gray, *et al* 1981).

On rare occasion, experiments have been devised to increase endogenous circulating TS. In one experiment, we took advantage of the findings cited earlier that young males experience acute increases in TS to the presence of receptive females. We first asked if the same would be observed in old rats, and the results confirmed a significant rise in TS in old males (Taylor, *et al* 1996). Using the same receptive female exposure paradigm, we compared chronic endogenous and exogenous TS increases on two groups of healthy 22-24 months rats. Old male rats were administered either exogenous (ExT) supplementations daily for 6 weeks or were exposed to brief daily exposures to an inaccessible estrous female for additional episodes of endogenous (EnT) hormone over the same time period. Neither treatment restored our healthy old male rats to levels of sexual behavior approximating those of untreated young adults. Nonetheless, EnT males showed greater increases in sexual motivation and performance than ExT males. Our conclusions included that aged sexual behaviors of healthy old rats retain notable capacity, particularly, for endogenous TS activation of sociosexual behaviors (Taylor, *et al* 1996).

III.2.5. Testosterone to Hypogonadal Young Males Increases Sexual Behavior

Success is often reported with chronic TS supplementation in young hypogonadal men. Insufficient production of TS results in various sexual deficits affecting both sexual interest and sexual performance. Testosterone therapy commonly improves both significantly.

For example, men 25 – 40 yrs of age were diagnosed with severe hypogonadism by having a mean TS level of 35 ng/ dl, compared to the minimal level of 300 ng/ dl in eugonadal males (Burris, *et al* 1992). Patients were injected with 200 mg TS enanthate intramuscularly every 2 weeks for up to a year. Results were striking. Nocturnal erections in the hypogonadal men increased steadily during hormone replacement and were in the normal range with 6 to 12 months of treatment. The hypogonadal men also reported increases in several aspects of sexual activity, including sexual interest and the number of spontaneous erections.

It is interesting to highlight that this was clearly a genomic effect of the steroids. Serum TS concentration increased immediately and finally reached the upper range of normal levels. Yet, the behaviors only gradually changed with the immediate changes in circulating TS (Burris, *et al* 1992).

Other studies have reported similarly significant improvements in sexual function in hypogonadal young men treated with testosterone (Arver, *et al* 1996, Ashmed, *et al* 1988). A recent meta-analysis (Isidori, *et al* 2005) of men with TS levels below 300 ng/ dl receiving chronic TS therapy concluded that hormone treatment was moderately effective, likely because some were moderately hypogonadal. Even with this analysis, the men reported improvements in the number of nocturnal erections, sexual thoughts and motivation, number of successful intercourses, erectile function and overall sexual satisfaction.

Adolescent boys with delayed puberty also appear to benefit from TS supplementation, however, the benefits are not as clear as in young men. Depo-testosterone was administered to delayed pubertal boys in 3-month blocks alternating with placebo. Although there were modest increases in measures of sexuality, there were significant hormone effects on physical aggressive behaviors and aggressive impulses. A causal correlation is difficult to dispute because numerous studies have shown that withdrawal of exogenous TS to hypogonadal or castrated males is followed by a rapid and marked decrease in sexual interest and activity that is reinstated in a few weeks with TS replacement therapy (Meston and Frohlich 2000).

Nonetheless, there are data to jolt us back to the recognition that sexuality is dependent on factors other than normal androgens in circulation (OCarroll and Bancroft 1984). Hormonal supplementation that results in normal TS values does not always restore libido and erectile function in hypogonadal males. Moreover, many hypogonadal men are capable of sexual erections. Almost a third of men receiving effective anti-androgen therapy for prostate disease can develop erections when tested with erotic stimulation (Morales and Heaton 2003).

Previous findings with normal males may provide a clue to understanding at least some of the exceptions. In one experiment, we treated gonadally intact male rats to increase TS levels in one group by exogenous TS injections and decreased TS effectiveness by administering an antiandrogen to a second group. We found that decreased TS potency had minimal effects on sexual and aggressive behaviors despite profound suppressive effects on reproductive organs and glands (Taylor, *et al* 1985).

In an elegant experiment with healthy young men (Buena, *et al* 1993), two groups were treated with a GnRH agonist that suppresses endogenous TS production. Both groups also received TS replacement by a sustained release, long-acting microcapsule formulation to restore serum TS levels at low and high ends of the normal male range, respectively. There were no differences between the two groups on any measure of libido or copulatory performance. The most plausible explanation is that the threshold for sexual behavior is considerably below the circulating TS value of normal males (Bhasin, *et al* 2001). This may explain why some partially hypogonadal men continue to have normal sexual function and the absence of correlation between sexuality in males with serum T levels either in the high or low normal ranges.

III.2.6. Supplements that Produce Supraphysiological Increases in Testosterone do not Change Behaviors of Healthy Young Males

Inspired by the upsurge in abuse of anabolic steroids there is now a substantial literature on the behavioral outcomes of supraphysiological increases in TS in gonadally intact young males. Here, we are defining supraphysiological as being in the highest values (circa 1000 ng/ dl), or slightly above these levels, of TS found in untreated, healthy men.

There are various reasons to predict that additional TS to men with normal endocrine function, the so-called eugonadal condition, would not change sociosexual behaviors. One is that androgen receptors in most tissues are either saturated or downregulated at physiological TS concentrations (Antonio, *et al* 1999). Additional TS would have no more binding sites.

Also, as cited in the previous section, the evidence points to the level of TS required for sexual interest and activity in adult males is lower than normal males' circulating levels of TS. The suggestion is that most males already are at high functional levels of circulating TS. Finally, the threshold model discussed earlier certainly predicts that exogenously induced TS changes above the threshold level would not be expected to influence sexual interest or behavior (Schiavi and Segraves 1995).

The data from men serving as subjects in biomedical experiments provide considerable support for the prediction. A meta-analysis concluded that supplements of TS had no effect on erectile function in eugonadal men compared to placebo (Isidori, *et al* 2005). In a similar paradigm, healthy young men with normal levels of TS were administered supplemental hormone to boost levels to supraphysiological TS values. The men showed an increased self-reported interest in sex during TS treatment. These changes, however, were not reflected in any change in overt sexual behavior, which in eugonadal men may be more determined by sexual relationship factors (Anderson, *et al* 1992).

Our work with gonadally intact male rats provides additional support. Additional hormone does not uniformly increase copulation in sexually experienced males, although TS therapy increased sexual performance of virgin males (Taylor, *et al* 1985).

The conclusion is that supplementation that increases TS to physiological, albeit high physiological, levels is unlikely to increase sexual performance. However, the treatment can increase sexual interest. Supplements that increase TS levels to pharmacologic levels may be quite another story.

III.2.7. Steroid Abuse Raises Testosterone to Pharmacological Levels with Increases in Aggressiveness and Perhaps Sexual Motivation

An important feature of the supraphysiological research cited above is that the TS supplements to eugonadal men were of minimal to modest dosages and of short durations. This is dictated by the consideration of human researchers bound by ethical considerations to keep the TS dosages to the participants in ranges that are unlikely to endanger their health. Even many researchers using animal models attempt to maintain as near physiological titers of steroid as possible to provide data that can be generalized to natural populations.

There are people outside the usual biomedical research protocols, however, who experience chronic, and greatly exaggerated, pharmacologic levels of circulating TS. These are, of course, professional or amateur athletes and others who abuse anabolic steroids. These compounds are more accurately identified as androgenic anabolic steroids (AAS) to indicate they have the significant androgenic effects of TS and muscle building (anabolic) features. AAS are synthetic derivatives of TS. Indeed, many AAS were developed by pharmaceutical firms as possible TS therapies with different characteristics (Clark and Henderson 2003).

The most potent AAS are injected to avoid the dangers of first-pass metabolism, with the result that androgen titers are chronically high and pharmacological. It is not uncommon for these values to be 20x or more of the highest, physiological values. Because these individuals are engaged in criminal activity, they are off-limits to responsible researchers. Thus, there are only informal, non-systematic data available on people abusing steroids.

Adding to the uncertainty of information on anabolic steroid abuse is that results of the supraphysiological biomedical studies cited in the previous section may not accurately reflect the outcomes of the high pharmacological dosages common among abusers of steroids (Yates, *et al* 1999). Fortunately, there are systematic data available from animal models administered high doses to mimic the pharmacological levels of steroid abusers (Blanco, *et al* 1997).

The behavioral results from these animal experiments suggest that AAS are more likely to elevate aggression than sexuality. For example, injection of TS propionate over 10 weeks to intact adult male rats increased inter-male aggression significantly with less effect on copulation (Lumia, *et al* 1994). Aggression was also increased toward the source of a tail pinch in intact male rats treated with high doses of TS for 12 weeks (McGinnis, *et al* 2002). Finally, a study of a highly strain of mice administered TS observed no further increases in their intact adults. Females of the strain, however, showed more aggression to the same dosage of TS (Bronson 1996). A recent review (Clark and Henderson 2003) of the animal literature concluded that AAS has minimal effects on sexual behavior of intact rats, although there were a few exceptions for animals treated chronically with very high dosages.

The available human data suggests that very high doses of TS may, in fact, increase both some aspects of sociosexual behaviors (Lukas 1993). Sexual performance in the form of impotency may be a significant risk factor of pharmacological dosages (Eklof, *et al* 2003), but heightened aggressiveness and libido may be increased. A 2-week, double-blind placebo-controlled crossover study administered high doses of methyltestosterone to 20 young, healthy volunteers. Results were statistically significant increases in sexual arousal, energy and irritability (Su, *et al* 1993). Self-reports by AAS abusing athletes have suggestion a similar conclusion (Clark and Henderson 2003). These results point to AAS agents that induce long-term pharmacologic elevation of systemic TS almost surely increase aggressive behaviors and also may increase sexual motivation. Sexual performance, however, is likely to suffer declines.

Conclusion

To summarize, we offer the following general principles of testosterone – sociosexual behavior relations. 1) The evidence is overwhelming that testosterone is critical for the organization and activation of sexual responses of the male. 2) In males, and likely also in females, testosterone is responsible for sexual motivation. 3) Probably the testosterone metabolites, DHT and especially E2, are ultimately responsible for much of the activation of brain system underlying the sociosexual behaviors of males. 4) Resting testosterone levels are unlikely to be related to individual differences in behavior, but momentary and, especially, chronic changes in testosterone in circulation are directly associated with changes in sociosexual behaviors. 5) Steroid supplements that increase circulating testosterone to high physiological levels are likely to improve the sexual well-being of hypogonadal and aged men, but anabolic steroids that produce pharmacologic testosterone levels are unlikely to produce beneficial behavioral outcomes. 6) The distribution of steroid receptors in brain areas unrelated to reproduction, along with the non-genomic effects of neuroactive steroids and neurosteroids, point to the likelihood that we have only scratched the surface of the impact steroids have on brain morphology and function, and behavior. The neuroendocrinology of testosterone and the other steroids are likely to have a most interesting future.

References

Abbud, R.A., Ameduri, R.K., Rao, J.S., Nett, T.M. & Nilson, J.H. (1999) Chronic hypersecretion of luteinizing hormone in transgenic mice selectively alters responsiveness of the alpha-subunit gene to gonadotropin-releasing hormone and estrogens. *Molecular Endocrinology, 13,* 1449-1459.

Adkins-Regan, E. (1981) Hormone specificity, androgen metabolism, and social behavior. *American Zoologist, 21,* 257-271.

Akingbemi, B.T. (2005) Estrogen regulation of testicular function. *Reproductive Biology and Endocrinology, 3,* doi: 10.1186/1477-7827-1183-1151.

Aluja, A. & Torrubia, R. (2004) Hostility-aggressiveness, sensation seeking, and sex hormones in men: Re-exploring their relationship. *Neuropsychobiology, 50,* 102-108.

Anderson, R.A., Bancroft, J. & Wu, F.C. (1992) The effects of exogenous testosterone on sexuality and mood of normal men. *Journal of Clinical Endocrinology & Metabolism, 75,* 1503-1507.

Antonio, J., Wilson, J.D. & George, F.W. (1999) Effects of castration and androgen treatment on androgen-receptor levels in rat skeletal muscles. *Journal of Applied Physiology, 87,* 2016–2019.

Archer, J. (1994) Testosterone and aggression. In: *The Psychobiology of Aggression* (ed. by M. Hillbrand & N.J. Pallone), pp. 3-25. The Haworth Press, New York.

Arlt, W., Haas, J., Callies, F., Reincke, M., Hubler, D., Oettel, M., Ernst, M., Schulte, H. & Allolio, B. (1999) Biotransformation of oral dehydroepiandrosterone in elderly men: significant increase in circulating estrogens. *Journal of Clinical Endocrinology & Metabolism, 84,* 2170-2176.

Arnold, A.P. & Gorski, R.A. (1984) Gonadal steroid induction of structural sex differences in the central nervous system. *Annual Review of Neuroscience, 7,* 413-442.

Arver, S., Dobs, A.S., Meikle, A.W., Allen, R.P., Sanders, S.W. & Mazer, N.A. (1996) Improvement of sexual function in testosterone deficient men treated for 1 year with a permeation enhanced testosterone transdermal system. *Journal of Urology, 155,* 1604-1608.

Ashmed, S.F., Boucher, A., Manni, A., Santen, R., Bartholomew, M. & Demers, L. (1988) Transdermal testosterone therapy in the treatment of male hypogonadism. *Journal of Clinical Endocrinology & Metabolism, 66,* 546-551.

Bachmann, G.A. (2002) The hypoandrogenic woman; pathophysiologic overview. *Fertility and Sterility, 77,* S72-S76

Ball, G.F. & Balthazart, J. (2006) Androgen metabolism and the activation of male sexual behavior: It's more complicated than you think! *Hormones and Behavior, 49,* 1-3.

Balthazart, J. & Ball, G.F. (1998) New insights into the regulation and function of brain estrogen synthase (aromatase). *Trends in Neuroscience, 21,* 243-249.

Bancroft, J. (2005) The endocrinology of sexual arousal. *Journal of Endocrinology, 186,* 411-427.

Bartke, A. & Dalterio, S. (1975) Episodic secretion of testosterone in laboratory mice. *Science., 100,* 1-5.

Baulieu, E.E. (1997) Neurosteroids: of the nervous system, by the nervous system, for the nervous system. *Recent Progress in Hormone Research, 52,* 1-32.

Baulieu, E.E. (1998) Neurosteroids: a novel function of the brain. *Psychoneuroendocrinology, 23,* 963-987.

Baum, M., Melamed, E. & Globus, M. (1986) Dissociation of the effects of castration and testosterone replacement on sexual behavior and neural metabolism of dopamine in the male rat. *Brain Research Bulletin, 16,* 145-148.

Baum, M.J. (2002) Neuroendocrinology of sexual behavior in the male. In: *Behavioral Endocrinology, 2nd Edition* (ed. by J. Becker, M. Breedlove & D. Crews), pp. 153-203. The M.I.T. Press, Cambridge, MA.

Beach, F.A. (1981) Historical origins of modern research on hormones and behavior. *Hormones & Behavior, 15,* 325-376.

Beck, S.G. & Handa, R.J. (2004) Dehydroepiandrosterone (DHEA): A misunderstood adrenal hormone and spine-tingling neurosteroid? *Endocrinology, 145,* 1039-1041.

Belelli, D. & Lamber, J.J. (2005) Neurosteroids: endogenous regulators of the GABA-A receptor. *Nature Reviews of Neuroscience 6,* 565-566.

Beyer, C., Larsson, K., Perez-Placios, G. & Morali, G. (1973) Androgen structure and male sexual behavior in the castrated rat. *Hormones & Behavior, 4,* 99-107.

Bhasin, S., Woodhouse, L., Dzekov, C. & Others, X. (2001) Testosterone dose-response relationships in healthy young men. *American Journal of Physiology: Endocrinology & Metabolism, 281,* E1172-E1181.

Bialek, M., Zaremba, P., Borowicz, K.K. & Czuczwar, S.J. (2004) Neuroprotective role of testosterone in the nervous system. *Polish Journal of Pharmacology, 56,* 509-518.

Birchard, K. (1999) Body-building supplement fails to strengthen muscle and may harm health. *Lancet, 353,* 1943-1944.

Birzniece, V., Backstrom, T., Johansson, M.A. & Others, X. (2006) Neuroactive steroid effects on cognitive functions with a focus on the serotonin and GABA systems. *Brain Research Reviews, 51,* 212-239.

Blanco, C.E., Popper, P. & Micevych, P. (1997) Anabolic-androgenic steroid induced alterations in choline acetyltransferase messenger RNA levels of spinal cord motoneurons in the male rat. *Neuroscience, 78,* 873-882.

Bonsall, R., Clancy, A. & Michael, R. (1992) Effects of the nonsteroidal aromatase inhibitor, fadrozole, on sexual behavior in male rats. *Hormones & Behavior, 26,* 240-254.

Bonsall, R.W., Rees, H. & Michael, R. (1985) The distribution, nuclear uptake and metabolism of (3H) dihydrotestosterone in the brain, pituitary gland and genital tract of the male rhesus monkey. *Journal of Steroid Biochemistry, 23,* 389-398.

Breedlove, S.M. & Hampson, E. (2002) Sexual differentiation of the brain and behavior. In: *Behavioral Endocrinology, Second Edition* (ed. by J.B. Becker, S.M. Breedlove, D. Crews & M.M. McCarthy), pp. 75-116. The MIT Press, Cambridge, MA.

Breedlove, S.M. & Jordan, C.L. (2001) The increasingly plastic, hormone-responsive adult brain. *Proceedings of the National Academy of Sciences, 98,* 2956-2957.

Bronson, F.H. (1996) Effects of prolonged exposure to anabolic steroids on the behavior of male and female mice. *Pharmacology Biochemistry & Behavior, 53,* 329–334.

Bronwyn, A.L., Crawford, C., Liu, P.Y., Kean, M.T., Bleasel, J.F. & Handelsman, D.J. (2003) Randomized placebo-controlled trial of androgen effects on muscle and bone in men requiring long- term systemic glucocorticoid treatment. *Journal of Clinical Endocrinology and Metabolism, 88,* 3167-3176.

Brown, W.A., Monti, P. & Corriveau, D. (1978) Serum testosterone and sexual activity and interest in men. *Archives of Sexual Behavior, 7,* 97-103.

Buena, F., Swerdloff, R.S., Steiner, B.S., Lutchmansingh, P., Peterson, M.A., Pandian, M.R., Galmarini, M. & Bhasin, S. (1993) Sexual function does not change when serum testosterone levels are pharmacologically varied within the normal male range. *Fertility & Sterility, 59,* 1118-1123.

Burris, A.S., Banks, S.M., Carter, S., Davidson, J.M. & Sherins, R.J. (1992) A long-term, prospective study of the physiologic and behavioral effects of hormone replacement in untreated hypogonadal men. *Journal of Andrology, 13,* 297-304.

Butera, P.C. & Czaja, J.A. (1989) Activities of sexual behavior in male rats by combined subcutaneous and intracranial treatments of 5 alpha-dihydrotestosterone. *Hormones & Behavior, 23,* 92-105.

Carlson, A.A., Young, A.J., Russell, A.F., Bennett, N.C., McNeilly, A.S. & Clutton-Brock, T. (2004) Hormonal correlates of dominance in meerkats (Suricata suricatta). *Hormones & Behavior, 46,* 141-150.

Carreau, S., Lambard, S., Delalande, C. & Others, X. (2003) Aromatase expression and role of estrogens in male gonad: a review. *Reproductive Biology and Endocrinology, 1,* 211-223.

Chambers, K.C. & Phoenix, C.H. (1992) Sexual behavior and serum levels of prolactin, testosterone, and estradiol in young and old rhesus males. *Physiology & Behavior, 52,* 13-16.

Chambers, K.C., Thornton, J. & Roselli, C. (1991) Age-related deficits in brain androgen binding and metabolism, testosterone, and sexual behavior of male rats. *Neurobiology of Aging, 12,* 123-130.

Chen, F., K., K., E., B., J., F. & Others, X. (2005) Direct agonist/antagonist functions of dehydroepiandrosterone. *Endocrinology, 146,* 4568-4576.

Chen, T. & Tu, W. (1992) Sex differences in estrogen and androgen receptors in hamster brain. *Life Sciences, 50,* 1639-1647.

Chubb, C. & Desjardins, C. (1984) Testicular function and sexual activity in senescent mice. *American Journal of Physiology, 247,* 569-573.

Clark, A.S. & Henderson, L.P. (2003) Behavioral and physiological responses to anabolic-androgenic steroids. *Neuroscience and Biobehavioral Reviews, 27,* 413-436.

Cooke, B., Hegstrom, C.D., Villeneuve, L.S. & Breedlove, S.M. (1999a) Sexual differentiation of the vertebrate brain: principles and mechanisms. *Frontiers in Neuroendocrinology, 20,* 323-362.

Cooke, B.M., Breedlove, S.M. & Jordan, C.L. (2003) Both estrogen receptors and androgen receptors contribute to testosterone-induced changes in the morphology of the medial amygdala and sexual arousal in male rats. *Hormones & Behavior, 43,* 336-346.

Cooke, B.M., Tabibnia, G. & Breedlove, S.M. (1999b) A brain sexual dimorphism controlled by adult circulating androgens. *Proceedings of the National Academy of Sciences (U.S.A.), 96,* 7538-7540.

Cooke, P.S., Buchanan, D.L., Lubahn, D.B. & Cunha, G.R. (1998) Mechanism of estrogen action: Lessons from the estrogen receptor-alpha knockout mouse. *Biology of Reproduction, 59,* 470-475.

Corona, G., Mannucci, E., Mansani, R. & Others, X. (2004) Aging and pathogenesis of erectile dysfunction. *International Journal of Impotence Research, 16,* 395-402.

Corpechot, C., Robel, P., Axelson, M., Sjovall, J. & Baulieu, E. (1981) Characterization and measurement of dehydroepiandrosterone sulfate in the rat brain. *Proceedings of the National Academy of Science, 78,* 4704-4707.

Craigen, W. & Bronson, F. (1982) Deterioration of the capacity for sexual arousal in aged male mice. *Biology of Reproduction, 26,* 869-874.

Dabbs, J. & Hargrave, K.R. (1997) Age, testosterone, and behavior among female prison inmates. *Psychosomatic Medicine, 59,* 477-480.

Damassa, D.A., Smith, E.R., Tennent, B. & Davidson, J.M. (1977) The relationship between circulating testosterone levels and male sexual behavior in rats. *Hormones & Behavior, 8,* 275-286.

Davidson, J.M. (1966) Characteristics of sex behaviour in male rats following castration. *Animal Behaviour, 14,* 266-272.

Davidson, J.M., Kwan, M. & Greenleaf, W.J. (1982) Hormonal replacement and sexuality in men. *Journal of Clinical Endocrinology and Metabolism, 11,* 599-623.

Davis, S.R. (1999) The therapeutic use of androgens in women. *Journal of Steroid Biochemistry & Molecular Biology, 69,* 177-184.

Davis, S.R., Goldstat, R., Papalia, M.A., Shah, S., Kulkarni, J., Donath, S. & Bell, R.J. (2006) Effects of aromatase inhibition on sexual function and well-being in postmenopausal women treated with testosterone: a randomized, placebo-controlled trial. *Menopause, 13,* 37-45.

Davis, S.R., McCloud, P., Strauss, B.J. & Burger, H. (1995) Testosterone enhances estradiol's effects on postmenopausal bone density and sexuality. *Maturitas, 21,* 227-236.

Dennerstein, L.M.B., Randolph, J., Taffe, J., Dudley, E. & Burger, H. (2002) Hormones, mood, sexuality, and the menopausal transition. *Fertility and Sterility, 77,* S42-S48.

Dewsbury, D.A. (1981) Effects of novelty on copulatory behavior: The Coolidge effect and related phenomena. *Psychological Bulletin, 89,* 464-482.

Dhatariya, K. (2005) Self-reported sexual function in women and androgen levels. *JAMA, 294,* 2167-2168.

Dobs, A.S., Nguyen, T., Pace, C. & Roberts, C.P. (2002) Differential effects of oral estrogen versus oral estrogen-androgen replacement therapy on body composition in postmenopausal women. *Journal of Clinical Endocrinology & Metabolism, 87,* 1509-1516.

Dominguez, J.M. & Hull, E.M. (2005) Dopamine, the medial preoptic area, and male sexual behavior. *Physiology & Behavior, 86,* 356-368.

DonCarlos, L.L., Garcia-Ovejero, D., Sarkey, S., Garcia-Segura, L.M. & Azcoitia, I. (2003) Androgen receptor immunoreactivity in forebrain axons and dendrites in the rat. *Endocrinology, 144,* 3632-3638.

Dougherty, D.M., Bjork, J.M., Moeller, F.G. & Swann, A.C. (1997) The influence of menstrual-cycle phase on the relationship between testosterone and aggression. *Physiology & Behavior, 62,* 431-435.

Eklof, A.C., Thurelius, A.M., Garle, M., Rane, A. & Sjoqvist, F. (2003) The anti-doping hot-line, a means to capture the abuse of doping agents in the Swedish society and a new service function in clinical pharmacology. *European Journal of Clinical Pharmacology, 59,* 571-577.

Engel, S.R. & Grant, K.A. (2001) Neurosteroids and behavior. *International Review of Neurobiology, 46,* 321-348.

Everitt, B.J. (1990) Sexual motivation: A neural and behavioral analysis of the mechanisms underlying appetitive and copulatory responses in male rats. *Neuroscience and Biobehavioral Reviews, 14,* 217-232.

Ewing, L., Gorski, R., Sbordane, R., Tyler, J., Desjardins, C. & Robaire, B. (1979) Testosterone-estradiol filled polydimethylsiloxane subdermal implants: Effect on fertility and masculine sexual and aggressive behavior of male rats. *Biology of Reproduction, 21,* 765-772.

Federman, D.D. (2004) Three facets of sexual differentiation. *New England Journal of Medicine, 350,* 323-324.

Fernandez-Guasti, A., Kruijver, F.P., Fodor, M. & Swaab, D.F. (2000) Sex differences in the distribution of androgen receptors in the human hypothalamus. *Journal of Comparative Neurology, 425,* 422-435.

Frankel, E. (1984) Plasma testosterone levels are higher in old mating rats than in old non-mating rats. *Experimental Gerontology, 16,* 345-348.

Frye, C.A. (2001) The role of neurosteroids and non-genomic effects of progestins and androgens in mediating sexual receptivity of rodents. *Brain Research Reviews, 37,* 201-222.

Frye, C.A. & McCormick, C.M. (2000) Androgens are neuroprotective in the dentate gyrus of adrenalectomized female rats. *Stress, 3,* 185-194.

Fukada, S., Nagashima, H., Marioka, K. & Aoki, J. (1988) Fluctuation in peripheral serum testosterone levels within a day with age and by sexual stimulation in male beagle dogs bred indoors. *Experimental Animals, 37,* 381-386.

Goldstein, I., Traish, A., Kim, N. & Munarriz, R. (2004) The role of sex steroid hormones in female sexual function and dysfunction. *Clinical Obstetrics And Gynecology, 47,* 471-484.

Goldstein, J.S. & Sites, C.K. (2002) Selective modulation of sex steroids. *Ageing Research Reviews, 1,* 17-28.

Gordon, R.J., Breedlove, M.S., Bernstein, S. & Lichtman, J.W. (1990) Neuromuscular junctions shrink and expand as muscle fiber size is manipulated: in vivo observations in the androgen-sensitive bulbocavernosus muscle of mice. *Journal of Neuroscience, 10,* 2660-2671.

Gray, G.D., Smith, E., Dorsa, D. & Davidson, J.M. (1981) Sexual behavior and testosterone in middle-aged rats. *Endocrinology, 109,* 1597-1604.

Gray, P.B., Singh, A.B., Woodhouse, L.J. & Others, X. (2005) Dose-dependent effects of testosterone on sexual function, mood, and visuospatial cognition in older men. *Journal of Clinical Endocrinology & Metabolism, 90,* 3838-3846.

Greenstein, A., Plymate, S.R. & Katz, P.G. (1995) Visually stimulated erection in castrated men. *Journal of Urology, 153,* 650-652.

Gruber, C.J., Tschugguel, W., Schneeberger, C. & Huber, J.C. (2002) Production and actions of estrogens. *New England Journal of Medicine, 346,* 340-352.

Guay, A., Munarriz, R., Jacobson, J., Talakoub, L., Traish, A., Quirk, F., Goldstein, I. & Spark, R. (2004) Serum androgen levels in healthy premenopausal women with and without sexual dysfunction: Part A. Serum androgen levels in women aged 20-49 years with no complaints of sexual dysfunction. *International Journal of Impotence Research, 16,* 112-120.

Hall, C.M., Jones, J.A., Meyer-Bahlburg, H.F., Dolezal, C., Coleman, M., Foster, P., Price, D.A. & Clayton, P.E. (2004) Behavioral and physical masculinization are related to genotype in girls with congenital adrenal hyperplasia. *Journal of Clinical Endocrinology & Metabolism, 89,* 419-424.

Haller, J., Millar, S., van de Schraaf, J., de Kloet, R.E. & Kruk, M.R. (2000) The active phase-related increase in corticosterone and aggression are linked. *Journal of Neuroendocrinology, 12,* 431-436.

Hamann, S. (2005) Sex differences in the responses of the human amygdala. *Neuroscientist, 11,* 288-293.

Haren, M.T., Morley, J.E., Chapman, I.M., O'Loughlin, P.D. & Wittert, G.A. (2002) Defining 'relative' androgen deficiency in aging men: how should testosterone be measured and what are the relationships between androgen levels and physical, sexual and emotional health?. *Climacteric, 5,* 15-25.

Hayes, F.J. (2000) Testosterone - fountain of youth or drug of abuse? *Journal of Clinical Endocrinology & Metabolism, 85,* 3020-3023.

Hijazi, R.A. & Cunningham, G.R. (2005) Andropause: Is androgen replacement therapy indicated for the aging male? . *Annual Review of Medicine, 56,* 117-137.

Hodes, G.E. & Shors, T.J. (2005) Distinctive stress effects on learning during puberty. *Hormones and Behavior, 48,* 163-171.

Howell, S. & Shalet, S. (2001) Testosterone deficiency and replacement. *Hormone Research, 56 (Suppl. 1),* 86-92.

Huang, J., Chang, L., Ho, D. & Ho, L. (1989) The effect of sexual activity on androgen metabolism, androgen-receptor translocation and glandular weight of ventral prostates of rats. *Endocrinology, 120,* 505-510.

Huhtaniemi, I. (2000) Mutations of gonadotrophin and gonadotrophin receptor genes: what do they teach us about reproductive physiology? *Journal of Reproduction and Fertility, 119,* 173–186.

Hull, E.M., Lorrain, D.S., Du, J., Matuszewich, L., Lumley, L., Putnam, S.K. & Moses, J. (1999) Hormone-neurotransmitter interactions in the control of sexual behavior. *Behavioural Brain Research, 105,* 105-116.

Isidori, A.M., Giannetta, E., Gianfrilli, D. & Others, X. (2005) Effects of testosterone on sexual function in men: results of a meta-analysis. *Clinical Endocrinology, 63,* 381-394.

Johannsson, G., Burman, P., Wiren, L. & Others, X. (2002) Low dose dehydroepiandrosterone affects behavior in hypopituitary androgen-deficient women: a placebo- controlled trial. *Journal of Clinical Endocrinology & Metabolism, 87,* 2046–2052.

Johnston, P. & Davidson, J.M. (1972) Intracerebral androgens and sexual behavior in the male rat. *Hormones & Behavior, 3,* 345-357.

Jones, K.J., Coers, S., Storer, P.D., Tanzer, L. & Kinderman, N.B. (1999) Androgenic regulation of the central glia response following nerve damage. *Journal of Neurobiology, 40,* 560-573.

Kalantaridou, S.N. & Calis, K.A. (2006) Testosterone therapy in premenopausal women. *Seminars in Reproductive Medicine, 24,* 106-114.

Keast, J.R. (1999) The autonomic nerve supply of male sex organs--an important target of circulating androgens. *Behavioural Brain Research, 105,* 81-92.

Kelliher, K.R., Liu, Y.C., Baum, M.J. & Sachs, B.D. (1999) Neuronal Fos activation in olfactory bulb and forebrain of male rats having erections in the presence of inaccessible estrous females. *Neuroscience, 92,* 1025-1033.

King, D.S., Sharp, R.L., Vukovich, M.D., Brown, G.A., Reifenrath, T.A., Uhl, N.L. & Parsons, K.A. (1999) Effect of oral androstenedione on serum testosterone and adaptations to resistance training in young men: a randomized controlled trial. *The Journal of the American Medical Association (JAMA), 281,* 2020-2028.

Knussmann, R., Christiansen, K. & Couwenbergs, C. (1986) Relations between sex hormone levels and sexual behavior in men. *Archives of Sexual Behavior, 15,* 429-445.

Kohl, J.V., Atzmueller, M., Fink, B. & Grammer, K. (2001) Human pheromones: Integrating neuroendocrinology and ethology. *Neuroendocrinology Letters, 22,* 309-321.

Kruger, T.H., Haake, P., Chereath, D., Knapp, W., Janssen, O.E., Exton, M.S., Schedlowski, M. & Hartmann, U. (2003) Specificity of the neuroendocrine response to orgasm during sexual arousal in men. *Journal of Endocrinology, 177,* 57-64.

Labrie, F., Belanger, A., Luu-The, V., Labrie, C., Simard, J., Cusan, L., Gomez, J. & Candas, B. (1998) DHEA and the intracrine formation of androgens and estrogens in peripheral target tissues: Its role during aging. *Steroids, 63,* 322-328.

Labrie, F., Luu-The, V., Belanger, A., Lin, S.X., Simard, J., Pelletier, G. & Labrie, C. (2005) Is dehydroepiandrosterone a hormone? *Journal of Endocrinology, 187,* 169-196.

Leranth, C., Hajszan, T. & MacLusky, N.J. (2004a) Androgens increase spine synapse density in the CA1 hippocampal subfield of ovariectomized female rats. *Journal of Neuroscience, 24,* 495- 499.

Leranth, C., Prange-Kiel, J., Frick, K.M. & Horvath, T.L. (2004b) Low CA1 spine synapse density is further reduced by castration in male non-human primates. *Cerebral Cortex, 14,* 503-510.

Lieberman, S. & Prasad, V. (1990) Heterodox notions on pathways of steroidogenesis. *Endocrine Rev., 11,* 469-493.

Linkowski, P., Mendlewicz, J., Leclercq, R. & Others, X. (1985) The 24-hour profile of adrenocorticotropin and cortisol in major depressive illness. *Journal of Clinical Endocrinology & Metabolism, 61,* 429-438.

Lu, S.F., McKenna, S.E., Cologer-Clifford, A., Nau, E.A. & Simon, N.G. (1998) Androgen receptor in mouse brain: sex differences and similarities in autoregulation. *Endocrinology, 139,* 1594-1601.

Lukas, S.E. (1993) Current perspectives on anabolic-androgenic steroid abuse. *Trends in Pharmacological Science, 14,* 61-68.

Lumia, A.R., Thorner, K.M. & McGinnis, M.Y. (1994) Effects of chronically high doses of the anabolic androgenic steroid, testosterone, on intermale aggression and sexual behavior in male rats. *Physiology & Behavior, 55,* 331-335.

Lupo-DiPrisco, C. & Dessi-Fulgheri, F. (1980) Endocrine and behavioral modifications in aging male rats. *Hormone Research, 12,* 149-160.

Mantzoros, C., Georgiadis, E. & Trichopoulos, D. (1995) Contribution of dihydrotestosterone to male sexual behaviour. *British Medical Journal, 310,* 1289-1291.

Martini, L., Celotti, F., Lechuga, M., Melcangi, R., Motta, M., Negri-Cesi, P., Poletti, A. & Zoppi, S. (1990) Androgen metabolism in different target tissues. *Annals New York Academy of Sciences, 595,* 184-198.

Matthews, K.A., Berga, S.L., Owens, J.F. & Flory, J.D. (1998) Effects of short-term suppression of ovarian hormones on cardiovascular and neuroendocrine reactivity to stress in women. *Psychoneuroendocrinology, 23,* 307-322.

Mazur, A., Mueller, U., Krause, W. & Booth, A. (2002) Causes of sexual decline in aging married men: Germany and America. *International Journal of Impotence Research, 14,* 101-106.

McEwen, B.S. (2001) Estrogens effects on the brain: multiple sites and molecular mechanisms. *Journal of Applied Physiology, 91,* 2785-2801.

McEwen, B.S., Gould, E., Orchinik, M., Weiland, N. & Woolley, C.S. (1995) Oestrogens and the structural and functional plasticity of neurons: implications for memory, ageing and neurodegenerative processes. In: *Non-reproductive actions of sex steroids* (ed. by C.R. Brock & J.A. Goode), pp. 52-73. John Wiley, New York.

McGinnis, M.Y., Lumia, A.R., Breuer, M.E. & Possidente, B. (2002) Physical provocation potentiates aggression in male rats receiving anabolic androgenic steroids. *Hormones & Behavior, 41,* 101-110.

McGivern, R.F., Handa, R.J. & Raum, W.J. (1998) Ethanol exposure during the last week of gestation in the rat: inhibition of the prenatal testosterone surge in males without long-term alterations in sex behavior. *Neurotoxicology & Teratology, 20,* 483-490.

Meisel, R.L. & Sachs, B.D. (1994) The physiology of male reproductive behavior. In: *The Physiology of Reproduction, Volume 2* (ed. by E. Knobil & J. Neill), pp. 3-106. Raven Press, Inc., N.Y.

Mellon, S.H. (1994) Neurosteroids: Biochemistry, modes of action, and clinical relevance. *Journal of Clinical Endocrinology & Metabolism, 78,* 1003-1008.

Meston, C.M. & Frohlich, P.F. (2000) The neurobiology of sexual function. *Archives of General Psychiatry, 57,* 1012-1030.

Meston, C.M. & Heiman, J.R. (2002) Acute dehydroepiandrosterone effects on sexual arousal in premenopausal women. *Journal of Sex & Marital Therapy, 28,* 53-60.

Michael, R.P., Bonsall, R.W. & Zumpe, D. (1987) Testosterone and its metabolites in male cynomologus monkeys (Macaca fascicularis behavior and biochemistry. *Physiology & Behavior, 40,* 527-537.

Michael, R.P., Clancy, A.N. & Zumpe, D. (1995) Distribution of androgen receptor-like immunoreactivity in the brains of cynomolgus monkeys. *Journal of Neuroendocrinology, 7,* 713-719.

Michael, R.P., Zumpe, D. & Bonsall, R.W. (1984) Sexual behavior correlates with the diurnal plasma testosterone range in intact male rhesus monkeys. *Biology of Reproduction, 30,* 652-657.

Miller, K., Sesmilo, G., Schiller, A., Schoenfeld, D., Burton, S. & Klibanski, A. (2001) Androgen deficiency in women with hypopituitarism. *Journal of Clinical Endocrinology & Metabolism, 86,* 561-567.

Miller, K.K. (2002) The androgen deficiency syndrome in women. *Endocrinology Rounds, 1,* 1-8.

Moffat, S.D., Zonderman, A.B., Metter, E.J., Kawas, C., Blackman, M.R., Harman, S.M. & Resnick, S.M. (2004) Free testosterone and risk for Alzheimer disease in older men. *Neurology, 62,* 188-193.

Morales, A. & Heaton, J.P. (2003) Hypogonadism and erectile dysfunction: pathophysiological observations and therapeutic outcomes. *BJU International, 92,* 896-899.

Nakamura, N., Fujita, H. & Kawata, M. (2002) Effects of gonadectomy on immunoreactivity for choline acetyltransferase in the cortex, hippocampus, and basal forebrain of adult male rats. *Neuroscience, 109,* 473-485.

Nottebohm, F. & Arnold, A.P. (1976) Sexual dimorphism in vocal control areas of the songbird brain. *Science, 194,* 211–213.

Nyunt, A., Stephen, G., Gibbin, J., Durgan, L., Fielding, A.M., Wheeler, M. & Price, D.E. (2005) Androgen status in healthy premenopausal women with loss of libido. *Journal of Sex & Marital Therapy, 31,* 73-80.

O'Carroll, R.E. & Bancroft, J. (1984) Testosterone therapy for low sexual interest and erectile dysfunction in men: a controlled study. *British Journal of Psychiatry, 145,* 146-151.

O'Connor, D.B., Archer, J. & Wu, F.C.W. (2004) Effects of testosterone on mood, aggression, and sexual behavior in young men: a double-blind, placebo- controlled, cross-over study. *Journal of Clinical Endocrinology & Metabolism, 89*, 2837-2845.

Occhiato, E.G., Guarna, A., Danza, G. & Serio, M. (2004) Selective non-steroidal inhibitors of 5alpha-reductase type 1. *Journal of Steroid Biochemistry & Molecular Biology, 88,* 1-16.

Payne, A.H. & Hales, D.B. (2004) Overview of steroidogenic enzymes in the pathway from cholesterol to active steroid hormones. *Endocrine Reviews, 25,* 947-970.

Penny, R. (1985) Episodic secretion of melatonin in pre-and post-pubertal girls and boys. *Journal of Clinical Endocrinology & Metabolism, 60,* 751-756.

Pfaus, J.G. (1996) Homologies of animal and human sexual behaviors. *Hormones & Behavior, 30,* 187-200.

Phoenix, C.H. & Chambers, K.C. (1986) Threshold for behavioral response to testosterone in old castrated male rhesus macaques. *Biology of Reproduction. 35,* 918-926.

Phoenix, C.H., Dixson, A.F. & Resko, J.A. (1977) Effects of ejaculation on levels of testosterone, cortisol, and luteinizing hormone in peripheral plasma of rhesus monkeys. *Journal of Comparative & Physiological Psychology, 91,* 120-127.

Phoenix, C.H., Goy, R.W., Gerall, A.A. & Young, W.C. (1959) Organizing action of prenatally administered testosterone propionate on the tissues mediating mating behavior in the female guinea pig. *Endocrinology, 65,* 369-382.

Piroli, G.G., Pietranera, L., Grillo, C.A. & DeNicola, A.F. (2002) Dehydroepiandrosterone regulation of prolactin gene expression in the anterior pituitary does not depend on galanin induction. *Neuroendocrinology Letters, 23,* 321-324.

Resko, J.A. & Roselli, C.E. (1997) Prenatal hormones organize sex differences of the neuroendocrine reproductive system: observations on guinea pigs and nonhuman primates. *Cellular & Molecular Neurobiology, 17,* 627-648.

Roselli, C.E. & Resko, J.A. (1997) Sex differences in androgen-regulated expression of cytochrome P450 aromatase in the rat brain. *Journal of Steroid Biochemistry & Molecular Biology, 61,* 365-374.

Rosler, A. & Witztum, E. (1998) Treatment of men with paraphilia with a long-acting analogue of gonadotropin-releasing hormone. *New England Journal of Medicine, 338,* 416-422.

Rupprecht, R. & Holsboer, F. (1999) Neuropsychopharmacological properties of neuroactive steroids. *Steroids, 64,* 83-91.

Sachs, B.D. (1997) Erection evoked in male rats by airborne scent from estrous females. *Physiology & Behavior, 62,* 921-924.

Sachs, B.D., Glater, G.B. & O'Hanlon, J.K. (1984) Morphology of the erect penis in rats under various gonadal hormone conditions. *Anatomical Record, 210,* 45-52.

Saltzman, E. & Guay, A. (2006) Dehydroepiandrosterone therapy as female androgen replacement. *Seminars in Reproductive Medicine, 24,* 97-105.

Samuels, M., Veldhuis, J., Henry, P. & Ridgway, E. (1990) Pathophysiology of pulsatile and copulsatile release of thyroid-stimulating hormone, luteinizing hormone, follicle-stimulating hormone, and alpha-subunit. *Journal of Clinical Endocrinology & Metabolism, 71,* 425-432.

Sarkola, T., Makisalo, H., Fukunaga, T. & Eriksson, C.J. (1999) Acute effect of alcohol on estradiol, estrone, progesterone, prolactin, cortisol, and luteinizing hormone in premenopausal women. *Alcoholism: Clinical & Experimental Research, 23,* 976-982.

Sarrel, P., Dobay, B. & Wiita, B. (1998) Estrogen and estrogen-androgen replacement in postmenopausal women dissatisfied with estrogen-only therapy. Sexual behavior and neuroendocrine responses. *Journal of Reproductive Medicine, 43,* 847-856.

Schiavi, R.C., Schreiner, P., White, D. & Mandeli, J. (1991) The relationship between pituitary-gonadal function and sexual behavior in healthy aging men. *Psychosomatic Medicine, 53,* 363-374.

Schiavi, R.C. & Segraves, R.T. (1995) The biology of sexual function. *Psychiatric Clinics of North America, 18,* 7-23.

Schiavi , R.C. & White, D. (1976) Androgens and male sexual function: a review of human studies. *Journal of Sex & Marital Therapy, 2,* 214-228.

Schiavi, R.C., White, D., Mandeli, J. & Levine, A.C. (1997) Effect of testosterone administration on sexual behavior and mood in men with erectile dysfunction. *Archives of Sexual Behavior, 26,* 231-241.

Scott, C., Kuehl, D., Ferreira, S. & Jackson, G. (1997) Hypothalamic sites of action for testosterone, dihydrotestosterone, and estrogen in the regulation of luteinizing hormone secretion in male sheep. *Endocrinology, 138,* 3686-3694.

Scott, C.J., Tilbrook, A.J., Rawson, J.A. & Clarke, I.J. (2000) Gonadal steroid receptors in the regulation of GnRH secretion in farm animals. *Animal Reproduction Science, 60-61,* 313-326.

Seidman, S.N. (2003) Testosterone deficiency and mood in aging men: pathogenic and therapeutic interactions. *World Journal of Biological Psychiatry, 4,* 14-20.

Sharpe, R.M. (1998) The roles of oestrogen in the male. *Trends in Endocrinology & Metabolism, 9,* 371-377.

Sherwin, B.B., Gelfand, M.M. & Brender, W. (1985) Androgen enhances sexual motivation in females: a prospective, crossover study of sex steroid administration in the surgical menopause. *Psychosomatic Medicine, 47,* 339-351.

Shifren, J.L. (2004) The role of androgens in female sexual dysfunction. *Mayo Clinic Proceedings, 79 (Supplement),* S19-S24.

Shors, T.J., Chua, C. & Falduto, J. (2001) Sex differences and opposite effects of stress on dendritic spine density in the male versus female hippocampus. *Journal of Neuroscience, 21,* 6292-6297.

Shughrue, P.J., Scrimo, P.J. & Merchenthaler, I. (2000) Estrogen binding and estrogen receptor characterization (ERalpha and ERbeta) in the cholinergic neurons of the rat basal forebrain. *Neuroscience, 96,* 41-49.

Simerly, R.B. (2002) Wired for reproduction: organization and development of sexually dimorphic circuits in the mammalian forebrain. *Annual Review of Neuroscience, 25,* 507-536.

Sodersten, P., Enertoh, P. & Petersson, A. (1983) Episodic secretion of luteinizing hormone and androgen in male rats. *Journal of Endocrinology, 97,* 145-153.

Somboonporn, W., Davis, S., Seif, M.W. & Bell, R. (2005) Testosterone for peri- and postmenopausal women. *Cochrane Database of Systematic Reviews, 2005,* DOI: 10.1002/14651858.CD14004509.pub14651852.

Southworth, M.B., Matsumoto, A., Gross, K., Soules, M. & Bremner, W. (1991) The importance of signal pattern in the transmission of endocrine information: Pituitary gonadotropin responses to continuous and pulsatile gonadotropin-releasing hormone. *Journal of Clinical Endocrinology and Metabolism, 72,* 1286-1289.

Stalenheim, E.G., Eriksson, E., von Knorring, L. & Wide, L. (1998) Testosterone as a biological marker in psychopathy and alcoholism. *Psychiatry Research, 77,* 79-88.

Sternbach, H. (1998) Age-associated testosterone decline in men: Clinical issues for psychiatry. *American Journal of Psychiatry, 155,* 1310-1318.

Stoffel-Wagner, B. (2001) Neurosteroid metabolism in the human brain. *European Journal of Endocrinology, 145,* 669-679.

Stone, T.H., Winslade, W.J. & Klugman, C.M. (2000) Sex offenders, sentencing laws and pharmaceutical treatment: a prescription for failure. *Behavioral Sciences & the Law, 18,* 83-110.

Su, T.P., Pagliaro, M., Schmidt, P.J., Pickar, D., Wolkowitz, O. & Rubinow, D.R. (1993) Neuropsychiatric effects of anabolic steroids in male normal volunteers. *JAMA The Journal of the American Medical Association, 269,* 2760-2764.

Swerdloff, R.S. & Wang, C. (2004) Androgens and the ageing male. *Best Practice & Research Clinical Endocrinology & Metabolism, 18,* 349-362.

Taylor, G., Bardgett, M., Farr, S., Humphrey, W., Womack, S. & Weiss, J. (1996) Aging of the brain-testicular axis: Reproductive systems of healthy old males with or without endocrine stimulation. *Proceedings of the Society of Experimental Biology & Medicine, 211,* 69-75.

Taylor, G.T. (1980a) Fighting in juvenile rats and the ontogeny of agonistic behavior. *Journal of Comparative & Physiological Psychology, 94,* 953-961.

Taylor, G.T. (1980b) Sex pheromones and aggressive behavior in male rats. *Animal Learning & Behavior, 8,* 485-490.

Taylor, G.T., Bardgett, M.E., Griffin, M.G. & Weiss, J. (1989) Reproductive behavior and physiology of nulliparous female rats after sexual experience. *Behavioural Processes, 19,* 31-46.

Taylor, G.T., Griffin, M.G. & Bardgett, M.E. (1991) Search for a male contraceptive: the effect of gossypol on sexual motivation and epididymal sperm. *Journal of Medicine, 22,* 29-44.

Taylor, G.T., Haller, J. & Regan, D. (1982) Female rats prefer an area vacated by a high testosterone male. *Physiology & Behavior, 28,* 953-958.

Taylor, G.T., Haller, J., Rupich, R. & Weiss, J. (1984) Testicular hormones and intermale aggressive behaviour in the presence of a female rat. *Journal of Endocrinology, 100,* 315-321.

Taylor, G.T. & Pitha, J. (1988) Hormone-cyclodextrin complexes in behavioral endocrinology: Simulating natural episodic release during therapy. *Biomaterials, Artificial Cells & Artificial Organs, 15,* 759-760.

Taylor, G.T., Scherrer, J., Weiss, J. & Pitha, J. (1994) Endocrine interactions: Adrenal steroids and precursors. *American Journal of Physiology, 266,* E676-E681.

Taylor, G.T. & Weiss, J. (1987) Behaviour and fecundity of female rats mated with preferred and non-preferred males. *Animal Behaviour, 35,* 115-121.

Taylor, G.T., Weiss, J. & Rupich, R. (1985) Suprathreshold manipulations of testosterone and reproductive functioning in gonadally intact sexually experienced and inexperienced male rats. *Physiology & Behavior, 35,* 735-739.

Timiras, P. & Cons, J.M. (1982) Hormones during prenatal and neonatal development. In: *Hormones in Development and Aging* (ed. by A. Vernadakis & P. Timiras), pp. 25-79. Spectrum Publications: Medical & Scientific Books, New York.

Tuiten, A., Van Honk, J., Koppeschaar, H., Bernaards, C., Thijssen, J. & Verbaten, R. (2000) Time course of effects of testosterone administration on sexual arousal in women. *Archives of General Psychiatry, 57,* 149-153.

VandePoll, N.E., Taminiau, M.S., Endert, E. & Louwerse, A.L. (1988) Gonadal steroid influence upon sexual and aggressive behavior of female rats. *International Journal of Neuroscience, 47,* 271-286.

Vanderschueren, D. & Bouillon, R. (2000) Estrogen deficiency in men is a challenge for both the hypothalamus and pituitary. *Journal of Clinical Endocrinology & Metabolism, 85,* 3604-3606.

Wade, J. (2006) Relationships among hormones, brain and behavior: Exceptions in search of a rule? *Hormones and Behavior, 49,* 577-579.

Weiss, J., Taylor, G.T., Zimmermann, F. & Nebenahl, K. (2000) Collection and analyses of biological fluids. In: *Handbook of experimental laboratory animals* (ed. by F. Zimmermann), pp. 485-510. Academic Press, New York.

Welt, C.K., Jimenez, Y., Sluss, P.M., Smith, P.C. & Hall, J.E. (2006) Control of estradiol secretion in reproductive ageing. *Human Reproduction, 21,* 2189-2193.

Wespes, E. & Schulman, C.C. (2002) Male andropause: myth, reality, and treatment. *International Journal of Impotence Research, 14,* S93-98.

Wickham, L.A., Gao, J., Toda, I., Rocha, E.M., Ono, M. & Sullivan, D.A. (2000) Identification of androgen, estrogen and progesterone receptor mRNAs in the eye. *Acta Ophthalmologica Scandinavica, 78,* 146-153.

Widstrom, R.L. & Dillon, J.S. (2004) Is there a receptor for dehydroepiandrosterone or dehydroepiandrosterone sulfate? *Seminars in Reproductive Medicine, 22,* 289-298.

Williams, J.R. (2000) The effects of dehydroepiandrosterone on carcinogenesis, obesity, the immune system, and aging. *Lipids, 35,* 325-331.

Wilson, J.D. (2000) Endocrinology: Survival as a discipline in the 21st century? *Annual Review of Physiology,* 947–950.

Wilson, J.D., Leihy, M.W., Shaw, G. & Renfree, M.B. (2002) Androgen physiology: unsolved problems at the millennium. *Molecular & Cellular Endocrinology, 198,* 1-5.

Woolley, C.S. (1998) Estrogen-mediated structural and functional synaptic plasticity in the female rat hippocampus. *Hormones & Behavior, 34,* 140-148.

Woolley, C.S., McEwen, B.S. & Beatty, W.W. (1993) Roles of estradiol and progesterone in regulation of hippocampal dendritic spine density during the estrous cycle in the rat. *Journal of Comparative Neurology, 336,* 293-306.

Xiao, L. & Jordan, C.L. (2002) Sex differences, laterality, and hormonal regulation of androgen receptor immunoreactivity in rat hippocampus. *Hormones & Behavior, 42,* 327-336.

Yates, W.R., Perry, P.J., MacIndoe, J., Holman, T. & Ellingrod, V. (1999) Psychosexual effects of three doses of testosterone cycling in normal men. *Biological Psychiatry, 45,* 254-260.

Young, E.A., Midgley, A.R., Carlson, N.E. & Brown, M.B. (2000) Alteration in the hypothalamic-pituitary-ovarian axis in depressed women. *Archives of General Psychiatry, 57,* 1157-1162.

Zhang, J.Q., Cai, W.Q., Zhou de, S. & Su, B.Y. (2002) Distribution and differences of estrogen receptor beta immunoreactivity in the brain of adult male and female rats. *Brain Research, 935,* 73-80.

Zitzmann, M. & Nieschlag, E. (2001) Testosterone levels in healthy men and the relation to behavioural and physical characteristics: facts and constructs. *European Journal of Endocrinology, 144,* 183-197.

Index

A

B

D

E

F

G

H

I

J

K

L

M

N

O

P

Q

R

S

T

U

V

W

X

Y

Z